Your Brain on Drugs

A Clinician's Guide to Medications, Substances, and Confounded QEEG Brain Maps

by Andrew Hill, PhD

Peak Brain Press LLC
Los Angeles, California

2026

Copyright

Peak Brain Press, LLC
www.peakbrainpress.com

ISBN: 979-8-951466-63-1
eISBN: 978-1-971402-07-9

First edition, 2026

Published by Peak Brain Press, LLC

Dedication

For the clients who taught me that the brain in front of us is never a textbook brain, and for the clinicians who keep asking better questions when the map does not fit the person.

Contents

Medical Disclaimer and Notice to Readers

Your Brain on Drugs: A Clinician's Guide to Medications, Substances, and Confounded QEEG Brain Maps is an educational reference for licensed clinicians with training in quantitative EEG (QEEG). It is not intended as a substitute for professional medical advice, diagnosis, or treatment. Nothing in this book should be used to start, stop, change the dose of, or substitute any medication for any person.

This book does not authorize clinical decisions. All prescribing, deprescribing, dose adjustment, and pharmacologic substitution decisions must be made by a licensed prescribing clinician who has evaluated the individual patient. The presence of a QEEG finding described in this book does not, by itself, constitute clinical grounds for any medication change.

QEEG is an interpretive tool, not a prescribing instrument. QEEG must not be used to recommend stopping, changing dose, or switching drugs. That principle is stated throughout this book because it is clinically important, legally significant, and scientifically accurate.

Benzodiazepine, opioid, alcohol, and stimulant tapers carry medical risk. Benzodiazepine and alcohol withdrawal can cause seizures and death. Opioid discontinuation carries overdose risk on resumption. These processes require medical supervision and are outside the scope of QEEG practice. Nothing in this book describes a taper protocol.

If you or someone you know is in distress or danger, contact a licensed prescribing clinician, an emergency department, or emergency services (911 in the United States). This book is not a clinical resource for emergencies.

The publisher, Peak Brain Press, and the author, Andrew Hill, PhD, disclaim all liability for any clinical outcome arising from use or misuse of the information in this book. Readers accept full responsibility for the clinical application of information presented here. Clinicians using this book as an educational reference remain bound by all applicable professional licensing, ethical, and legal requirements.

Preface

This book came from a recurring clinical problem. A client arrives for QEEG assessment, and the map looks ready to explain the client's symptoms. Then the medication list arrives: stimulant in the morning, SSRI at night, benzodiazepine as needed, cannabis on weekends, caffeine before the appointment, antihistamine for sleep, recent concussion, poor sleep, chronic pain, or a medication taper that no one mentioned during scheduling.

At that point, the QEEG is still useful, but it is no longer simple. The map records a brain in a medication state, a sleep state, a pain state, a developmental state, a hormonal state, a substance state, and a measurement pipeline, not an isolated trait portrait. If the clinician ignores those facts, the interpretation can become elegant and wrong.

The goal of this book is to help clinicians avoid that mistake.

Medication effects on EEG are not new. Pharmaco-EEG has a long history, and practitioners have had access to class-level descriptions for decades. Kerson's work, standard clinical EEG texts, and the pharmaco-EEG literature all show that medications can change power spectra, vigilance, sleep architecture, task response, and seizure risk. Yet the clinical neurofeedback setting adds a different problem. The practitioner often sees clients not in controlled laboratory conditions, but in real life: medicated, under-slept, comorbid, polypharmacy-exposed, and recorded on clinical systems with their own reference, filter, artifact, and database conventions.

This book is written for that setting.

This is not a prescribing guide, and it does not use QEEG to select or change medications. It teaches a medication-aware way to read the map: how exposure and context change what the tracing means.

The book is organized around two complementary questions:

Forward direction: Can an active medication, substance, condition, recording state, or pipeline factor plausibly produce the same direction of QEEG finding?

Inverse direction: Given a detected QEEG phenotype, what does the literature suggest about the client's likely response to specific medications or intervention modalities?

The forward question dominates Parts I, II, IV, V, and VI. If the answer is yes, confidence in the phenotype interpretation should be reduced. The finding may still matter. It may still guide training. It may still be worth tracking longitudinally. But the report should say what else could be producing it.

The inverse question is the subject of Part III. It asks whether a phenotype pattern carries predictive information about treatment response, drawing on research lineages from Suffin and Emory through the Brainmarker-I framework. The evidence base for inverse-direction inference is thinner than for forward-direction effects, and the gap between group-level association and individual-level prediction remains the central limitation. Part III states that limitation repeatedly and treats its entries as hypothesis-generating, not prescriptive.

The book uses three named claim types (spectral effect, phenotype inference, and workflow heuristic), defined fully in Chapter 4. The labels name what kind of statement is being made, not how strong the evidence is, which keeps useful clinical reasoning from becoming overclaiming.

The book also treats non-drug confounders as central, not peripheral. Sleep deprivation, drowsiness, TBI, obstructive sleep apnea, Long COVID, ME/CFS, fibromyalgia, migraine, chronic pain, menstrual cycle, pregnancy, hormonal contraception, adolescence, aging, withdrawal, paradoxical response, and pipeline choices can all alter QEEG interpretation. Medication effects rarely appear in isolation from these contexts.

Several chapters are deliberately gap-heavy. Some agents have no human resting-QEEG evidence. Some medication stacks have never been studied. Some claims that circulate in practitioner culture are plausible but unverified. When the evidence is absent, the book says so. An explicitly labeled gap is better than a confident sentence without a source.

The book is paired conceptually with a live database and lookup tool. A print book can teach the framework, but the evidence base keeps moving. Newer medications, formulations, pharmacogenomic data, aperiodic metrics, and clinical registry work all change what a defensible row in the table has to say. The live database is intended to carry row-level claim types, update dates, citation links, and clinical-portability notes so the framework can stay current after publication.

This book is part of a larger system. The *QEEG Field Guide* asks "what am I looking at?" It covers recording, artifacting, pattern recognition, normative databases, and phenotypes. This book asks "what changed it from baseline?" It covers medications, substances, supplements, formulations, kinetics, withdrawal, and the non-drug states that practitioners routinely confuse for drug effects. A future companion, *The Dynamic Brain*, will ask "what does the brain do on its own?" and will cover development, aging, endogenous state shifts, and illness trajectories. This book assumes the reader already cares about raw EEG quality, artifact, reference, montage, normative databases, and clinical context. It extends those concerns into medication-aware interpretation.

The person in front of the clinician is always more important than the category. A medication class does not determine an individual response. A diagnosis is not an EEG phenotype. A developmental variant is not a pathology label. A QEEG map is not a treatment plan by itself. Good interpretation is not the elimination of uncertainty; it is the disciplined handling of it.

Medication effects are easy to underestimate because clinicians often learn QEEG through clean phenotype examples. Real recordings are less tidy. A client may show a finding that is biologically real, medication-amplified, sleep-contaminated, and pipeline-sensitive at the same time. The practical question is how much confidence the clinician should place in the attribution, not only whether the map is valid.

This book keeps returning to confidence for that reason. Confidence is not certainty. A finding can be present while its cause remains uncertain. The clinical task is to separate observation from attribution, document the factors that matter, and revise the formulation when physiology or medication state changes.

The Posture of This Book

This book holds five positions that distinguish it from a standard drug-effects reference and that deserve naming at the outset.

The client exists as a composite. A recording measures a person at a specific moment under specific biological conditions, not a stable, isolated brain. Medications, substances, sleep, pain, hormonal state, age, recent illness, and the technical pipeline used to process the signal are all part of the measurement. A QEEG report that ignores these factors captures an artifact that looks like the client's brain, not the client's brain under documented conditions.

The recording is a moment, not a trait. Traits are stable across time and state. Moments are not. Much of what QEEG practice calls a "phenotype" is better understood as a measurement-context-specific pattern. A "theta excess" on a sleep-deprived, stimulant-withdrawn, caffeinated Tuesday morning is not the same clinical object as the same z-score under stable, controlled conditions. This book takes that difference seriously and builds it into every confidence judgment.

The claim-type system is a position on knowledge. The three claim types in this book are not a ranking of studies. They are a position on what kinds of statements are epistemically defensible given the literature available. A spectral-effect claim makes a different kind of assertion than a workflow heuristic. The clinician who uses workflow-heuristic language as if it were a spectral effect has made an error of scope, not just confidence.

The report is a small piece of writing with consequences. A QEEG report can influence prescribing indirectly. A client who reads "masked ADHD phenotype" may ask about stopping a medication; a prescriber who receives "beta-excess phenotype" may consider an additional prescription. The report's language has downstream effects the clinician cannot fully control, which is why the language has to be disciplined.

The framework is a discipline, not an algorithm. The ten-step workflow in Chapter 26 orders the questions; it does not answer them. What this book provides is a way of thinking: what might be producing this pattern, how confident should I be, what would change my confidence, and how should I write the limit. That is a framework for judgment, not a substitute for it.

Three Reading Paths

Path 1: First-year clinician. Read Chapters 1, 4, 5, 6, 8, 25, and 26 in order. Then read Appendix B (decision aid), Appendix C (intake form), Appendix F (the minimum method record), and Appendix H (worked reports). This gives you the framework, the three most common drug classes that will distort your readings, the most important differential chapter, and the operational tools. Come back to the other Part II chapters as specific cases require. Do not read Part III (Ch.19–21) until you have at least six months of clinical QEEG practice; the prediction entries will be more useful once you have phenotype experience to anchor them to.

Path 2: Experienced clinician. Read Chapter 26 (decision framework) and Chapter 18 (patterns across substances) first. These are the two chapters that compress the book's framework most efficiently. Then read Chapter 25 (when it's not the drug) and Chapter 22 (polypharmacy) for the clinical scenarios most likely to create interpretation errors. Use Part II chapters as drug-specific references when a client's regimen raises a specific question.

Path 3: Peer reviewer / researcher. Read Chapters 1, 4, and 19. These establish the book's epistemological commitments. Chapter 19 states the limits of inverse-direction inference explicitly; if those limits are not explicit, the book is not doing its job. Chapter 4 (claim types) includes the aperiodic-decomposition caveat that contextualizes the entire spectral-effect empirical base. For the inverse-direction chapter-by-chapter entries, Appendix G (phenotype crosswalk) is the most intellectually testable artifact.

What This Book Is Not

This book is a pharmaco-EEG interpretation framework, not a medication reference. It does not provide dosing ranges, prescribing indications, taper schedules, adverse-event management, or substitution strategies. It does not replace pharmacology texts, psychiatry references, or medical consultation.

Part III is designed to inform the clinician-prescriber conversation, not to replace it. The phenotype-by-phenotype entries describe group-level associations between EEG patterns and medication response. Those associations do not translate directly to individual prediction. Effect sizes are typically small to moderate, replication has been uneven across frameworks, and polypharmacy, comorbidity, state confounds, and pipeline variability all reduce real-world applicability.

A medicated recording is often clinically meaningful because it shows the client as they present under current treatment. The problem is not that medication is present. The problem is interpreting a medicated recording as if medication were absent. This book is an attempt to help clinicians avoid that mistake, not a criticism of any clinical approach that preceded it.

How to Use This Book

This book can be read straight through, but most clinicians will use it in layers.

If you are new to pharmaco-EEG, begin with Part I (Mechanisms). The opening chapters explain how drugs reach the EEG through receptor-to-spectrum pathways, how pharmacology shapes brain exposure, and how the claim-type framework works. Do not skip the claim-type framework. It is the logic that keeps the rest of the book from becoming a list of overconfident drug effects.

If you are trying to interpret a specific medication class, go to Part II (Patterns). Those chapters cover stimulants, antidepressants, benzodiazepines, antipsychotics, anticonvulsants, anesthesia, ketamine, opioids, sleep medications, OTC agents, and supplements. The synthesis chapter at the end of Part II shows cross-substance patterns that repeat across classes.

If the clinical question is the inverse one, where a detected phenotype raises the question of which medications or modalities might work best, use Part III (Phenotype Patterns). Chapter 19 frames the epistemic ground rules for inverse-direction inference, reviews replication issues across the five major prediction frameworks, names known failure modes, and closes with validation standards the field has not yet met. Chapter 20 traces the prediction research lineages. Chapter 21 provides 45 entries (41 phenotypes shared with the *Field Guide* taxonomy plus 4 medication-prediction constructs unique to this book) with claim types, framework attributions, and cross-references back to the forward-direction drug chapters. Every Part III entry should be read as hypothesis-generating, not prescriptive.

If the case involves polypharmacy, paradoxical responses, comorbidity, or a finding that might not be a drug effect at all, use Part IV (Complex Cases). The "When It's Not the Drug" chapter covers TBI, post-viral fatigue, OSA, sleep deprivation, and other states that mimic drug effects. The decision framework chapter is the one to return to before writing a report.

If the clinical question involves formulation, kinetics, timing, withdrawal, tolerance, or hormonal modifiers of drug response, use Part V (Time).

If the client uses caffeine, alcohol, nicotine, cannabis, or psychedelics, use Part VI (Substances). These exposures are often missing from medication lists but present in the EEG. Last-use timing matters.

Appendix A contains the medication-phenotype interaction matrix. Use it as a quick confidence-adjustment tool, not as a diagnostic algorithm.

Appendix B contains the decision aid. Use it when you are deciding whether a phenotype finding should be considered high-confidence, reduced-confidence, substantially reduced, or not interpretable for phenotype attribution.

Appendix C contains a pre-recording intake form template. Use it before acquisition, not after interpretation. The most important medication fact is often the one that was never asked.

Appendix D is a glossary. Use it to keep terminology consistent across QEEG, pharmaco-EEG, clinical pharmacology, and confounder language.

Appendix E covers pharmacogenetics and individual differences. Use it when the response seems unusually strong, weak, delayed, paradoxical, or inconsistent with dose.

Appendix F covers recording and pipeline considerations. It carries the minimum acquisition and processing record this book asks you to keep with every map: hardware, reference and montage, filters, usable minutes, vigilance segmentation, artifact method, band edges, and database name and version, along with the matching rule for comparing one recording to another. Use it when you write the method block, and to remember that a pipeline change between sessions can mimic a medication effect.

Appendix G is a cross-book phenotype name crosswalk. Use it to translate phenotype names between this book, the *QEEG Field Guide*, and the consumer titles.

Appendix H contains worked complete reports, each with a weak version followed by a stronger one. Use it to see the framework applied end to end in report language.

Appendix I is written for prescribers. Use it to explain what a QEEG can and cannot do, either in collaboration or by handing it to the prescriber directly.

Clinicians reading under time pressure can use this sequence:

1. Review the client's medication, substance, sleep, and condition inventory.
2. Identify the dominant QEEG findings.
3. Ask whether any active factor can produce the same direction of finding.
4. Assign an interaction mode: masking, mimicry, exaggeration, or transformation.
5. Adjust confidence.
6. Write the caveat directly.
7. Coordinate medication questions with the prescriber when needed.

Do not use this book to justify unsupervised medication discontinuation. For prescribed psychotropics, recording the client as they usually present is the right call. For habitual substance patterns (caffeine, cannabis, nicotine), the person's ordinary functional state is the default recording condition; timing information for all exposures serves interpretation, not imposition (see the governing rule in Appendix C).

New clinicians should treat this book as a checklist of questions rather than a catalog of answers. Before deciding that a finding means ADHD, anxiety, hyperarousal, underarousal, trauma, executive dysfunction, or medication effect, ask what else could move the signal in the same direction. Experienced clinicians may want to start with the decision framework (Chapter 26), then work backward through the class and confounder chapters. Prescribers and collaborating clinicians can use the framework to understand why a QEEG report lowers confidence in a finding without using QEEG to direct medication management.

A Suggested Intake Workflow

Use the intake form before scheduling when possible. Ask for prescriptions, dose, timing, duration, prescriber, over-the-counter agents, supplements, recreational substances, caffeine, nicotine, sleep, recent sedation or anesthesia, menstrual and pregnancy context when relevant, chronic conditions, head injury history, and current symptom severity. Ask again on the recording day. Medication lists change, and clients often remember details only when prompted.

At acquisition, record eyes-open and eyes-closed conditions explicitly and note drowsiness, movement, muscle tension, medication timing, caffeine timing, sleep deprivation, pain flare, acute illness, withdrawal, or unusual stress. At interpretation, begin with raw EEG and data quality, then examine phenotype, medication context, and confounders. At report writing, separate observation from attribution. At follow-up, treat response as new data.

EEG Bands, Electrode Sites, and Abbreviations

This page collects the shorthand the book uses most often. For full conceptual definitions, see the glossary in Appendix D.

Frequency Bands

The table below gives conventional broad-band ranges as an orientation. Alpha (8-12 Hz) and SMR (12-15 Hz) are the two ranges stated explicitly in this book. Delta, theta, and gamma are used throughout but are not assigned fixed edges here; formal band definitions are covered in the companion *QEEG Field Guide*. Band edges vary between normative databases and processing pipelines (Appendix F), and that variation is one reason this book does not fix a single set.

Individual chapters narrow to sub-bands for specific findings, which is ordinary practice rather than a discrepancy: clinicians train particular ranges for particular purposes. When a chapter names a range, that range governs. Beta covers the widest family. The book uses roughly 14 to 30 Hz for beta broadly, and narrows by context: spindling patterns are described at 15 to 20 Hz and at 18 to 25 Hz, and excess or high beta at 20 to 30 Hz and 22 to 28 Hz. None of these is the beta range.

Band	Conventional range
Delta	below 4 Hz
Theta	4-8 Hz
Alpha	8-12 Hz
SMR	12-15 Hz
Beta	~13-30 Hz (sub-ranges vary)
Gamma	above 30 Hz

Electrode Sites

This book uses the international 10-20 system. The letter indicates the scalp region: F frontal, C central, T temporal, P parietal, O occipital. Odd numbers mark left-hemisphere sites, even numbers mark right-hemisphere sites, and z marks the midline.

Sites named in this book: Fz, F3, F4, F7, F8, Cz, C3, C4, T3, T4, T5, T6, Pz, P3, P4, O1, O2. Reference schemes named include linked ears and linked mastoid; Appendix F asks you to record which one you used, because a power map and a coherence estimate taken under different references are not comparable.

Abbreviations

Abbreviation	Meaning
CPAP	continuous positive airway pressure
CYP	cytochrome P450; drug-metabolizing enzyme family
FAA	frontal alpha asymmetry
GABA-A	GABA type A receptor; benzodiazepine target
GLP-1	glucagon-like peptide 1
iAPF	individual alpha peak frequency
IR / XR	immediate release / extended release
LAI	long-acting injectable (depot formulation)
LVF	low-voltage fast; an EEG phenotype
M1	O-desmethyltramadol, tramadol's active metabolite. Not an electrode site
ME/CFS	myalgic encephalomyelitis / chronic fatigue syndrome
NFB	neurofeedback
NMDA	N-methyl-D-aspartate; a glutamate receptor subtype
OCP	oral contraceptive pill
OSA	obstructive sleep apnea
PK / PD	pharmacokinetics / pharmacodynamics
PRN	as needed (pro re nata)
QHS	at bedtime (quaque hora somni)
SMR	sensorimotor rhythm; 12-15 Hz at central sites

Abbreviation	Meaning
SNRI	serotonin-norepinephrine reuptake inhibitor
SSRI	selective serotonin reuptake inhibitor
TBR	theta/beta ratio

Part I

Mechanisms

Ch 1: Introduction

1.1 Why Medication Effects Matter in NFB Practice

The client is forty-three years old, works as a high school teacher, and has been on escitalopram for nine months. She scheduled the QEEG because her attention has been getting worse since she started the medication, not better. Before she sits down, she mentions she has been sleeping about five hours a night, drinks two large coffees before arriving, and takes a half-dose alprazolam most evenings because the anxiety "doesn't fully respond to the SSRI." She also used an antihistamine last night for a sinus headache.

The eyes-closed segment produces elevated frontal theta, reduced posterior alpha amplitude, mild diffuse slowing, and a theta/beta ratio at the high end of normative limits. The map looks like an underarousal phenotype. It may be exactly that. It may also be escitalopram at nine months producing sedation and alpha shifts, alprazolam residual from last evening suppressing alpha reactivity, sleep restriction elevating frontal theta, antihistamine contributing to diffuse slowing, caffeine partially offsetting all of the above, and the clinician reading a composite of those interactions as a stable trait pattern.

The question is not which of these is true in isolation. The clinician is rarely looking at a clean trait marker; more often, the map is a layered measurement.

That is the problem this book was written to address. In U.S. adults, roughly one in six uses at least one psychiatric medication (Moore & Mattison, 2017), and psychiatric polypharmacy has become common enough that single-drug assumptions routinely miss the actual clinical picture (Mojtabai & Olfson, 2010). The medicated QEEG records the client as they present clinically: under current medication exposure, sleep, pain, substance use, hormonal state, and the choices the clinician made about acquisition and processing. Those conditions are the measurement context, and ignoring them does not make them disappear. It makes the interpretation wrong in a direction the report will not name.

The practical question behind most chapters is therefore this: when a QEEG finding appears in a medicated client, how much confidence should the clinician place in the phenotype reading? Sometimes the answer is high confidence: the medication has little relation to the detected feature, or the feature persists across recordings under different exposure states. Sometimes the answer is low confidence: a medication, substance, sleep state, illness, or pipeline factor can produce the same direction of change. Most of the time the answer sits between those poles, which is where this book does its work.

The book also addresses a second, complementary question. Once a phenotype is identified with reasonable confidence, does it carry information about how the client might respond to particular medications or intervention modalities? This is the inverse direction, and Part III takes it up explicitly. The evidence for inverse-direction prediction is thinner than for forward-direction effects, the gap between group-level association and individual-level application is wide, and the entries in Part III are framed as hypothesis-generating rather than prescriptive. Both directions use the same claim-type framework (Chapter 4), but confidence in inverse-direction claims is generally lower because the translation from group to individual has not been reliably achieved by any current framework.

1.2 The Four Interaction Modes

Masking occurs when a medication suppresses the same feature the clinician is trying to detect. A stimulant can reduce theta activity in a client whose unmedicated baseline might otherwise show a theta-dominant attention phenotype. A recording obtained near peak stimulant exposure may therefore look more "normalized" than the client's untreated physiology.

Mimicry occurs when a medication creates a pattern that resembles a phenotype. Benzodiazepines can increase beta activity enough to resemble endogenous beta excess. Antipsychotics, opioids, sedating antidepressants, anticonvulsants, and untreated sleep disorders can all contribute to slowing that may resemble underarousal, encephalopathic change, or a frontal theta pattern.

Exaggeration occurs when an endogenous tendency and a medication effect point in the same direction. A client with untreated sleep apnea and a sedating medication may show more slowing than either factor would produce alone. A chronic-pain client on gabapentinoids and opioids may show a composite signature that cannot be cleanly assigned to one source.

Transformation occurs when the medication changes the meaning of the phenotype rather than merely changing its magnitude. For example, a high beta pattern under benzodiazepine exposure may not carry the same implication as a high beta pattern in an unmedicated anxious client. The surface measurement looks similar, but the clinical reading changes.

These modes are not mutually exclusive. A single recording can show masking in one band, mimicry in another, and exaggeration in a third. That is why medication effects cannot be handled as a short footnote at the end of a report. They belong inside the interpretive model.

These four modes are presented here as an integrated taxonomy. Earlier texts catalogued drug effects by class; this book organizes them by the type of interpretive error they generate. The taxonomy is the working framework behind every chapter that follows, not decorative scaffolding.

1.3 What This Book Is, and Is Not

This book is a practitioner-oriented pharmaco-EEG interpretation framework, not a systematic review, meta-analysis, or guide to prescribing or medication management. The literature base was assembled through targeted searches, citation chasing, textbook anchors, and focused review rounds across psychotropics, substances, anesthetics, chronic medical confounders, developmental stage, reproductive hormone state, methodology, and withdrawal. The goal is clinical interpretive discipline: knowing when a QEEG feature is likely to be endogenous, when it may be pharmacological, when it may be condition-driven, and when the honest answer is that the available literature cannot separate the layers.

Kerson's edited volume on drug effects on the EEG provides an important practitioner anchor for class-level pharmaco-EEG patterns (Kerson, 2023). This book has a different job. It organizes the literature around clinical QEEG phenotype interpretation: not just what a drug does to the EEG, but how that effect can change a neurofeedback clinician's confidence in a phenotype label. A benzodiazepine beta signature, for example, is also a warning about interpreting beta excess,

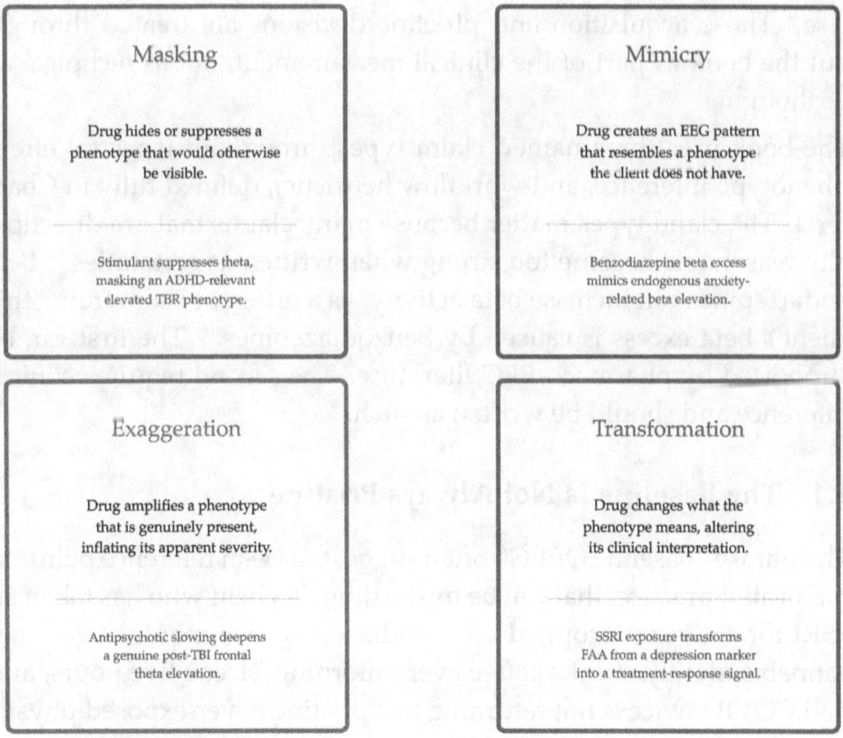

Figure 1.1: Four interaction modes: masking, mimicry, exaggeration, and transformation with representative drug-phenotype examples.

SMR targets, arousal state, and medication timing, not merely a benzodiazepine fact.

The International Pharmaco-EEG Society guidelines also matter because they remind the reader that pharmaco-EEG is a measurement discipline, not just a list of drug effects (International Pharmaco-EEG Society, 2012). Recording state, eyes-open or eyes-closed condition, timing, artifact handling, and signal processing determine whether a drug effect is visible, attenuated, or mistaken for something else. Those acquisition and pipeline decisions are treated throughout the book as part of the clinical measurement, not as technical afterthoughts.

The book uses three named claim types throughout (spectral effect, phenotype inference, and workflow heuristic), defined fully in Chapter 4. The claim types matter because many claims that are directionally reasonable become too strong when written as certainties. "Benzodiazepines can increase beta activity" is a different claim from "this client's beta excess is caused by benzodiazepines." The first can be supported by pharmaco-EEG literature. The second requires clinical inference and should be written as such.

1.4 The Baseline Is Not Always Pristine

The phrase "baseline QEEG" often suggests a clean reference point. In medicated practice, that can be misleading. A client who has taken an SSRI for six years, stopped a benzodiazepine two months ago, uses cannabis nightly, drinks coffee every morning, sleeps five hours, and had COVID twice is not returning to a pristine never-exposed physiological baseline just because the eyes are closed for five minutes.

This does not make the recording invalid. It makes documentation essential. Time since last dose, formulation, chronicity, recent titration, discontinuation, sleep, illness, pain, developmental stage, reproductive hormone status, and pipeline parameters all become measurement variables. The recording is still clinically meaningful, but its meaning depends on knowing what has shaped it.

The same principle applies to technical processing. Reference montage, filters, artifact rejection, ICA, ASR, segment selection, and normative database choice can shift the apparent phenotype. Modern spectral interpretation also has to separate periodic oscillatory power

(Buzsaki & Draguhn, 2004; Klimesch, 1999) from the aperiodic background of the EEG, because a drug can change apparent band power by changing the overall spectral slope rather than a discrete rhythm (Cole & Voytek, 2017; Donoghue et al., 2020; He, 2014). The instrument is the full acquisition and processing pipeline, not just the amplifier. A z-score, for instance, is a comparison between the client's processed data and a reference distribution built under specific assumptions. If the client's recording is heavily shaped by medication timing, sleep loss, chronic illness, or a different processing pipeline, the z-score can still be mathematically correct while being clinically easy to overread.

The phrase "baseline" should therefore be used with care. In this book, baseline usually means "the client's recorded state under documented conditions," not "the client's untouched trait physiology." When a pristine baseline is not available, the goal is not to pretend otherwise. The goal is to say exactly what is known, what is likely, and what cannot be separated.

This book is the second volume of a three-part clinical system: the *perturbation engine*. The *QEEG Field Guide* is the perception engine ("what am I looking at?"). *Your Brain on Drugs* is the perturbation engine ("what changed it from baseline, and how?"). *The Dynamic Brain* is the baseline engine ("what does the unperturbed brain do on its own?"). Each volume answers a different question, and together they cover the ground. This one does not depend on the other two to be usable. The method a clinician needs to record and read a medicated map at the standard this book asks for is in Appendix F, inside this volume, and nothing in these pages waits on a book that has not shipped. The companion volume *Dynamic Brain* takes up the baseline question directly: how the resting EEG matures across childhood, stabilizes through adulthood, drifts in late life, and varies across hormone state, sleep, and circadian phase. This book treats those normative arcs as background context and assumes the reader has access to age-appropriate norms. When a medicated recording is read against a normative database, the developmental, sex-typed, and aging contributions to "normal" are not in the medication list. They belong in the baseline engine, and *Dynamic Brain* is the reference for that side of the trilogy.

1.5 A Composite Opening Case

A client in her late thirties presents for QEEG-guided neurofeedback because of poor attention, fatigue, and mood instability. Her medication list includes an SSRI, low-dose quetiapine (Seroquel) for sleep, occasional clonazepam (Klonopin), daily caffeine, and nightly cannabis. She had COVID twice, sleeps six hours on weeknights, and reports possible sleep apnea but has not completed a sleep study. Her eyes-closed QEEG shows frontal theta elevation, diffuse slowing, reduced posterior alpha organization, and intermittent beta excess.

This recording invites two common misreads. One would be to call the frontal theta pattern an ADHD phenotype and train it as if the recording were unmedicated. Another would be to dismiss the entire QEEG as "just medication." Both responses are too crude. The more useful interpretation is layered: frontal theta is present, but confidence that it reflects an endogenous attention phenotype is reduced by sedating medication exposure, chronic sleep restriction, possible OSA, Long COVID history, and cannabis use. The beta excess may be endogenous arousal, recent caffeine, benzodiazepine effect, cannabis withdrawal, or artifact. The correct clinical move is to document the competing explanations, adjust confidence, and decide whether the current-state recording is sufficient for training or whether a second recording under more stable documented conditions would change the interpretation.

1.6 How to Use This Book

The front matter contains a full reading guide. In brief: Part I (Chapters 1–4) builds the interpretive frame. Part II (Chapters 5–18) covers medication classes for targeted lookup. Part III (Chapters 19–21) reverses the question: given a detected phenotype, what does the literature suggest about treatment response? This is the inverse-direction axis, built from research lineages spanning Suffin and Emory through the Brainmarker-I framework, and every entry is hypothesis-generating rather than prescriptive. Part IV (Chapters 22–26) addresses polypharmacy, paradoxical responses, comorbidity, non-drug confounders, and the decision framework for reading a medicated QEEG. Part V (Chapters 27–29) covers formulation, kinetics, withdrawal, and hormonal modifiers. Part VI (Chapters 30–34) covers common substances. The appendices (interaction table, decision aid, intake form, glossary, pharmacogenetics) turn the prose into tools.

1.7 What to Do With Uncertainty

Uncertainty in medicated QEEG interpretation is part of the result, not a defect to hide. A report that states uncertainty explicitly is often more useful than one that presents every phenotype as equally stable. The clinician can usually sort findings into high-confidence features (stable across recordings and weakly explained by the medication list), reduced-confidence features (real measurements with plausible medication or confounder overlap), and deferred features (unstable recording conditions such as acute withdrawal, intoxication, severe sleep deprivation, recent complicated anesthesia, or a major medical flare).

The distinction between reduced confidence and deferral matters. Reduced confidence does not mean the clinician throws away the recording. It means the report carries a caveat and the treatment plan should not depend too heavily on that one feature. Deferral means the recording may still document the current state, but it should not be used as the main basis for phenotype selection until the state stabilizes.

This language also helps with client communication. Clients often want to know whether a finding is "real." The better answer is that the measurement is real, but its source may not be singular. Frontal theta can be real and still have multiple plausible contributors. Beta excess can be real and still be medication-shaped. A slow iAPF can be real and still depend on age (Babiloni et al., 2024), hormonal state, substance use, and recording condition. Clinical maturity means resisting the pressure to reduce every real finding to one cause.

1.8 The Three Deliverables

This book is the full clinical reference: reasoning, caveats, worked examples, and breadth across drug, substance, condition, and methodological coverage. The companion article extracts the main framework and decision aid. The live database carries row-level claim types that can be updated as the literature moves. A print book can teach the model in depth but cannot stay current forever; a database can stay current but cannot teach judgment; an article can anchor the work academically but cannot carry every class and caveat. The three formats divide that labor.

1.9 A Note on Clinical Responsibility

The interpretation model in this book is deliberately conservative. It asks the clinician to document more, claim less, and preserve uncertainty when the literature does not support a stronger statement. That restraint is a safety principle, not an academic nicety. Clients may interpret QEEG language as evidence that a medication is helping, harming, masking, or causing their symptoms. A careless report can therefore influence medication behavior even when the clinician never intended to give medication advice. I have seen a client taper an SSRI because a report used the word "masked" without explaining what that meant. The prescriber never saw the report. The client acted on the language.

The safer report separates observation from inference. The observation is the measured EEG pattern. The inference is the possible relationship between that pattern and the client's medications, substances, conditions, and recording state. What you recommend from the QEEG is usually measurement, not prescribing: better timing, repeat under stable conditions, sleep-apnea workup, an explicit withdrawal history. Medication changes to suit a QEEG question are not part of a neurofeedback report.

This distinction protects the client, the prescriber, and the neurofeedback clinician. It also produces better science. Clear medication documentation supports later work on phenotype stability, misclassification, treatment response, and protocol safety. Vague or absent documentation does not.

1.10 Interpretation traps

- **Treating the medication list as administrative background.** The medication list is part of the signal context. Read it before interpreting the phenotype map.
- **Citing a drug-class effect as a client-specific cause.** A known class effect lowers or changes confidence; it does not prove causality in a single recording.
- **Ignoring non-drug confounders.** TBI, untreated OSA, Long COVID, ME/CFS, fibromyalgia, pain, sleep deprivation, adolescence, aging, pregnancy, cycle phase, OCP status, and chronic pain can overlap with or outweigh drug signatures.

- **Assuming stopped medication means clean baseline.** Withdrawal, discontinuation, rebound, and long-term trait-like changes may persist after a drug is stopped.
- **Comparing across pipelines as if they were the same instrument.** A drug effect measured under one reference / filter / artifact pipeline may not transfer cleanly to another.
- **Forgetting paradoxical responders.** Some clients respond opposite to the population-level expectation. A sedating medication can activate, and a stimulant can sedate. The client's report matters.

1.11 Intake questions

At minimum, every medicated QEEG intake should ask:

- **What prescription medications are you taking, at what dose, and when was the last dose?** Record drug, dose, formulation, last-dose time, and duration on the current regimen.
- **What over-the-counter medications, supplements, cannabis products, nicotine products, caffeine, alcohol, or other substances have you used in the last week?** Include timing, amount, and usual pattern.
- **Have any medications been started, stopped, increased, decreased, or skipped in the last month?** Mark titration, discontinuation, withdrawal, drug holidays, and adherence problems.
- **Have you had recent anesthesia, procedural sedation, outpatient ketamine/esketamine, concussion, major illness, severe sleep loss, or pain flare?** These can change the recording independent of daily medications.
- **For female clients, what is the current reproductive-hormone context?** Document pregnancy, postpartum month, cycle day if known, hormonal contraceptive use, perimenopause, menopause, and hormone therapy.
- **Have you ever had an unexpected or opposite reaction to a medication or supplement?** This includes stimulation from antihistamines, sedation from stimulants, agitation from benzodiazepines, or mood activation from antidepressants.

1.12 Clinical recommendations

The safest default is to record the client as they usually present, document the conditions precisely, and interpret with confidence adjustments. A second recording under a different medication state can be useful when that change is already clinically appropriate and coordinated with the prescriber. QEEG must not be used to recommend stopping, changing dose, or switching drugs; those decisions rest with the prescriber, and the map is not a back-door to medication management.

When a medication effect and a phenotype overlap, the report should say so directly. "Frontal theta elevation is present, but confidence that this is an endogenous attention phenotype is reduced by current antipsychotic/opioid exposure and poor sleep" is more useful than either ignoring the medication or dismissing the finding outright.

A clinician should also distinguish three possible goals before recommending any repeat recording. The first is **current-state training**, where the client is expected to remain on the same regimen and the QEEG is used to guide intervention under real-world conditions. The second is **state comparison**, where a second recording is obtained after a clinically appropriate medication, sleep, or substance-use change to clarify which findings are stable. The third is **deferral**, where the recording conditions are too unstable for phenotype interpretation, such as acute withdrawal, recent anesthesia with complicated recovery, severe sleep deprivation, intoxication, or an active medical flare.

For prescribed pharmacology, the book favors current-state interpretation with transparent caveats. It does not favor casual medication discontinuation. Medication changes can destabilize mood, sleep, seizure threshold, pain, blood pressure, or safety. When off-medication recordings are clinically appropriate, they should be planned with the prescriber and documented as a measurement strategy, not a treatment recommendation. For habitual substance patterns (caffeine, cannabis, nicotine), the same principle applies: the person's ordinary functional state is the default recording condition, not a "clean" state manufactured by enforced abstinence. Timing information for all exposures remains clinically useful for interpretation (see Appendix C).

The report language should make the confidence level visible. A high-confidence statement might read, "The posterior alpha slowing is present across conditions and is not strongly explained by the current medication list." A reduced-confidence statement might read, "The diffuse slowing overlaps with current sedating medication exposure and untreated OSA risk, so interpretation as an endogenous underarousal phenotype is tentative." A deferred statement might read, "Because the recording occurred during acute benzodiazepine withdrawal, phenotype interpretation should be deferred until the client is clinically stable."

1.13 Evidence summary

- **Spectral effect:** Many major medication and substance classes have reproducible EEG effects, but the strength and specificity vary by class and recording condition.
- **Phenotype inference:** Medication, substance, condition, developmental, hormonal, and pipeline effects can mimic, mask, exaggerate, or transform common QEEG phenotype readings.
- **Workflow heuristic:** Treat every medicated QEEG as an interpreted measurement under documented exposure conditions, not as an unqualified trait baseline.

Ch 2: EEG Signals as Readouts of Pharmacology

2.1 Why This Chapter Exists

Medication effects make more sense when the clinician remembers what the EEG measures at the scalp. A QEEG map is a scalp-level estimate of synchronized electrical fields shaped by cortical populations, thalamocortical loops, neuromodulatory tone, and the analysis pipeline, not a direct picture of brain activity (Schomer & Lopes da Silva, 2017).

Medications do not push isolated frequency buttons. They change excitability, inhibition, arousal, synchrony, receptor gain, vigilance, and network coupling. The bands are the visible surface of those deeper mechanisms. This chapter provides the minimal receptor-to-spectrum map needed for the rest of the book. General EEG interpretation, band definitions, recording technique, source localization, and microstate theory are covered in the *QEEG Field Guide*.

2.2 Receptor Systems and Spectral Signatures

The rest of this book repeatedly connects receptor systems to EEG signatures. The mapping is not one-to-one, but it is clinically useful.

GABA-A positive allosteric modulation often organizes faster rhythmic activity and sedation-related changes. Benzodiazepines can produce prominent beta activity while also impairing cognition, reactivity, and vigilance. The beta does not mean the client is "more activated." It can be the spectral face of pharmacological inhibition and altered cortical synchrony.

Glutamatergic modulation can produce broad effects because glutamate is the major excitatory transmitter in cortex. NMDA antagonism, especially ketamine, can change broadband activity, gamma-related measures, and the aperiodic spectrum. These changes reflect disinhibition, altered recurrent excitation, and state-dependent network effects.

Dopaminergic and noradrenergic agents often affect arousal, attention, theta/beta balance, and task engagement. Classic stimulants may reduce excess slow activity and increase faster activity in some ADHD samples, but the effect depends on age, baseline, dose, formulation, timing, and task condition.

Serotonergic agents can affect alpha, theta, sleep architecture, emotional processing, and reactivity. SSRIs and SNRIs are not uniformly activating or sedating in EEG terms. Their effects vary by compound, duration, responder status, sex, baseline, and discontinuation state.

Cholinergic systems are central to cortical activation, attention, sensory gating, and desynchronization. Anticholinergic burden can push interpretation toward slowing, impaired vigilance, or cognitive inefficiency. Cholinergic differences in developmental variants such as Down syndrome populations may explain paradoxical responses to anticholinergic medications.

Adenosine, histamine, orexin, cannabinoid, opioid, and neurosteroid systems regulate arousal, sleep pressure, pain, sedation, and network stability. Caffeine antagonizes adenosine and can shift arousal and beta. Antihistamines can sedate and slow. Orexin antagonists change sleep-wake stability. Cannabinoids produce acute and chronic effects that differ sharply. Opioids can slow and interact with other depressants. Neurosteroids such as brexanolone act through GABA-A modulation.

2.3 The Aperiodic Background

Traditional QEEG emphasizes oscillatory bands, but the spectrum contains both periodic peaks and an aperiodic background. The aperiodic component is often described as the 1/f-like slope. Donoghue and colleagues formalized a method for separating periodic and aperiodic components (Donoghue et al., 2020). The clinical implication for drug interpretation: apparent band-power change can reflect a shift in the background slope rather than a specific rhythm.

A drug that flattens the aperiodic slope can make higher frequencies look stronger and lower frequencies look weaker, even if no narrow beta or gamma generator has changed. Ketamine and esketamine are the clearest examples in later chapters. Stimulants, sedatives, aging, and sleep deprivation can also interact with the aperiodic background.

2.4 Why Mechanism Does Not Equal Interpretation

Mechanism helps, but mechanism is not client-level causality. Knowing that benzodiazepines can increase beta does not prove that a given client's beta excess is benzodiazepine-driven. Mechanism gives the clinician plausible alternatives. Interpretation still depends on timing, dose, duration, state, repeated recordings, symptoms, and fit with the rest of the QEEG. If a client is on a drug class known to move a band in the same direction as a phenotype, confidence should drop. If the literature is absent, the report should say so.

2.5 Drug-Dosing Across the Lifespan

Developmental stage and aging change how drugs reach the brain and what they do when they arrive.

Adolescent and emerging-adult PK/PD: CYP enzyme maturation continues into early adulthood. Hepatic and renal clearance differs from adult values in early adolescence. Body composition, receptor density, and neural pruning change the pharmacodynamic context. Drug doses calibrated for adults may produce different exposure levels and spectral effects in younger populations. Stimulant holidays, cannabis onset, caffeine loading, and polypharmacy initiation concentrate in this age window.

Aging PK/PD: Hepatic and renal clearance decline. Body fat increases. Albumin may decrease. The blood-brain barrier may become more permeable. The net result is higher effective exposure at standard doses, longer time to clearance, and greater sensitivity to sedation, anticholinergic burden, and drug interactions. Polypharmacy is the norm, not the exception. Anticholinergic burden is a cumulative interpretive factor that grows with age and medication count.

Both of these shifts matter because they change the spectral signature of a given drug dose. An SSRI in a 16-year-old and the same SSRI in a 75-year-old do not produce the same exposure, the same receptor occupancy, or the same EEG consequence, even at the same milligram dose.

2.6 Case Vignette

A clinician reviews an eyes-closed QEEG from a client taking clonazepam (Klonopin) at night, methylphenidate most mornings, and caffeine before the appointment. The report shows elevated beta, modest frontal theta, and weak posterior alpha reactivity. A quick interpretation: hyperarousal with attention-related slowing. A better interpretation asks how the spectrum was generated. The beta may relate to benzodiazepine exposure, stimulant timing, caffeine, muscle tension, or true arousal. The frontal theta may reflect attention physiology, partial stimulant masking, drowsiness, or state drift. The weak alpha reactivity may be medication-related or vigilance-related.

The useful report states the observed pattern, identifies competing generators, and lowers confidence where the medication and state history overlap with the phenotype.

2.7 Interpretation traps

- **Treating band names as mechanisms.** Theta, alpha, beta, and gamma are summaries, not causes. Interpret the generator context before assigning meaning.
- **Reading beta as activation in every case.** Benzodiazepine-related beta can accompany sedation and cognitive slowing.
- **Ignoring aperiodic slope.** A broadband change can masquerade as a band-specific effect.
- **Forgetting reactivity.** A normal resting alpha value may hide abnormal alpha blocking or medication-related reactivity changes.

2.8 Intake questions

- **What was the time since last dose for stimulants, sedatives, caffeine, nicotine, cannabis, and sleep medications?** Timing determines whether the recording captures peak effect, trough, withdrawal, or steady state.
- **Was the client alert throughout the recording?** Vigilance drift can create slow activity and alpha changes that resemble medication effects.
- **Does the apparent band change look narrowband or broadband?** Broadband changes should raise the possibility of aperiodic-slope effects or artifact.

2.9 Evidence Summary

- **Spectral effect:** EEG rhythms arise from synchronized cortical and thalamocortical population activity; periodic rhythms and aperiodic background are separable and both drug-sensitive (Donoghue et al., 2020; Schomer & Lopes da Silva, 2017; Steriade et al., 1993).
- **Phenotype inference:** Medication and condition effects can alter the generator, state, or spectral background that produces a phenotype-like finding. Drug-dosing differences across the lifespan change spectral signatures at equivalent milligram doses.
- **Workflow heuristic:** Treat every QEEG phenotype as a generator hypothesis under documented state and pipeline conditions, not as a direct label for trait physiology.

Ch 3: Pharmacology Primer for Clinicians

3.1 Why Pharmacology Matters in QEEG Practice

A QEEG recording does not know whether a medication is prescribed for attention, depression, sleep, pain, seizures, blood pressure, allergies, or hormone symptoms. It only reflects the brain state present during the recording. For the clinician interpreting that recording, the medication list is useful only if it is translated into exposure: what drug, what dose, what formulation, when taken, how long used, whether the client is titrating or withdrawing, and whether metabolism makes the exposure higher or lower than expected. This chapter gives the pharmacology needed for that translation. A client taking methylphenidate at peak blood level is not in the same recording state as a client who skipped the morning dose. A client taking extended-release medication is not in the same state as a client taking immediate-release medication. A CYP2D6 poor metabolizer taking atomoxetine (Strattera) may have a different exposure than a normal metabolizer taking the same nominal dose (Clinical Pharmacogenetics Implementation Consortium, 2019; Kim et al., 2018). A client discontinuing a benzodiazepine is not the same as being "off benzodiazepines." The withdrawal state can have its own physiology.

3.2 Pharmacokinetics: What the Body Does to the Drug

Pharmacokinetics describes how the body absorbs, distributes, metabolizes, and eliminates a drug. For QEEG interpretation, the most important terms are route, Tmax, Cmax, half-life, steady state, active metabolites, and formulation.

Route determines how the drug enters the body. Oral medications pass through absorption and first-pass metabolism before reaching systemic circulation. Sublingual, buccal, transdermal, intranasal, intramuscular, and intravenous routes can produce different timing profiles. Intranasal esketamine, transdermal nicotine, long-acting injectable antipsychotics, and oral extended-release stimulants are not interchangeable from a QEEG timing standpoint.

Tmax is the time to peak concentration. A drug with peak effect one to two hours after dosing may shape a morning recording differently from an afternoon recording. The clinician does not need a pharmacokinetic curve for every client, but should know whether the recording occurred near expected peak, trough, steady exposure, or withdrawal.

Cmax is the peak concentration. Higher peaks often produce stronger acute effects, more side effects, and more visible state changes. Immediate-release formulations usually create sharper peaks than extended-release formulations. This matters for stimulants, sedatives, analgesics, and rescue medications. A sharp peak may produce a visible effect that a smoother formulation does not.

Half-life describes how long it takes the concentration to fall by half. Short half-life medications create more within-day fluctuation. Long half-life medications produce smoother exposure and may remain relevant even when the last dose was not recent. Fluoxetine (Prozac), diazepam (Valium), methadone (Dolophine), long-acting injectables, and some anticonvulsants cannot be understood only by asking, "Did you take it today?"

Steady state occurs after repeated dosing has produced a relatively stable concentration pattern. A client on day two of a medication is often not physiologically equivalent to the same client after several weeks. Pharmaco-EEG studies often use single-dose designs, while clinical clients are frequently at steady state, titrating, skipping doses, or tapering. That mismatch is one reason many chapter recommendations are labeled as clinical heuristics rather than controlled findings.

Active metabolites can extend or alter drug effects. A parent compound may clear while an active metabolite remains. This is clinically relevant for benzodiazepines, antidepressants, antipsychotics, opioids, and some anticonvulsants. A client may report that a medication was taken "yesterday" while the brain is still under meaningful exposure.

3.3 Pharmacodynamics: What the Drug Does to the Brain

Pharmacodynamics describes how a drug acts at receptors, transporters, enzymes, ion channels, and network systems. Standard psychopharmacology texts organize these actions by neurotransmitter systems, receptor families, and circuit effects (Nestler et al., 2020; Stahl, 2021). For QEEG interpretation, the clinician does not need to memorize every receptor subtype. The useful question is: what kind of state does this mechanism tend to create?

Full agonists activate a receptor. Partial agonists activate it less strongly and can sometimes stabilize a system by preventing both underactivation and overactivation. Antagonists block receptor activity. Inverse agonists reduce constitutive receptor activity. Positive allosteric modulators do not directly activate the receptor in the same way as an agonist; they change how strongly the receptor responds to its natural ligand. These distinctions matter because drugs in the same broad clinical category can produce different EEG patterns.

The section below maps receptor systems to their QEEG implications. The mapping is probabilistic: it points toward likely directions, not certainties (Mohler, 2006; Traynelis et al., 2010).

3.4 Receptor Systems as QEEG Clues

GABAergic medications often raise questions about sedation, inhibition, beta activity, reactivity, tolerance, and withdrawal. Benzodiazepines, Z-drugs, barbiturates, alcohol, neurosteroids, and some anticonvulsants are not identical, but they all touch the broad inhibitory side of the system. A QEEG recorded under GABAergic exposure should be interpreted with special attention to beta, vigilance, alpha reactivity, and slow activity.

Glutamatergic medications raise different questions. Ketamine and memantine are direct glutamate (NMDA) antagonists; topiramate (Topamax) has multi-mechanism action including AMPA/kainate antagonism; lamotrigine (Lamictal) is primarily a voltage-gated sodium channel blocker whose effect on excitatory transmission is downstream of presynaptic glutamate release reduction. Their QEEG signatures cannot be reduced to one glutamate pattern. The common interpretive issue is that they may change excitability, plasticity, and network stability in ways that alter both narrowband rhythms and broadband spectral shape.

Dopamine and norepinephrine medications raise arousal and attention questions. Stimulants, atomoxetine, bupropion (Wellbutrin), modafinil (Provigil)-like agents, some antidepressants, and some wake-promoting agents can affect alertness, effort, task performance, sleep, appetite, anxiety, and sympathetic tone. Their resting EEG effects may be smaller than task-related effects. The clinician should not expect every clinically effective stimulant to produce a dramatic resting map.

Serotonergic medications raise mood, sleep, alpha, activation, and discontinuation questions. SSRIs and SNRIs are often treated as a single category, but compounds differ in half-life, receptor profile, noradrenergic action, anticholinergic burden, sedation, and discontinuation risk. Psychedelics act through serotonergic systems but do not resemble daily SSRIs. A serotonin label alone is too broad to interpret a QEEG.

Cholinergic medications and anticholinergic burden matter because acetylcholine supports attention, cortical activation, memory, and sensory gating. First-generation antihistamines, TCAs, bladder medications, some antipsychotics, and many OTC products can add anticholinergic load. In older adults, anticholinergic burden can be clinically consequential even when no single medication looks dramatic on the list.

Histamine and orexin systems regulate wakefulness. Sedating antihistamines can produce drowsiness-related slowing and reduced reactivity. Orexin antagonists alter sleep-wake stability. These classes matter because clients may not think of them as "brain medications." They may appear as allergy medication, sleep aids, or routine nighttime pills.

Adenosine, cannabinoid, opioid, and neurosteroid systems often enter through everyday exposures: caffeine, cannabis, pain medication, alcohol, sleep aids, and postpartum depression treatments. Their EEG relevance is often mediated by arousal, pain, sleep, withdrawal, and sedation rather than a single clean spectral fingerprint.

3.5 Exposure States for QEEG Reports

A medication list becomes clinically useful when each medication is assigned an exposure state at the time of recording. The categories do not need to be complicated.

Peak exposure means the recording likely occurred near the expected maximum effect. This is most relevant for immediate-release stimulants, caffeine, nicotine, sedatives, rescue medications, intranasal esketamine, and acute substance use. Peak exposure can exaggerate a drug's visible QEEG effect.

Trough exposure means the recording likely occurred near the end of the dosing interval. A trough recording may show less of the medication effect, more rebound, or more underlying symptoms. For some drugs, trough is still meaningful exposure because of long half-life or active metabolites.

Steady exposure means the medication is taken consistently and the recording likely reflects the ordinary treated state. This is often the most clinically useful condition when the client will remain on the regimen during neurofeedback. The report should still say that the phenotype is interpreted under current medication exposure.

Titration exposure means the dose or drug was recently changed. This is a less stable state. Symptoms and QEEG features may reflect side effects, adaptation, or unstable sleep rather than eventual treatment response.

Discontinuation or withdrawal exposure means the client is stopping, reducing, skipping, or recovering from a drug. This state deserves its own label. It is not the same as being unmedicated. For sedatives, alcohol, stimulants, caffeine, nicotine, cannabis, antidepressants, antipsychotics, and anticonvulsants, discontinuation can change sleep, arousal, seizure threshold, mood, and spectral features.

Unknown exposure means the medication list lacks enough timing or adherence information to interpret confidently. Unknown exposure is common. It should not be silently converted into an assumption of stable dosing.

These categories are simple enough to use in ordinary clinical reports. A sentence such as "QEEG was recorded under steady SSRI exposure, peak caffeine exposure, and uncertain cannabis-withdrawal status" gives the reader more interpretive information than a medication list alone.

3.6 Dose Does Not Equal Exposure

Clinicians often ask what dose a client takes. Dose is necessary, but it is not sufficient. A dose is what was prescribed or swallowed. Exposure is what reached the brain over time.

A low dose can produce high exposure in a poor metabolizer, an older adult, a client with hepatic impairment, or a client taking an inhibitor. A high dose can produce lower exposure in an ultrarapid metabolizer, a smoker for some CYP1A2-metabolized drugs, a pregnant client with increased clearance, or a client with inconsistent adherence. Two clients can report the same dose and show different side effects, different symptom response, and different QEEG state.

Exposure is also shaped by behavior. A client may take a medication differently from the label, split tablets, skip weekends, take extra doses before demanding work, use caffeine to offset sedation, use cannabis to sleep, or combine OTC sleep aids with prescription sedatives. These patterns often matter more for QEEG interpretation than the formal prescription.

The intake form should therefore ask both prescribed use and actual use. "How do you usually take it?" is often more informative than "What is prescribed?"

3.7 Chronic Adaptation, Tolerance, and Sensitization

The same medication can have different EEG implications after one dose, after six weeks, and after years. Acute pharmaco-EEG studies are useful because they isolate short-term drug effects under controlled conditions. Clinical QEEG clients often arrive after long exposure. The brain may have adapted.

Tolerance means the same dose produces less of a subjective or physiological effect over time. A client on long-term benzodiazepines, cannabis, opioids, caffeine, or sleep medication may not look like a healthy volunteer after one acute dose. The medication can still shape the EEG, but the shape may be mixed with adaptation, dependence, rebound between doses, and sleep effects.

Sensitization is the opposite pattern: repeated exposure can make some responses stronger or more unstable. Stimulants, substances, antidepressant activation, akathisia, and withdrawal-kindling phenomena can all raise this question. The QEEG clinician does not diagnose sensitization from a resting map, but should document exposure history when the client reports escalating reactivity, agitation, paradoxical responses, or loss of predictable effect.

Chronic adaptation is one reason this book keeps separating drug signatures from phenotype causality. A drug class may have a known acute direction, but a long-treated client can show a different pattern because treatment response, tolerance, sleep, comorbidity, and discontinuation history have accumulated. The report should reflect the actual exposure history rather than assuming that an acute study maps perfectly onto a chronic outpatient.

3.8 Medication Timing and Neurofeedback Decisions

The timing question depends on the clinical goal. If neurofeedback will be delivered while the client remains medicated, the most relevant QEEG is often the medicated current-state recording. A second recording to compare states is a medical decision the prescriber leads, not something you schedule by treating the QEEG as a medication plan.

For stimulants, the timing question is often direct: record on usual dose, off dose, or both? The answer depends on whether treatment will occur on medication, whether off-dose functioning matters, and whether skipping medication is safe and clinically appropriate. For SSRIs, timing is less about same-day peak and more about steady state, recent changes, and discontinuation. For benzodiazepines and sleep medications, last dose, chronic use, tolerance, and withdrawal risk matter. For antipsychotics and anticonvulsants, steady-state and safety considerations usually dominate.

For ketamine, esketamine, procedural sedation, and anesthesia, the recording window can be the whole question. A QEEG recorded during the acute effect answers a different question than one recorded days later. The report should specify whether the recording was intended to capture acute drug effect, recovery, or ordinary baseline after the treatment window.

For cannabis, alcohol, nicotine, and caffeine, "usual routine" is often safer than sudden abstinence. Abstinence can create withdrawal or rebound that is less representative than the ordinary exposure state. The point is not to encourage use. The point is to avoid confusing withdrawal physiology with trait physiology.

3.9 Report Language Examples

The pharmacology primer becomes useful when it changes report language.

Weak language: "The client has elevated beta consistent with hyperarousal."

Better language: "Elevated beta is present. Interpretation as endogenous hyperarousal is reduced by benzodiazepine exposure, recent caffeine use, and possible muscle artifact."

Weak language: "The QEEG was recorded off stimulant."

Better language: "The QEEG was recorded after the client skipped the usual morning extended-release stimulant dose. This may capture an off-medication state but should not be treated as a never-medicated baseline."

Weak language: "Medication effects were considered."

Better language: "The recording occurred under steady SSRI exposure, recent caffeine exposure, and nightly cannabis use. These factors overlap with alpha, beta, sleep, and vigilance interpretation; phenotype confidence is adjusted accordingly."

This style is more defensible because it separates observation, exposure, inference, and confidence. It also makes repeat recordings more useful. If the next report changes, the clinician can ask whether the client, medication state, or recording conditions changed.

3.10 Formulation and Route

Formulation is easy to miss and critical for QEEG timing.

Immediate-release medications produce sharper exposure windows. An immediate-release stimulant taken shortly before a recording may show a stronger acute effect than the same medication taken the previous afternoon. Extended-release and sustained-release formulations flatten the curve and can keep the client in an on-drug state across much of the day. A clinician who records "methylphenidate" without IR versus ER has lost important information.

Long-acting injectable antipsychotics create a different problem. The medication is not merely present or absent. The client moves through an injection cycle. The date of last injection, dose, interval, and whether the client is near loading, plateau, or end-of-cycle trough may matter. Direct QEEG studies across LAI cycles are sparse, so most interpretation remains a workflow heuristic. The intake form should still capture the cycle position.

Transdermal formulations create steadier exposure but can still vary with patch timing, skin absorption, heat, removal time, and adherence. Transdermal nicotine has EEG and sleep effects distinct from combustible nicotine timing. Transdermal stimulants and hormones require the same logic, even when direct QEEG evidence is limited.

Intranasal, sublingual, buccal, IM, and IV routes can produce rapid or distinctive exposure windows. Intranasal esketamine has a treatment-session timing profile that differs from daily oral antidepressants. Intranasal benzodiazepine rescue medications create acute exposure in a clinical context that is not comparable to nightly oral sedative use. Outpatient ketamine, emergency sedation, and procedural anesthesia all require timing documentation.

The practical rule is that drug name alone is insufficient. Record route, formulation, dose, last-dose time, duration, and recent changes.

3.11 Metabolism, Pharmacogenomics, and Drug Interactions

Two clients can take the same dose and have different exposure. Body size, age, liver function, kidney function, pregnancy, inflammation, smoking status, and genetic metabolism all matter. For the QEEG clinician, the practical implication is that a reported dose does not equal an experienced dose. CYP2D6 status can produce markedly higher atomoxetine exposure in poor metabolizers than the nominal dose implies (Clinical Pharmacogenetics Implementation Consortium, 2019; Kim et al., 2018); the same enzyme governs many antidepressants, opioids, and antihistamines. CYP1A2 is induced by smoking, which is why tobacco cessation can raise levels of medications like olanzapine and caffeine. Appendix E covers pharmacogenomics in more detail.

Drug interactions compound this variability. Pharmacokinetic interactions (one drug changing the concentration of another) and pharmacodynamic interactions (two drugs converging on the same physiological pathway) both change what the QEEG captures. An SSRI inhibiting CYP2D6 can raise levels of CYP2D6-metabolized opioids such as oxycodone and of many antipsychotics, and can lower active-metabolite exposure for prodrugs such as codeine and tramadol; opioids and benzodiazepines together produce more sedative-spectral impact than either alone. A client whose medication list shows "SSRI + opioid + benzo" is not three separate pharmacological inputs. They are a composite exposure with interactions the individual chapters cannot fully capture. See Chapter 22 for common polypharmacy stacks and their interaction modes.

3.12 Titration, Withdrawal, and Drug Holidays

A client starting, stopping, increasing, decreasing, skipping, or cycling medication is in a different interpretation state than a client on stable dosing.

During titration, the brain may not yet reflect the eventual steady-state pattern. Side effects may be stronger than later therapeutic effects. Sleep, anxiety, appetite, pain, and adherence may be unstable. A QEEG during titration can be useful as a current-state measurement, but it should not be treated as stable phenotype evidence.

Withdrawal and discontinuation are not the absence of a drug. Benzodiazepine withdrawal, alcohol withdrawal, stimulant abstinence, caffeine withdrawal, cannabis withdrawal, and nicotine withdrawal can each produce EEG-relevant changes. SSRI/SNRI discontinuation may produce strong symptoms even without a validated resting-QEEG signature. Antipsychotic discontinuation can carry relapse and supersensitivity concerns. The clinician should document discontinuation state explicitly and avoid treating it as a clean baseline.

Drug holidays require the same discipline. Weekend stimulant holidays are common in pediatric ADHD (Ibrahim & Donyai, 2015; Martins et al., 2004), but direct QEEG evidence for on-day versus off-day phenotype interpretation is sparse. A Sunday recording may not represent a never-medicated baseline, and a Monday pre-dose recording may still reflect chronic treatment effects, sleep changes, or rebound.

Generic and brand switching is usually handled by prescribers and pharmacists, but it can matter when clients report abrupt changes. Lamotrigine bioequivalence studies suggest that approved generic formulations generally meet pharmacokinetic expectations (Privitera et al., 2017; Ting et al., 2015). That does not mean every subjective report is irrelevant. It means the QEEG clinician should document the switch and avoid making medication claims outside scope.

3.13 Phenotype Interaction Effects

The four interaction modes defined in Chapter 1 (masking, mimicry, exaggeration, and transformation) apply directly to the pharmacology covered here. Formulation adds another layer: a phenotype observed at peak immediate-release exposure may not appear at trough, a long-acting injectable may create stable chronic exposure rather than a discrete post-dose window, and a skipped dose may reflect rebound rather than baseline.

3.14 Case Vignette

A college student presents for QEEG-guided neurofeedback because of attention problems and anxiety. He takes extended-release mixed amphetamine salts most mornings, an SSRI at night, caffeine before class, and occasional diphenhydramine for sleep. He skipped the stimulant on the day of recording because he wanted the QEEG to show his "real brain." He slept poorly and drank a large coffee on the way to the appointment.

The recording shows elevated frontal theta, elevated beta, and weak posterior alpha reactivity. A simple interpretation might call this ADHD with hyperarousal. The pharmacology history complicates that reading. The skipped stimulant may reveal re-emergent attention physiology, but it may also introduce a rebound or off-medication state that differs from his usual functioning. Caffeine may contribute to beta. Diphenhydramine use and poor sleep may contribute to slow activity and weak reactivity. The SSRI may affect alpha-related findings. The more defensible report states that the recording captures an off-stimulant, caffeine-exposed, sleep-restricted state rather than a clean trait baseline.

3.15 Interpretation traps

- **Recording drug name without formulation.** IR, ER, transdermal, LAI, intranasal, and IV exposures produce different timing profiles.
- **Treating skipped medication as clean baseline.** Skipping can create rebound, withdrawal, or sleep disruption.

- **Ignoring metabolism.** CYP status, smoking, pregnancy, interacting drugs, and organ function can make the same dose produce different exposure.
- **Forgetting titration state.** Starting or changing a medication is more unstable than steady dosing.
- **Confusing pharmacodynamic and pharmacokinetic interactions.** One changes concentration; the other changes effect.

3.16 Intake questions

When reviewing medication exposure, ask:

- **What exact formulation are you taking?** Record IR, ER, XR, SR, patch, injection, nasal, sublingual, or other route.
- **When was the last dose, and is this your usual timing?** Document whether the recording reflects peak, trough, skipped dose, or routine exposure.
- **How long have you been on this dose?** Separate new starts, titration, steady state, taper, and discontinuation.
- **Have you had pharmacogenomic testing or unusual medication reactions?** Record CYP findings and paradoxical responses when known.
- **Have any interacting substances changed recently?** Include smoking, caffeine, cannabis, alcohol, supplements, antibiotics, and new prescriptions.

3.17 Clinical Recommendations

Medication timing should be treated as a measurement variable. If the goal is everyday functioning, record under ordinary stable conditions and document the exposure. If the goal is state comparison, plan it explicitly and coordinate any medication-state change with the prescriber. Do not let a client skip or stop medication casually for a QEEG because they believe it will reveal a purer baseline. Reports should describe exposure state in plain language: "recorded three hours after extended-release stimulant dose," "recorded near end of LAI cycle," "recorded during SSRI taper," or "recorded under stable nightly medication regimen." These phrases make the interpretation safer and more reproducible. The map does not justify recommending discontinuation, dose changes, or switching agents. Those decisions stay with the prescriber.

3.18 Evidence Summary

- **Spectral effect:** Pharmacokinetics, pharmacodynamics, receptor action, and route determine brain exposure and therefore the timing and plausibility of EEG effects.
- **Phenotype inference:** Last-dose timing, formulation, metabolism, titration, withdrawal, and drug interactions can change whether a phenotype-like finding is endogenous, pharmacological, or state-dependent.
- **Workflow heuristic:** Treat drug name, dose, formulation, last-dose timing, duration, and recent changes as mandatory QEEG metadata rather than optional intake details.

Ch 4: Methods, Claim Types, and Scope

4.1 Why the Evidence Framework Matters

This book asks clinicians to make practical decisions in an evidence base that is uneven. Some drug effects on the EEG are supported by controlled pharmaco-EEG studies. Some phenotype implications are reasonable but indirect. Some clinical recommendations are necessary in practice but have not been validated as formal algorithms. If those categories are blurred, the book becomes more confident than the literature allows.

The claim-type framework exists to prevent that error. It separates what the literature has directly measured from what the clinician can infer and what remains a clinical heuristic.

This matters because QEEG-based neurofeedback practice often operates at the edge of several literatures: clinical EEG, pharmaco-EEG, psychopharmacology, sleep medicine, neurology, psychiatry, developmental neuroscience, and signal processing. A stimulant study in children with ADHD, a ketamine study in treatment-resistant depression, a benzodiazepine study in healthy volunteers, and a pipeline study on artifact rejection do not answer the same kind of question. They can all inform interpretation, but they do not carry equal weight for a single clinical claim.

4.2 Scope of the Search and Audit

The literature base for this book was assembled as a targeted narrative review and citation audit. The project did not attempt a formal systematic review, meta-analysis, or quality-appraisal protocol. Instead, it used repeated focused searches and audit rounds across medication classes, substances, anesthetics, chronic medical confounders, developmental stage, reproductive hormone state, paradoxical responses, methodology, and withdrawal. Key sources were checked against PubMed, Crossref, article metadata, and the project's reference audit before entering the master bibliography.

The scope is intentionally clinical. The book asks how drug, substance, condition, and pipeline effects may alter QEEG phenotype interpretation in neurofeedback practice. It does not attempt to review all EEG effects of every medication, all sleep-EEG literature, all event-related potential studies, all seizure-risk literature, or all psychopharmacology. When a topic matters but lacks direct resting-QEEG evidence, the chapter labels it as a gap or heuristic rather than filling the space with invented specificity.

Several source types appear throughout the book. Controlled pharmaco-EEG studies are the strongest anchors for drug-specific spectral effects. Clinical EEG reviews and guidelines provide safety and methodology context (International Pharmaco-EEG Society, 2012; Tatum et al., 2016). Practitioner-oriented EEG drug-effect resources provide class-level clinical framing (Kerson, 2023). Mechanistic psychopharmacology and neuroscience sources help explain why a spectral effect may occur. Chronic-condition and developmental literature identify non-drug confounders that can overlap with medication signatures.

The audit was a filter as much as a search. It removed unsupported numerical claims, rejected misassigned citations, corrected fabricated or misapplied PMIDs, and downgraded class effects when the literature did not support strong claims. Those corrections are not incidental. They shaped the way the book handles uncertainty.

4.3 Source Hierarchy

The book uses a practical source hierarchy. At the top are controlled human EEG or QEEG studies that measure the relevant drug, dose context, and recording condition. A double-blind acute pharmaco-EEG study in healthy volunteers can be strong for acute spectral direction. A clinical sample study can be strong for treated-patient relevance. Neither is automatically strong for every clinical use.

Next are repeated observational EEG findings, clinical EEG safety studies, and guideline-level sources. These often matter for antipsychotics, anticonvulsants, anesthesia, and paroxysmal abnormality risk. A clinical EEG study may not map perfectly onto resting QEEG phenotyping, but it can still warn the clinician about slowing, epileptiform risk, sedation, or state instability.

Mechanistic psychopharmacology sits below direct EEG evidence for spectral claims but above pure speculation. Mechanism is useful when compound-specific resting-QEEG data are absent. It can justify cautious expectations, such as anticholinergic burden raising concern for slowing or GABAergic modulation raising concern for beta and sedation. Mechanism alone should not be written as if it directly measured the QEEG pattern.

Textbook and practitioner sources are used as orientation, not as substitutes for direct evidence. Kerson's drug-effect text is valuable for clinical framing (Kerson, 2023). IPEG recommendations help anchor measurement discipline (International Pharmaco-EEG Society, 2012). ACNS-oriented clinical EEG sources help with safety and terminology (Tatum et al., 2016). These sources help define the conversation, but drug-specific claims still need drug-specific support when available.

Finally, expert clinical heuristics are used when practice requires a decision and the literature is incomplete. The book does not hide those heuristics. It labels them.

4.4 Numerical Claims and Why Many Were Removed

Numbers can make a clinical statement sound stronger than it is. That is useful when the number is real and traceable. It is dangerous when the number was inferred, remembered loosely, or imported from the wrong context.

The audit for this project found several numerical or specific claims that could not be defended. Some cited papers reported categorical abnormality rates rather than continuous power changes. Some were review articles rather than primary data. Some were the wrong topic. The revision rule is strict: no percentage, Hz shift, band-power magnitude, prevalence, or washout interval appears unless the source directly supports it.

When the literature supports direction but not magnitude, the book uses qualitative language. "Associated with increased slow activity" is acceptable when the source supports direction. "Increases theta by 20-35%" is not acceptable unless the source directly reports that magnitude under relevant conditions. Range language is not a workaround. An unsupported range is still unsupported.

The same rule applies to washout and timing guidance. A recommendation to wait one week after uncomplicated elective anesthesia, for example, should be framed as a cautious clinical heuristic based on available recovery-window evidence, not as a validated universal rule. If a client is older, medically complicated, cognitively changed, or recovering from major surgery, the timing question belongs to clinical judgment and medical coordination.

4.5 Pure Gaps

Some categories have little or no direct human resting-QEEG evidence. This includes several newer psychiatric agents, metabolic medications, hormone-related interventions, wellness supplements, and off-label compounds. The book calls these pure gaps when the audit could not identify defensible resting-QEEG data.

A pure gap is not the same as no effect. It means the book cannot responsibly describe a signature. For example, if a medication has central nervous system effects but no direct resting-QEEG study, the chapter may describe mechanism, clinical state effects, or related-compound cautions. It should not invent a band pattern.

Pure gaps are useful for the live database. A database that includes explicit "no direct resting-QEEG evidence found" rows will be more honest than one that leaves rows empty or fills them with speculation. The gap itself becomes information for clinicians, researchers, and future update rounds.

4.6 How the Claim Types Map to the Database

The book's tables and future lookup database should preserve the same claim-type logic. A drug row should not say "increases beta" without a field for source type, population, recording condition, confidence, and phenotype implication. A phenotype row should separate measured feature from interpretation. An interaction row should identify whether the claim is a spectral effect, a phenotype inference, or a workflow heuristic.

This structure keeps the database from becoming an overconfident checklist. A clinician looking up benzodiazepines should see that beta effects are relatively well supported, that beta-excess interpretation is reduced in confidence, and that repeat-recording guidance is a clinical workflow rule. A clinician looking up a newer medication with no direct QEEG data should see a gap row rather than a false signature.

The database should also carry negative constraints. If a source was rejected for a claim, that should be visible in the audit notes. If a compound has evidence only in sleep EEG, anesthesia EEG, animal work, ERP tasks, or source-localized research, the row should not be upgraded to resting-QEEG evidence. The source context travels with the claim.

4.7 Boundary Conditions

Several boundary conditions recur across the book.

First, pediatric, adolescent, adult, and older-adult findings do not automatically generalize. EEG maturation and medication metabolism change across development. The book is especially cautious with late adolescents and young adults, because EEG maturation is still underway through adolescence (Tarokh & Carskadon, 2010) and their theta / beta interpretation can sit between pediatric and adult assumptions.

Second, sex and reproductive-hormone state matter. Resting alpha frequency varies with menstrual cycle phase, estradiol level, and oral contraceptive use (Brötzner et al., 2014). iAPF, alpha (Mazaheri & Jensen, 2010), sleep, mood, medication metabolism, pregnancy, postpartum state, menstrual cycle, hormonal contraception, perimenopause, and menopause can all affect QEEG interpretation. A finding cannot always be treated as a stable trait without that context.

Third, acute, chronic, and withdrawal states are different. A single-dose pharmaco-EEG study may not predict a client on years of treatment. A skipped dose may not reveal a clean baseline. Withdrawal can create its own EEG-relevant state.

Fourth, pipeline effects are not mere technical noise. Reference, filtering, artifact rejection (Bigdely-Shamlo et al., 2015), ICA, ASR, epoch selection, normative database, aperiodic modeling, and source localization (Mahjoory et al., 2017; Pascual-Marqui, 2002) can all change what the clinician sees. The pipeline is part of the instrument.

Fifth, vigilance state during the recording is itself a boundary condition. Eyes-closed paradigms invite sleep-onset physiology before the client is aware of it (Santamaria & Chiappa, 1987), and the spectral signatures of drowsiness (theta increase, individual alpha peak deceleration, beta decrease, slow rolling eye movements) overlap several of the most clinically important resting phenotypes. Standard amplitude-threshold artifact rejection does not catch drowsiness, and ICA does not remove it because it is not an artifact at all. Operational detection criteria and a working prevalence estimate for undetected drowsiness in clinical eyes-closed recordings are described in Hill (2026, manuscript submitted to *NeuroRegulation*; see (Hill, 2026)); Chapter 25 carries the clinical recognition guidance.

These boundary conditions are why the book repeatedly says "confidence is reduced" rather than "the phenotype is invalid." A finding can remain clinically useful while its source remains uncertain.

4.8 How to Read Chapter Claims

Each later chapter should be read in layers. The opening sections describe why the medication or confounder matters in practice. The mechanism section gives a plausible biological route from exposure to EEG effect. The spectral section describes what has been reported directly, with no invented magnitudes. The phenotype interaction section translates those effects into masking, mimicry, exaggeration, or transformation. The case vignette shows how the logic sounds in clinical prose. The evidence summary then states the claim-type bottom line.

Readers should resist skipping directly to the recommendation line. A recommendation can be sensible only when the preceding evidence level is understood. The same applies to tables: a table cell is a compressed statement, not the full evidence. If the table says "reduced confidence," the reader should return to the chapter text to see whether the confidence adjustment comes from a spectral-effect finding, a phenotype inference, or a workflow heuristic.

4.9 The Three Claim Types

This book labels every claim as one of three named types. The names describe what kind of statement is being made, not how strong the evidence behind it is. A replicated double-blind trial and a single cross-sectional naturalistic sample can both support a spectral-effect claim, and a phenotype inference can rest on a stronger body of work than the spectral-effect claim it was built from. The types do not rank against each other on quality, and reading them as a strength ladder is the most common way to misuse them. Evidence quality lives in the chapter text: the gap labels, the "limited evidence" notes, the sentences that say which population and which recording condition a finding came from. Read those, not the label, when the question is how much to trust a claim.

In tables and figure columns, the short forms "spectral," "phenotype," and "heuristic" appear where space is limited. They refer to these same three claim types.

Spectral effect. A spectral-effect claim concerns what a drug, substance, condition, or method does to the EEG or QEEG itself. The evidence behind these claims is typically direct and replicated: controlled pharmaco-EEG studies, repeated clinical EEG findings, or guideline-level sources. That said, the range is wide. A spectral-effect claim can rest on a single well-conducted study, and a large body of band-power replications may carry less weight than it appears once the aperiodic-decomposition gap is considered. Examples include benzodiazepine-associated beta effects, stimulant-related changes in slow and fast activity in some ADHD samples, ketamine-related broadband and aperiodic effects, and anesthesia-related EEG state changes. A spectral-effect label does not mean every individual client will show the effect. It means the direction is grounded in direct EEG evidence.

Phenotype inference. A phenotype-inference claim translates a spectral effect into a QEEG phenotype implication. If benzodiazepines can increase beta, then benzodiazepine exposure can reduce confidence that beta excess reflects endogenous hyperarousal. If stimulants can reduce excess theta in some ADHD samples, then stimulant exposure can mask an unmedicated theta phenotype. These claims are clinically important, but they are often not directly tested as phenotype-misclassification studies. They are careful extrapolations. The underlying spectral evidence is often solid; what makes the claim indirect is the inferential step from a measured EEG change to a confidence adjustment on a phenotype label.

Workflow heuristic. A workflow-heuristic claim is a practical rule for interpretation or workflow. Examples include documenting last-dose time for all relevant medications, preferring stable current-state recordings over casual washout, considering repeat recordings when exposure states differ, and lowering confidence when several confounders point in the same direction. These rules are rarely the subject of formal outcome studies, so the evidence behind them is typically clinical consensus or expert practice rather than comparative trial data. Workflow heuristics may be wise and clinically necessary, but they should not be written as if they were validated prediction rules.

A chapter may have spectral-effect evidence for a direction, phenotype-inference logic for confidence, and workflow-heuristic guidance for intake or repeat recording. The reader should keep those layers separate.

4.10 How These Claim Types Translate to Standard Evidence Grading

Clinicians trained in evidence-based medicine often work with GRADE, Cochrane, or US Preventive Services Task Force grading systems. The three claim types in this book are not a substitute for those frameworks and do not map onto them cleanly. A short translation may help readers used to the standard grading vocabulary.

A spectral-effect claim in this book is not the same as GRADE "high quality evidence." A spectral-effect claim asserts that a drug reliably moves a measurable EEG feature in a stated direction under stated conditions. That claim can be supported by controlled pharmaco-EEG studies, repeated clinical EEG observations, or guideline-level sources. It does not assert a clinical outcome, a treatment recommendation, or a population-level efficacy estimate. In GRADE terms, a spectral-effect claim is closer to a well-characterized intermediate biomarker finding than to a clinical-effectiveness rating.

A phenotype-inference claim is an inferential bridge. It takes a spectral effect and asks what it means for confidence in a phenotype label. In GRADE terms, this is the kind of claim that would typically be downgraded for indirectness: the spectral evidence answers a measurement question, the phenotype claim answers an interpretive question, and the gap between them depends on clinical reasoning rather than direct study.

A workflow heuristic is a practice rule. It is not graded in the standard sense because it is rarely the subject of comparative studies. A workflow heuristic may still be wise (record under documented conditions, do not adjust prescriptions to suit a QEEG question), but it is wisdom-as-discipline rather than wisdom-as-trial-evidence.

Readers who want to translate this book's claims into GRADE language should expect that even the strongest claims here would carry multiple GRADE-style downgrades for indirectness, imprecision, and applicability to individual clients. That limitation reflects the honest position of pharmaco-EEG as a field, not a weakness in the framework. The claim-type system in this book is built to keep the clinician from overreading; it is not built to replace formal evidence grading where such grading applies.

4.11 Extending the Claim Types to Inverse-Direction Claims

The claim types above were designed for forward-direction reasoning: given a drug, what does it do to the EEG? Part III asks the inverse question: given a phenotype, what does the literature suggest about treatment response? The same three types apply, but the confidence ceiling is generally lower because the evidence base is thinner and the translation from group-level association to individual-level prediction introduces additional uncertainty.

The axis also changes, and a reader moving between the two halves of the book should know it. In the forward direction the label names the kind of claim: measured spectral effect, phenotype inference, or workflow rule. In the inverse direction every entry is the same kind of claim, so the label grades the strength of the prediction evidence instead. That is why a forward-direction workflow heuristic can be a sound piece of practice discipline while an inverse-direction workflow heuristic is an untested hypothesis about someone's treatment. Same label, different work.

An inverse-direction **spectral-effect** claim would require a pre-registered, multi-site, prospectively validated prediction framework that reliably stratifies individual patients to treatments with clinically meaningful effect sizes. The Brainmarker-I iAPF stratification model (Voetterl et al., 2023) is the best-designed study the field has produced: it is pre-registered and its sertraline (Zoloft) contrast was tested out-of-sample against a randomized dataset, which is unusual here. But that contrast rests on a single study, with no independent laboratory having published a pharmacological replication, so it sits at phenotype-inference level. No inverse-direction claim in this book currently reaches spectral-effect level.

An inverse-direction **phenotype-inference** claim is a group-level association between a phenotype and treatment outcome that has been replicated at least once, with effect sizes that are real but modest. Examples include elevated frontal theta predicting moderate stimulant response in ADHD (Suffin & Emory, 1995; Arns et al., 2008), frontal alpha asymmetry showing sex-dependent associations with SSRI response (Bruder et al., 2001), and frontal QEEG patterns predicting relapse risk in chronic alcohol dependence (Winterer et al., 1998). Most Part III entries sit at phenotype-inference level.

An inverse-direction **workflow-heuristic** claim is a hypothesis derived from mechanism, clinical observation, or a single unreplicated study. Many phenotypes in Part III carry workflow-heuristic treatment-response hypotheses because direct prediction studies have not been conducted.

An additional distinction matters for inverse-direction claims: **individual-level confidence**. Even a well-replicated group-level association (phenotype inference) does not automatically translate to individual-level prediction. Within-group heterogeneity is always larger than between-group differences, comorbidity and polypharmacy add noise that controlled studies managed but individual clients do not, and recording conditions vary. The Part III entries carry this caveat explicitly. When a clinician uses a Part III entry to inform a prescriber conversation, the language should reflect group-level association, not individual certainty.

4.12 What Counts as Direct Evidence

Direct evidence means the study measured the relevant EEG feature under conditions close enough to the claim being made. A resting EEG study in adults taking a specific medication is closer to a neurofeedback QEEG claim than a cognitive ERP study in healthy volunteers. A controlled acute-dose study is strong for acute spectral effect, but weaker for chronic steady-state outpatient interpretation. A sleep-EEG study may be strong for sleep architecture and weaker for eyes-closed resting QEEG.

Direct evidence also requires the correct citation. A paper about cocaine dependence cannot support an opioid claim. A paper that reports categorical EEG abnormality rates cannot support invented continuous band-power percentages. A paper about lamotrigine (Lamictal) reducing delta and theta cannot be paraphrased as increasing alpha power. Each of those is a real failure mode in this literature, and the book is written to avoid them.

The highest-confidence chapters rely on direct EEG or QEEG evidence for the class or compound. Lower-confidence chapters may rely on mechanism, related compounds, clinical EEG safety literature, or condition-overlap evidence. When that happens, the chapter should say so.

4.13 What Counts as a Phenotype Claim

A phenotype claim goes beyond the EEG measurement and assigns clinical meaning. "Theta is elevated" is a measurement. "This is an ADHD-related underarousal phenotype" is a phenotype interpretation. "Current stimulant exposure may mask the unmedicated theta phenotype" is a medication-phenotype interaction claim.

This distinction matters because many clinical QEEG errors occur at the translation step. A finding may be real, clean, and statistically unusual, while the phenotype explanation remains uncertain. A beta z-score can be real and still be medication-shaped. A slow alpha peak can be real and still depend on age, hormone state, cannabis use, drowsiness, or recording condition. A frontal theta pattern can be real and still have multiple plausible generators.

The book therefore treats phenotype interpretation as a confidence judgment. The clinician is not asked to decide whether the finding is real or fake. The clinician is asked to decide how much confidence to place in a particular explanation.

4.14 Applying the Claim Types to the Four Interaction Modes

The four interaction modes from Chapter 1 (masking, mimicry, exaggeration, and transformation) each require claim-type discipline. A worked example: masking claims are strongest when a drug directly reduces the same feature the clinician is trying to detect. A stimulant may reduce slow activity in some ADHD samples. The spectral-effect claim is the direction itself. The phenotype-inference claim is

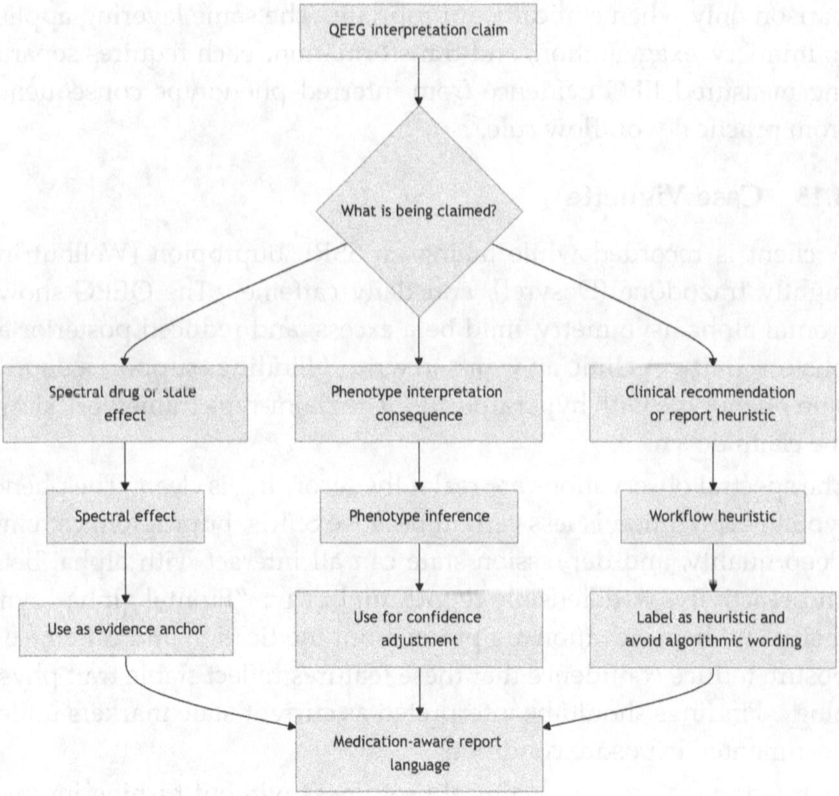

Figure 4.1: Claim-type framework: spectral effect, phenotype inference, and workflow heuristic.

that stimulant exposure can lower confidence in an unmedicated theta-phenotype reading. The workflow-heuristic recommendation is to document dose timing and consider prescriber-coordinated state comparison only when clinically appropriate. The same layering applies to mimicry, exaggeration, and transformation: each requires separating measured EEG evidence from inferred phenotype consequence from practical workflow rule.

4.15 Case Vignette

A client is recorded while taking an SSRI, bupropion (Wellbutrin), nightly trazodone (Desyrel), and daily caffeine. The QEEG shows frontal alpha asymmetry, mild beta excess, and reduced posterior alpha reactivity. A clinician wants to write, "Findings support a depression phenotype with hyperarousal." The claim-type framework slows the claim down.

The spectral observations are real if the recording is clean. The phenotype interpretation is less certain because SSRIs, bupropion, caffeine, sleep quality, and depression state can all interact with alpha, beta, and reactivity. A defensible report might say: "Frontal alpha asymmetry and beta elevation are present, but medication and caffeine exposure reduce confidence that these features reflect stable trait physiology. Findings should be interpreted as current-state markers under documented exposure conditions."

That language preserves clinical usefulness without turning indirect evidence into certainty.

4.16 Interpretation traps

- **Treating a phenotype inference as a spectral effect.** A plausible phenotype consequence is not the same as a directly measured misclassification effect.
- **Treating a workflow heuristic as if it were validated.** Intake and timing rules are clinical heuristics unless tested.
- **Inventing numbers to sound precise.** Qualitative uncertainty is better than fabricated magnitude.
- **Using a citation outside its scope.** A valid paper can still be the wrong paper for a claim.
- **Forgetting pure gaps.** No direct resting-QEEG evidence means no direct signature, not permission to extrapolate confidently.

4.17 Intake questions

For every medication-QEEG claim, ask:

- **What is the measured EEG effect?** Separate observation from interpretation.
- **What source directly supports the spectral direction?** If none, label the claim as gap or heuristic.
- **Is the phenotype consequence directly tested or inferred?** Most are inferred and should be labeled as phenotype inferences.
- **Is the recommendation validated or a practical rule?** Label practical rules as workflow heuristics.
- **What would change confidence?** Consider dose timing, repeat recording, state stability, artifact review, or comparison initiated or explicitly designed by the treating prescriber.

4.18 Clinical recommendations

Use claim-type language in reports and manuscripts. When the evidence supports a spectral effect, say so. When the clinical implication is inferred, say that confidence is reduced or adjusted rather than claiming causality. When a workflow recommendation is a clinical heuristic, label it as such.

Do not recommend medication discontinuation to test a hypothesis. If a different medication state would be clinically informative, coordinate with the prescriber and ground the choice in the client's safety and treatment goals, not the map alone.

4.19 A Methodological Caveat: The Aperiodic-Decomposition Gap

One limit on the confidence ceiling of spectral-effect claims in this book deserves explicit naming, because it affects the entire empirical foundation.

Most of the controlled pharmaco-EEG literature on which this book's spectral-effect claims rest was conducted before aperiodic spectral decomposition became a standard analytical step. The key tools (FOOOF, now called *specparam*, and related aperiodic-extraction methods) allow researchers to separate the 1/f-like aperiodic "background" of the EEG from discrete oscillatory peaks (Donoghue et al., 2020; He,

2014). A related line of work shows that the shape of an oscillation, when it departs from a sine wave, also distorts what band power appears to measure (Cole & Voytek, 2017). Before these tools were widely applied, studies typically analyzed band-power values that combined both components. A drug-related "increase in frontal theta" might reflect a genuine theta oscillation change, an aperiodic slope shift that made the theta range appear elevated, or both in unknown proportions.

This gap is not a disqualifying problem for the book's framework, but it is a real limitation on the confidence level of specific magnitude claims. Several examples:

- The benzodiazepine-associated beta literature (some of the most replicated in pharmaco-EEG) was analyzed largely with band-power approaches. Whether benzodiazepines increase oscillatory beta, shift the aperiodic slope, or both has not been systematically disentangled.
- The stimulant-and-TBR literature is similarly pre-aperiodic. The apparent theta decrease and beta increase under stimulants may in part reflect a slope change rather than independent oscillatory movements.
- The antipsychotic slow-wave literature uses band-power methods that cannot separate 1/f background elevation from delta/theta oscillation increases.

What this means in practice: the **directional** claims in this book's spectral-effect evidence summaries are supported by the literature and remain the best available guidance for clinical interpretation. The **magnitude** claims (any specific percentages or absolute differences) should be held lightly, because the underlying measurements may combine aperiodic and periodic contributions. When the second edition of this book is produced, translating the spectral-effect empirical base into aperiodic-aware terms (offset, exponent, and oscillatory peak parameters) will be a priority. For now, the clinician's working assumption should be: drug effects on the EEG are real and directionally predictable; whether they reflect primarily periodic power, aperiodic changes, or both is often unresolved in the source literature.

The evidence summaries at the end of each Part II chapter include a one-line note when this gap matters for that drug class.

4.20 Evidence summary

- **Spectral effect:** Direct EEG/QEEG evidence can support drug, substance, condition, or pipeline effects on spectral features, but only within the source's actual scope. The label marks the claim as a measured spectral one rather than an inference; how much weight any single spectral-effect direction carries still depends on the study named in the chapter. Spectral-effect magnitude claims carry additional uncertainty from the aperiodic-decomposition gap described above.
- **Phenotype inference:** Translating spectral effects into phenotype-confidence adjustments is often clinically necessary but usually indirect.
- **Workflow heuristic:** Intake, timing, repeat-recording, and report-language rules are practical safeguards unless directly validated.

Part II

Patterns

Ch 5: Stimulants

5.1 Why this class matters in NFB practice

Stimulants sit close to the center of QEEG-guided neurofeedback because many referrals involve attention, executive function, school performance, fatigue, or ADHD. They also sit close to the center of the medication-confound problem. A stimulant can change the same spectral features clinicians often use to reason about attention phenotypes: theta, beta, theta/beta ratio, arousal state, vigilance, and sometimes alpha peak measures.

Strongest evidence	Pediatric methylphenidate studies and reviews support stimulant-related reductions in slow activity and increases in faster activity in subgroups.
Biggest interpretation trap	Treating skipped-dose recordings as clean: Skipping may create an atypical day with rebound, sleep disruption, or changed caffeine use.
Default clinical action	Record the medication state most relevant to treatment, document formulation and last-dose timing, and use comparison initiated or explicitly designed by the treating prescribers.

Stimulants do not "invalidate" QEEG. The issue is whether the QEEG is being interpreted as the client's ordinary treated state, the client's off-medication state, or a comparison between the two. A recording obtained near stimulant peak answers a different question than a recording obtained before the morning dose or after a skipped dose. A clinician who does not document timing may treat a state-dependent recording as a stable trait profile.

This chapter covers classic psychostimulants such as methylphenidate and amphetamine formulations, the non-stimulant attention medication atomoxetine (Strattera), and modafinil (Provigil)/armodafinil (Nuvigil) as a separate wake-promoting subgroup. These agents overlap clinically, but they should not be collapsed into one EEG signature.

5.2 Mechanism (clinician-level pharmacology)

Methylphenidate primarily increases catecholaminergic signaling by blocking dopamine and norepinephrine transporters. Amphetamine formulations increase catecholamine availability through transporter-related and vesicular mechanisms. The clinical result is often improved alertness, attention, response inhibition, and task engagement in appropriately selected clients, but the EEG effect depends on baseline physiology, age, diagnosis, dose, formulation, and timing.

Atomoxetine is a norepinephrine reuptake inhibitor used for ADHD and related attention problems, not a classic stimulant. Its exposure is strongly affected by CYP2D6 status, enough that pharmacogenomic dosing guidance exists (Clinical Pharmacogenetics Implementation Consortium, 2019). A poor metabolizer can have higher exposure than expected from the nominal dose, which matters when a QEEG is interpreted as if the medication effect were ordinary.

Modafinil and armodafinil are wake-promoting agents with mechanisms that differ from methylphenidate and amphetamine. They affect arousal systems, catecholamine signaling, and sleep-wake regulation, but their QEEG profile is better treated as a milder activator or vigilance-stabilizing pattern rather than as a direct copy of classic stimulants. There is enough distinct modafinil literature to warrant separating it from methylphenidate and amphetamine.

Stimulant interpretation is also a formulation problem. Immediate-release and extended-release preparations create different recording windows, as discussed in the Classic Stimulants section below.

5.3 Known spectral effects

The stimulant QEEG literature is strongest in pediatric ADHD and less complete in adults. Loo and Barkley's review summarizes the broader ADHD EEG and stimulant literature but should be read as a cautious review rather than a primary pharmaco-EEG trial (Loo &

Barkley, 2005). The safest phrasing is that stimulant medications are often associated with reductions in excess slow activity and increases in faster activity in some ADHD samples, with heterogeneity across studies and subgroups.

Clarke and colleagues provide a primary pediatric stimulant anchor: a six-month stimulant trial in children with ADHD was associated with EEG normalization that showed up mainly in the theta and beta bands (Clarke, Barry, Bond, et al., 2002). That supports the clinical concern that stimulant exposure can mask or reduce the theta features often used in attention-phenotype interpretation. It does not prove that every client on methylphenidate will show that pattern, and it should not be used to quote unsupported magnitudes.

QEEG phenotypes may also predict stimulant response rather than merely reflect stimulant exposure. Arns and colleagues reported that pretreatment EEG phenotypes, including slow alpha peak and other subgroup patterns, predicted differential response to stimulant treatment in children with ADHD (Arns et al., 2008). Arns later discussed iAPF as a predictor of stimulant nonresponse (Arns, 2012). These findings are clinically interesting, but they should not be conflated with direct stimulant-induced EEG changes. Prediction and acute effect are different claims.

Atomoxetine is covered in its own section below; it should not be collapsed into classic stimulant spectral expectations.

Modafinil and armodafinil are covered separately below.

5.4 Phenotype interaction effects

Stimulants most often create a masking problem. A client whose unmedicated recording might show frontal theta elevation or elevated TBR may show a more normalized pattern when recorded near stimulant peak. That can be clinically useful if the treatment question is current functioning on medication. It is misleading if the clinician interprets the medicated recording as a clean unmedicated phenotype. I see this pattern regularly in the stimulant-exposed adolescents who come through a clinical QEEG intake: a school-day recording, near-peak medication, nine hours of sleep forgone the night before, energy drink at breakfast. The "clean" map gets read as a phenotype. It is a measurement of a drugged, caffeinated, sleep-deprived brain at peak pharmacological effect. Those are not the same thing.

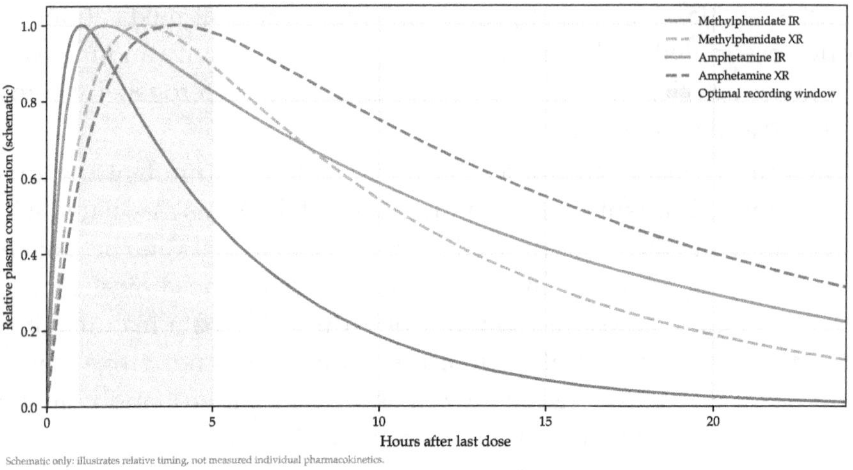

Figure 5.1: Stimulant formulation timing: IR vs. XR concentration curves with recording windows. Schematic only.

They can also create transformation. A lower theta pattern under stimulant exposure does not necessarily mean the client lacks an attention-related phenotype. It may mean the phenotype is medication-responsive. For neurofeedback planning, the key question is whether training is meant to support treated functioning, reduce residual symptoms despite medication, or understand off-medication physiology.

Exaggeration and mimicry are less central but still possible. Stimulants, caffeine, anxiety, sleep loss, and withdrawal states can all push arousal and beta-related features. A beta excess under stimulant plus caffeine exposure should not be interpreted the same way as beta excess in an unmedicated anxious client. Stimulants can also worsen sleep, and sleep loss can increase slow activity the next day, creating a mixed state in which the medication and its sleep consequences point in different directions.

The theta/beta ratio requires special caution in adolescents and young adults. TBR changes with age, and the 16-20 range is the most vulnerable to overinterpretation. A high TBR in a late adolescent may reflect incomplete maturation, sleep timing, cannabis exposure, stimulant timing, or ADHD-related physiology. The book therefore treats

TBR in adolescents as a confidence-weighted marker, not as a standalone diagnostic shortcut.

Adult ADHD also differs from pediatric ADHD. Adult samples may show theta-related features without the same beta-deficit pattern often emphasized in children. A clinician should not assume that pediatric stimulant normalization targets transfer directly to adult clients.

5.5 Classic Stimulants: Methylphenidate and Amphetamines

Methylphenidate and amphetamine formulations are the medications most likely to raise the on-medication versus off-medication QEEG question. Families, clients, and clinicians often believe that an off-medication recording is more authentic. Sometimes it is clinically useful. Sometimes it is less representative than the ordinary treated day. The choice depends on the question. If the client will train, work, and study while taking the medication, the treated recording may be the most relevant map for current-state neurofeedback planning. If the referral question is whether an attention phenotype exists independent of stimulant exposure, an off-medication comparison may be useful, but it should be planned carefully. A skipped dose after poor sleep, high caffeine, or weekend schedule change is not a clean trait baseline. Methylphenidate evidence supports the core masking concern. In pediatric ADHD, methylphenidate can reduce frontal / central theta and increase posterior beta (Clarke, Barry, Bond, et al., 2002). That direction overlaps directly with common QEEG ADHD phenotype language. The recording may show treated physiology rather than erasing ADHD.

Amphetamine formulations likely raise the same interpretive family of questions, but the chapter avoids pretending that methylphenidate data automatically quantify amphetamine effects. The two classes share catecholaminergic relevance but differ in mechanism, formulation options, clinical potency, duration, side-effect profile, and individual response. When direct EEG evidence is missing for a specific formulation, the report should use class-level caution rather than compound-specific certainty.

Newer stimulant formulations add timing complexity. Delayed-release, long-acting, extended-release, prodrug, and transdermal products can shift when the EEG is recorded relative to effect. A medication taken the night before may be designed to work the next morning. A patch may create different exposure than an oral tablet. A prodrug may produce smoother kinetics than immediate-release amphetamine. These formulation facts belong in the QEEG record.

5.6 Atomoxetine

Atomoxetine is usually grouped clinically with ADHD medications, but it should not be written as a stimulant in EEG prose. It is a norepinephrine reuptake inhibitor with delayed clinical onset compared with immediate stimulant effects. Its QEEG interpretation problem is less about a sharp same-day peak and more about steady exposure, dose, CYP2D6 metabolism, side effects, sleep, and activation.

Clarke's atomoxetine work gives the chapter a direct EEG anchor (Barry et al., 2009). The available evidence is more limited than for methylphenidate, and the book therefore treats atomoxetine conclusions cautiously. A clinician should not assume that atomoxetine will mask theta in the same way as methylphenidate or amphetamine. The mechanism and timing differ.

CYP2D6 status is unusually important for atomoxetine. Poor metabolizers can have higher exposure, and genotype-based dosing guidance exists (Clinical Pharmacogenetics Implementation Consortium, 2019). If a client reports unusual sedation, agitation, insomnia, or side effects at ordinary doses, CYP2D6 status becomes relevant context. The QEEG report should not diagnose metabolism, but it can record known pharmacogenomic results and flag exposure uncertainty.

The practical report phrase is: "Atomoxetine exposure may influence attention/arousal interpretation; confidence in theta/TBR conclusions is adjusted for stable dosing status, side effects, sleep, and CYP2D6 information when available." That phrasing is cautious enough for the evidence base.

5.7 Viloxazine (Qelbree) and Serdexmethylphenidate (Azstarys)

Two newer ADHD agents may appear on intake forms and deserve brief mention.

Viloxazine (Qelbree) is a selective norepinephrine reuptake inhibitor FDA-approved for ADHD in children (2021) and adults (2022). Its mechanism parallels atomoxetine (norepinephrine reuptake inhibition) with additional serotonergic modulation (5-HT2B agonism, 5-HT2A antagonism, 5-HT7 antagonism). Legacy pharmaco-EEG studies from the 1970s–80s, when viloxazine was marketed in Europe as an antidepressant, showed increased alpha and beta power and decreased theta, consistent with a noradrenergic-activating profile. No modern ADHD-focused resting-QEEG study exists. The QEEG clinician should interpret viloxazine as a norepinephrine-predominant agent with possible alpha/beta modulation, document timing and side effects, and avoid claiming a precise spectral fingerprint.

An important pharmacogenomic note: viloxazine is a strong CYP1A2 inhibitor. Clients taking viloxazine alongside CYP1A2 substrates (caffeine, clozapine (Clozaril), olanzapine (Zyprexa), theophylline) will have increased exposure to those drugs. A client on viloxazine who drinks the same amount of coffee as before may effectively be consuming far more caffeine from a pharmacokinetic standpoint. This can alter the arousal, beta, and sleep interpretation of the QEEG without any change in the client's reported behavior.

Serdexmethylphenidate (Azstarys) is a prodrug of d-methylphenidate combined with immediate-release d-methylphenidate, FDA-approved for ADHD in 2021. The prodrug component provides extended duration via enzymatic conversion. From a QEEG perspective, serdexmethylphenidate produces the same active metabolite (d-methylphenidate) as other methylphenidate formulations, so the spectral interpretation framework from the methylphenidate section applies. The main difference is timing: the prodrug creates a smoother, longer exposure curve than standard IR methylphenidate. No serdexmethylphenidate-specific QEEG data exist. Document the formulation and last dose.

5.8 Alpha-2 Agonists (Clonidine and Guanfacine)

Clonidine (Kapvay) and guanfacine (Intuniv) are alpha-2 adrenergic agonists used as first-line non-stimulant ADHD medications and commonly co-prescribed with methylphenidate or amphetamine in pediatric and adult ADHD. They appear in nearly every pediatric polypharmacy stack, yet their QEEG implications are rarely discussed.

The QEEG clinician will encounter them often enough to need a working framework, even though direct resting-state evidence is sparse.

Mechanism and pharmacologic differences. Both agents reduce presynaptic norepinephrine release and hyperpolarize locus coeruleus neurons, decreasing tonic arousal and enhancing prefrontal signal-to-noise. Guanfacine is relatively selective for alpha-2A receptors in prefrontal cortex, where postsynaptic alpha-2A stimulation strengthens working-memory network firing. Clonidine is less selective (alpha-2A, -2B, -2C, and imidazoline receptors), acts more broadly in brainstem and peripheral autonomic circuits, and produces more sedation and hypotension. Clonidine has a shorter half-life (6–10 hours) and is often used as a night-time sleep-settling agent alongside daytime stimulants. Guanfacine ER has a longer half-life (~17 hours), less peak-related sedation, and builds steady-state over several days.

Known spectral effects. Direct ADHD-focused resting-state QEEG data are limited. The strongest anchor is a 2024 pediatric RCT comparing d-methylphenidate, guanfacine, and their combination in children with ADHD: guanfacine monotherapy decreased global alpha power, while the combination produced broader reductions across slow and alpha bands, interpreted as a more normalized cortical engagement pattern. A companion task-related EEG study showed that guanfacine and combination treatment produced distinct oscillatory modulations in posterior visual-attentional networks during working memory. For clonidine, the available EEG data come from sedation, antihypertensive, and pain paradigms rather than ADHD treatment cohorts. In those contexts, clonidine at sedating doses produces increased slow-frequency power (delta / theta) and reduced higher-frequency activity, consistent with central sympatholysis.

Interaction with stimulants. When alpha-2 agonists are co-prescribed with methylphenidate or amphetamine, the expected net EEG effect is an intermediate arousal state: stimulant-associated frontal activation plus alpha-2-mediated smoothing of slow excess and alpha abnormalities. This is based on a single pediatric RCT, so the book frames it as plausible rather than established.

Timing. For QEEG recording purposes, testing at trough (morning, pre-dose) will show minimal acute sedative effect from a night-time clonidine IR dose. ER formulations taken twice daily can create a sustained low-level milieu that slightly increases slow activity across the day, especially in sensitive patients. Guanfacine ER produces more stable plasma levels with less pronounced peak-trough EEG fluctuation than clonidine IR.

Withdrawal and rebound. Abrupt clonidine discontinuation can cause rebound hypertension, tachycardia, and agitation; guanfacine carries similar warnings with a milder clinical profile. These autonomic rebounds could transiently increase cortical arousal and high-frequency activity on EEG, potentially mimicking anxiety or withdrawal states. A missed-dose QEEG should be interpreted in light of possible sympathetic overactivity.

Sedation versus endogenous vigilance. Drug-induced drowsiness from alpha-2 agonists will look like increased frontal and central theta/delta, reduced posterior alpha, and diminished alpha reactivity, similar to endogenous vigilance problems. Distinguishing factors are temporal linkage to dosing (within a few hours of clonidine) and corroborating subjective reports of sleepiness.

Evidence summary. The spectral-effect evidence is limited: the mechanism and sparse direct data support directional expectations (slowing, alpha reduction), but no systematic QEEG characterization in ADHD populations exists for clonidine, and guanfacine resting-state evidence rests on a single pediatric trial. Treat alpha-2 agonist QEEG interpretation as a confidence modifier (document dose, formulation, timing, and sedation state) rather than a precise spectral fingerprint.

5.9 Modafinil and Armodafinil

Modafinil and armodafinil deserve a separate subsection because they are wake-promoting agents, not simple copies of methylphenidate or amphetamine. Their clinical use often involves narcolepsy, residual sleepiness, shift-work sleep disorder, fatigue, OSA-related sleepiness, or off-label cognitive fatigue. These referral contexts already shape EEG interpretation.

Wang and colleagues studied modafinil after CPAP withdrawal in OSA and found increased EEG activation ratios along with improved vigilance (D. Wang et al., 2015). This is not the same as saying modafinil produces a universal beta increase in all resting QEEGs. It says that modafinil can alter activation and vigilance under sleepiness conditions.

Bodenmann and Landolt found that modafinil's sleep-EEG effects depend partly on COMT genotype (Bodenmann & Landolt, 2010). Linton and colleagues reported resting microstate changes in healthy adults (Linton et al., 2022). Saletu and colleagues' narcolepsy work suggests that modafinil treatment can normalize some of the EEG differences between people with narcolepsy and control subjects (M. T. Saletu et al., 2005). Together, these sources support a "wakefulness and network-state" framing rather than a simple theta/beta story.

For QEEG practice, modafinil raises two questions. First, is the recording capturing treated wakefulness, untreated sleepiness, or sleep-loss recovery? Second, is the apparent improvement in the map a medication effect, a vigilance effect, or both? In clients with OSA, narcolepsy, shift work, Long COVID, ME/CFS, or medication-related fatigue, modafinil may change the state being measured as much as it changes a band.

5.10 Pre-Recording Timing

The default is to record the client in the ordinary prescribed medication state (see the governing rule in Appendix C). A recording near stimulant peak answers a different question than one obtained before the morning dose, and documenting which state was captured is the essential step. The 48-hour interval sometimes cited as a stimulant clearance convention covers the duration of clinical effect for common formulations; extended-release methylphenidate runs about 10 to 12 hours of clinical effect, and methylphenidate's elimination half-life is roughly 3 to 4 hours whatever the formulation, because the extended-release delivery system lengthens absorption rather than elimination.

For clients who take stimulants daily, the ordinary medication state is typically the clinically relevant one, especially when the client will train, work, and attend sessions while taking the medication. Any deliberately altered medication-state comparison, such as an off-medication recording, must be initiated or explicitly designed by the prescriber. The QEEG clinician does not independently direct clients to stop stimulants.

Some clients should never be recorded off medication. Do not request any timing change when the stimulant treats narcolepsy or another hypersomnolence disorder, when the client drives to the appointment, or when the prescriber has flagged behavioral or cardiovascular instability. Record in the ordinary treated state and document the timing.

For all other daily psychotropics (SSRIs, SNRIs, antipsychotics, mood stabilizers), the same principle applies: record the client in the ordinary medication state and document last-dose timing. Whether the recording falls near peak, trough, or mid-cycle exposure affects interpretation and belongs in the report.

When the clinical goal is specifically to evaluate the medicated phenotype (for example, assessing whether stimulant treatment normalizes a theta pattern), a treated-state recording is appropriate and should be labeled as such.

5.11 Drug Holidays and Skipped Doses

Drug holidays are common in ADHD practice, especially for children and adolescents. They may be used for appetite, sleep, growth, side effects, school demands, family preference, or prescriber strategy. From a QEEG standpoint, a drug holiday is a documented exposure state, not a neutral default.

A weekend holiday may change sleep timing, caffeine use, activity level, mood, irritability, and family stress. A summer holiday may reflect a different routine from the school year. An off-dose day may include rebound symptoms, fatigue, or compensatory caffeine. Direct EEG evidence for drug-holiday interpretation is sparse, so the book treats drug-holiday QEEG decisions as workflow heuristics.

When an off-medication recording is needed, the clinician should document the reason, the duration off medication, last dose, sleep, caffeine, and whether the day was typical. The report should avoid phrases like "true baseline" unless the conditions justify it.

5.12 Report Language Examples

Weak language: "Stimulants normalized the QEEG."

Better language: "The recording was obtained near expected peak extended-release stimulant exposure. Frontal theta was not elevated under this treated condition, so confidence in the unmedicated theta phenotype cannot be determined from this recording alone."

Weak language: "Off medication, the QEEG proves ADHD."

Better language: "The skipped-dose recording shows elevated frontal theta and TBR, but interpretation is reduced by late-adolescent maturation, poor sleep, and caffeine exposure. Findings are compatible with an attention-related phenotype but are not specific."

Weak language: "Modafinil acts like other stimulants."

Better language: "Modafinil is treated as a wake-promoting agent with evidence for activation and vigilance effects; its QEEG interpretation should consider sleepiness, OSA/CPAP context, fatigue condition, and microstate/network findings."

Weak language: "Atomoxetine should not affect the QEEG because it is not a stimulant."

Better language: "Atomoxetine is not a classic stimulant, but norepinephrine reuptake inhibition and CYP2D6-dependent exposure can affect arousal, sleep, and attention-state interpretation."

5.13 Choosing the Recording State

For stimulant cases, the recording-state decision should be made before the appointment, not improvised at intake. The clinician should ask what the QEEG is supposed to guide.

If the goal is current-state treatment planning, record the client as they usually function. For many school, work, and executive-function referrals, that means the usual medication state. The report then says that the phenotype was interpreted under treated conditions.

If the goal is unmedicated phenotype exploration, an off-medication recording may be useful only when the comparison is prescriber-coordinated and the conditions are controlled enough to be meaningful. Document sleep, caffeine, nicotine, cannabis, exercise, illness, pain, and schedule.

If the goal is comparison, two recordings may be more useful than one: usual medication state and carefully documented alternative state. Even then, the comparison is descriptive. It shows how the client's measured EEG differs across states. It does not by itself prove the medication caused every difference.

If the goal is neurofeedback protocol selection while the medication regimen is unstable, deferral may be better than guessing. New stimulant start, recent dose increase, side effects, insomnia, appetite disruption, anxiety activation, or inconsistent adherence can make the current QEEG less stable. A current-state recording can still be informative, but it should not be overread as a durable phenotype.

5.14 Stimulants, Sleep, and Caffeine

Stimulant interpretation cannot be separated from sleep and caffeine. A stimulant can improve daytime attention while worsening insomnia in some clients. Caffeine may be used to extend stimulant effect, compensate for poor sleep, or manage withdrawal. The QEEG then captures a three-way interaction among medication, sleep pressure, and adenosine blockade.

The practical problem is that sleep loss can increase slow activity and reduce vigilance, while stimulants and caffeine can push alertness and faster activity. A recording can therefore contain mixed signals: treated attention, insufficient sleep, rebound fatigue, and compensatory caffeine. The clinician should not force that mixture into one label.

In adolescents and college-age clients, this is especially common. Late sleep timing, irregular dosing, energy drinks, cannabis, nicotine vaping, and academic stress can all appear in the same case. A TBR or frontal theta finding in that context remains interpretable, but at lower confidence unless the state variables are documented.

5.15 What Not to Claim

The stimulant chapter warrants four specific limits on what a QEEG clinician can claim:

- A medicated QEEG without elevated theta does not prove that an unmedicated attention phenotype is absent.
- An off-medication QEEG with elevated theta does not prove ADHD, especially in late adolescents, poor sleepers, cannabis users, or clients with chronic fatigue or concussion history.
- Stimulant response does not prove that the QEEG target was the cause of the symptoms.
- QEEG does not justify starting, stopping, or changing stimulant (or any) medication; coordinate any planned on/off comparison with the prescriber.

The more defensible claim is conditional: stimulant exposure, timing, age, sleep, caffeine, and formulation all change confidence in theta / TBR interpretation.

5.16 Case vignette

A seventeen-year-old client is referred for QEEG-guided neurofeedback because of persistent attention problems despite medication. He takes extended-release methylphenidate most school mornings, uses caffeine before exams, sleeps irregularly, and sometimes skips medication on weekends. The QEEG is scheduled on a Saturday because the family wants to see his "real baseline." He skips methylphenidate, sleeps late, drinks an energy drink before the appointment, and reports gaming until 2 AM.

The QEEG shows elevated frontal theta, elevated TBR, and scattered beta excess. A quick report might call this a classic ADHD phenotype with hyperarousal. A better report says that the recording captures a skipped-dose, sleep-restricted, caffeine-exposed adolescent state. Elevated theta and TBR may reflect ADHD-related physiology, but confidence is reduced by age, sleep, caffeine, and non-usual medication timing. The beta finding may reflect caffeine, arousal, muscle artifact, or an endogenous pattern.

The clinically useful next step is to decide what question matters, not to tell the family to stop medication. If neurofeedback will be delivered on school-day medication, a usual-dose recording may be more relevant. If the goal is state comparison, any off-medication recording should be planned safely and documented carefully.

5.17 Interpretation traps

- **Calling a medicated-normalized QEEG "normal baseline."** Stimulant response may mask a theta or TBR phenotype.
- **Treating skipped-dose recordings as clean.** Skipping may create an atypical day with rebound, sleep disruption, or changed caffeine use.
- **Collapsing atomoxetine into stimulants.** Atomoxetine has a distinct mechanism and CYP2D6 exposure issues.
- **Collapsing modafinil into classic stimulants.** Modafinil should be treated as a wake-promoting subgroup with its own evidence base.

- **Overreading adolescent TBR.** Late-adolescent TBR can reflect maturation and state, not only ADHD physiology.
- **Ignoring formulation.** IR, ER, delayed-release, transdermal, and actual-use patterns matter for recording timing.
- **Missing benzodiazepine interactions.** Stimulant clients may also take benzodiazepines for anxiety or sleep, creating competing arousal and sedation effects. A skipped stimulant dose with continued benzodiazepine use is a different state from a skipped stimulant dose without sedative exposure. See Chapter 8 for benzodiazepine tapering pitfalls.

5.18 Intake questions

When stimulant or attention medication appears on the intake form, ask:

- **What exact medication and formulation are you taking?** Record methylphenidate vs amphetamine, IR vs ER / XR / SR, atomoxetine, modafinil / armodafinil, patch, or delayed-release product.
- **When was the last dose, and is that usual for you?** Note peak, trough, skipped dose, weekend holiday, or unusual timing.
- **What caffeine, nicotine, cannabis, or sleep aids were used in the last 24 hours?** These can alter arousal and beta / theta interpretation.
- **How stable is the current regimen?** Separate new starts, dose changes, steady dosing, drug holidays, and discontinuation.
- **For adolescents and young adults, what is the sleep schedule?** Sleep timing can strongly influence theta and TBR interpretation.

5.19 Clinical recommendations

The safest default is to record the client under the medication state most relevant to treatment, document it precisely, and interpret phenotype confidence accordingly. If the client trains while taking medication, a usual-dose recording may be the best current-state guide. If the clinical question requires off-medication comparison, that comparison should be initiated or explicitly designed by the treating prescriber and planned so that sleep, caffeine, and adherence do not create a misleading state.

Reports should say whether the recording was on usual stimulant, off usual stimulant, near peak, near trough, or under uncertain timing. For atomoxetine, report steady-state and CYP2D6 information when known. For modafinil, report sleep-loss context, OSA/CPAP status, narcolepsy diagnosis, or shift-work context when relevant.

Use cautious language for stimulant effects. "Stimulant exposure may reduce confidence in an unmedicated theta/TBR phenotype" is safer than "the stimulant normalized the QEEG." "Elevated TBR in a late adolescent should be interpreted with developmental caution" is safer than using the ratio as a stand-alone diagnostic label.

When residual symptoms persist on medication, the medicated QEEG can be especially useful. It shows the physiology still present under the client's ordinary support system, which may be the most relevant state for neurofeedback planning and outcome tracking across real clinical visits.

5.20 Evidence summary

- **Spectral effect:** Pediatric methylphenidate studies and reviews support stimulant-related reductions in slow activity and increases in faster activity in some ADHD samples, with heterogeneity and limited adult generalization. *Aperiodic caveat: the underlying studies used band-power methods that do not separate periodic theta/beta changes from aperiodic slope shifts; directional claims hold, magnitude claims carry additional uncertainty.*
- **Phenotype inference:** Stimulant exposure can mask or transform theta/TBR-based attention phenotype interpretation, especially when dose timing, age, sleep, and caffeine are undocumented.
- **Workflow heuristic:** Record the medication state most relevant to treatment, document formulation and last-dose timing, and use comparison initiated or explicitly designed by the treating prescriber only when clinically appropriate.

Ch 6: SSRIs and SNRIs

6.1 Why this class matters in NFB practice

Antidepressants are among the most common medication exposures in QEEG-guided neurofeedback practice. Moore and Mattison's national estimate places prescription psychiatric medication use at roughly one in six U.S. adults, with antidepressants forming a large share of that exposure (Moore & Mattison, 2017). A clinician who treats adults will therefore see SSRIs, SNRIs, bupropion, trazodone (Desyrel), mirtazapine (Remeron), TCAs, and other antidepressant strategies frequently.

Strongest evidence	Antidepressants can alter EEG/QEEG measures, but directions vary by compound, state, responder status, sex, method, and the specific claim.
Biggest interpretation trap	Using FAA as a universal SSRI biomarker: FAA findings are sex-dependent and method-sensitive.
Default clinical action	Treat antidepressant dose stability, side effects, sleep, tapering, and hormone context as required metadata for QEEG interpretation.

The QEEG interpretation problem runs deeper than antidepressant EEG effects alone. Depression, anxiety, insomnia, trauma, chronic pain, reproductive hormone state, aging, caffeine, cannabis, and withdrawal can alter the same features clinicians may want to interpret: alpha power, iAPF, frontal alpha asymmetry, beta activity, theta cordance, sleep-related slowing, and reactivity. Antidepressant chapters therefore require more confidence language than most readers expect.

This chapter focuses on SSRIs and SNRIs while briefly noting adjacent antidepressant categories when they affect interpretation. Ketamine/esketamine, neurosteroid antidepressants, TCAs, bupropion, trazodone, mirtazapine, and sleep-focused antidepressant use receive fuller treatment in later chapters or cross-references.

6.2 Mechanism (clinician-level pharmacology)

SSRIs increase serotonergic signaling by blocking serotonin reuptake. SNRIs increase serotonergic and noradrenergic signaling, with the noradrenergic contribution varying by compound and dose. These mechanisms affect mood, anxiety, sleep, appetite, sexual function, autonomic tone, and emotional processing. They can also influence EEG indirectly through improved depression, worsened insomnia, activation, sedation, discontinuation, or changed sleep architecture.

The clinician should avoid thinking of SSRIs as a single EEG mechanism. Fluoxetine (Prozac) has a long half-life and active metabolite profile that differs from paroxetine (Paxil). Sertraline (Zoloft) differs from citalopram (Celexa), escitalopram (Lexapro), fluvoxamine, and vortioxetine (Trintellix). Venlafaxine (Effexor) and duloxetine (Cymbalta) are not interchangeable. Some antidepressants are more activating, some more sedating, and some carry more anticholinergic or histaminergic effects. The QEEG effect can reflect the compound, the clinical response, the side-effect state, and the disorder being treated.

Duration matters. Acute serotonergic changes, early side effects, steady-state adaptation, long-term symptom response, and discontinuation are different physiological states. A client recorded during week one of an SSRI trial may not resemble the same client after remission, partial response, emotional blunting, insomnia, or discontinuation symptoms.

6.3 Known spectral effects

Older pharmaco-EEG work from the Saletu group provides an important anchor for antidepressant EEG mapping. Saletu, Grunberger, and Linzmayer studied sertraline and zimelidine using EEG brain mapping and psychometry (B. Saletu et al., 1986). Later Saletu work also contributes to the broader antidepressant pharmaco-EEG background (B. Saletu et al., 2006). These studies support the idea that antidepressants can have measurable EEG effects, but they should not be used to invent precise modern QEEG phenotype magnitudes.

Newer SSRI/SNRI literature suggests that EEG patterns may predict or track response, but with inconsistent spectral directions across studies. A 2026 machine-learning response-prediction study in the bibliography is a useful emerging anchor (Li et al., 2026). Its clinical relevance is that high-frequency activity and connectivity measures may carry treatment-response information. The caution is that response prediction does not equal a simple drug-effect signature, and it does not separate activation-syndrome subgroups cleanly.

Prefrontal theta cordance studies, including Bares and colleagues, are relevant because they show that early EEG-derived measures can predict antidepressant response in some depressed samples (Bares et al., 2007; Bares et al., 2008). Cordance is not raw theta power, and those findings should not be rewritten as ordinary band-power claims. They are examples of response-prediction biomarkers, not direct evidence that all antidepressants produce the same resting theta effect.

Frontal alpha asymmetry is the antidepressant biomarker most likely to be overused clinically. Bruder and colleagues found the responder/nonresponder alpha asymmetry difference at occipital rather than frontal sites, and noted that in their earlier, more female samples the hemispheric difference was stronger among women (Bruder et al., 2008). However, a 2025 meta-analysis of resting FAA in depression found a small pooled effect (mean difference −0.03) with high heterogeneity and no subgroup that recovered a larger signal (Luo et al., 2025); resting FAA is better understood as a group-level association too small to carry an individual prediction. The book treats FAA as a constrained and method-sensitive marker. FAA should not be presented as a universal SSRI/SNRI response biomarker, and any extrapolation beyond the narrow Bruder sample conditions should be flagged.

Hormonal state matters for alpha interpretation. iAPF and alpha measures can vary with menstrual cycle and hormonal contraception (Brötzner et al., 2014). This matters because antidepressant response, depression symptoms, PMDD, perimenopause, postpartum state, and contraceptive use often appear in the same clinical context. A low iAPF or alpha change in a woman should not be assigned to medication without reproductive-hormone context.

Compound	Primary QEEG Vectors	Claim type	Interaction Modes	Confidence
SSRIs	faa context, serotonergic modulation	heuristic	exaggeration, mimicry, transformation	reduced, substantially reduced
SNRIs	serotonergic noradrenergic modulation	heuristic	exaggeration	substantially reduced
Tricyclic antidepressants	sedation anticholinergic context	heuristic	n/a	n/a
MAOIs	monoaminergic modulation	heuristic	n/a	n/a
Bupropion	seizure threshold context, activating profile	heuristic	n/a	n/a

Figure 6.1: SSRI/SNRI interpretation confidence: compounds by QEEG vectors, claim type, and interaction modes.

6.4 Phenotype interaction effects

SSRIs and SNRIs most often create masking and transformation, but all four interaction modes apply. Masking occurs when mood or anxiety symptoms improve under medication and the QEEG no longer shows the pattern that would have appeared in the acute state; this is clinically meaningful if treatment will occur under stable medication. Mimicry occurs when side effects produce patterns that resemble other phenotypes; the medication class label alone is not enough. Four side-effect clusters drive this: activation (insomnia, agitation, akathisia-like restlessness), caffeine compensation in response to SSRI sedation, frank sedation itself, and withdrawal-adjacent states during taper. Exaggeration occurs when antidepressant effects and comorbid conditions point the same direction: depression plus insomnia plus SSRI activation plus caffeine can look different from depression plus hypersomnia plus a sedating adjunct. Transformation is most visible in FAA and alpha interpretation, where an unmedicated depressed woman, a woman on an SSRI, a woman on oral contraceptives, and a postmenopausal woman should not be treated as the same clinical object even when the surface measure looks similar.

6.5 Activation, Switching, and Paradoxical Responses

SSRIs and SNRIs can be activating for some clients. Activation may present as anxiety, insomnia, agitation, irritability, restlessness, or hypomanic symptoms. In clients with unrecognized bipolar vulnerability, antidepressant-induced mood switching is a clinical safety concern. The QEEG clinician should not diagnose these states from a recording, but should document them because they alter arousal and beta / theta interpretation.

The paradoxical-response literature also warns against assuming population-average response. Some clients do not respond in the expected direction. If a client reports that an SSRI made them wired, emotionally flat, sedated, or cognitively slowed, that report is clinically relevant to the QEEG state. It should not be dismissed because it is not the modal effect.

For QEEG language, the safest phrasing is: "Current antidepressant exposure and reported activation/sedation symptoms reduce confidence that arousal-related findings reflect stable trait physiology." That statement is practical and does not claim causality beyond the evidence.

6.6 Discontinuation and the Pristine-Baseline Myth

SSRI and SNRI discontinuation is a major interpretive state even though direct resting-QEEG evidence is limited. A client tapering or recently stopping medication may experience dizziness, sensory symptoms, irritability, anxiety, insomnia, mood worsening, flu-like symptoms, or cognitive fog. The QEEG may reflect discontinuation, relapse, sleep disruption, stress, or baseline physiology.

Discontinued is not the same as never medicated. A client who stopped venlafaxine two weeks ago is not automatically a pristine unmedicated baseline. The report should document taper schedule, last dose, symptom state, sleep, and whether the prescriber is involved. If the recording occurs during discontinuation symptoms, phenotype interpretation should be cautious.

Discontinuation also complicates relapse interpretation. Worsening mood after stopping medication may represent relapse, discontinuation syndrome, situational stress, sleep disruption, or several factors. QEEG cannot reliably separate those causes by itself. The report should avoid causal claims and instead state the exposure state explicitly.

6.7 Case vignette

The intake form lists a single antidepressant: sertraline, recently increased. The conversation adds trazodone three nights per week, two coffees before noon, and irregular cycles consistent with perimenopause. The forty-two-year-old client is here for residual depression, poor concentration, and insomnia. The QEEG shows frontal alpha asymmetry, mild beta excess, and reduced posterior alpha organization.

A quick report might frame the FAA as a depression biomarker and the beta as hyperarousal. A better report is more conditional. FAA may be clinically relevant, but its antidepressant-response meaning is sex-dependent and method-sensitive. The beta excess may reflect anxiety, SSRI activation, caffeine, poor sleep, muscle artifact, or an endogenous arousal pattern. Posterior alpha interpretation requires attention to reproductive-hormone state and sleep.

The useful clinical statement replaces "the medication caused the pattern" or "the QEEG proves depression" with: "Current antidepressant exposure, recent dose increase, sleep disturbance, caffeine use, and perimenopausal context reduce confidence in assigning alpha and beta findings to stable trait physiology." Layered measurement requires honest confidence limits, not epistemic cowardice. The recording is still useful: it documents the current state, names the confidence limits, and gives the prescriber something more accurate than a single-cause story.

6.8 SSRIs Versus SNRIs

SSRIs and SNRIs overlap clinically, but the QEEG clinician should keep them separate when possible. SSRIs are primarily serotonergic reuptake inhibitors. SNRIs add clinically relevant norepinephrine reuptake inhibition, though the strength of that effect varies by compound and dose. A client on venlafaxine, desvenlafaxine (Pristiq), or duloxetine may therefore present more activation, blood-pressure, sleep, or arousal questions than a client on a low-dose SSRI, depending on the case.

This does not mean SNRIs have a simple beta signature. The evidence does not justify that shortcut. It means the exposure history should ask about activation, insomnia, sweating, tremor, agitation, blood pressure, pain indication, and discontinuation risk. Venlafaxine discontinuation, for example, is clinically notorious even though direct resting-QEEG evidence for discontinuation is sparse.

SSRIs also differ from one another. Fluoxetine's long half-life makes same-week discontinuation different from paroxetine or venlafaxine tapering. Fluvoxamine has interaction issues. Paroxetine carries more anticholinergic and discontinuation concerns than some other SSRIs. Sertraline and escitalopram are common enough that clinicians may stop noticing them, but common does not mean irrelevant.

The report should therefore avoid writing "on antidepressant" as if the class were uniform. The minimum useful phrase is compound, dose, duration, recent change, and side-effect state.

6.9 Adjacent Antidepressants

Many clients use medications with antidepressant indications or antidepressant-like roles that are not SSRIs or SNRIs. Bupropion is often activating and catecholaminergic. Mirtazapine and trazodone are often used for sleep and can shape drowsiness, alpha reactivity, and slow activity through sedation and sleep architecture. TCAs have anticholinergic and antihistaminergic properties that make them mechanistically different from SSRIs. MAOIs are less common but pharmacologically broad. Ketamine / esketamine and neurosteroid antidepressants receive separate treatment because their EEG mechanisms are different.

This matters because the medication list can say "antidepressant" while the QEEG issue is sleep medication, anticholinergic burden, activation, pain treatment, or postpartum neurosteroid exposure. A sedating antidepressant used at night should not be interpreted like a morning SSRI. A bupropion-stimulant combination should not be interpreted like SSRI monotherapy.

Those agents are cross-referenced in other chapters. Antidepressant indication still does not determine EEG mechanism.

6.10 Sleep, Pain, and Somatic Indications

Antidepressants are not always prescribed for depression. They may be used for anxiety, OCD, PTSD, pain, migraine, insomnia, PMDD, vasomotor symptoms, or functional somatic symptoms. The indication matters because the condition itself can shape QEEG interpretation.

A client on duloxetine for fibromyalgia and depression brings pain, fatigue, sleep, and noradrenergic exposure into the same recording. A client on amitriptyline (Elavil) for migraine has anticholinergic, sedating, and pain-related confounds. A client on trazodone for sleep may show medication-related sedation but also improved sleep continuity. A client on an SSRI for PMDD may use luteal-phase dosing, making cycle timing part of the medication exposure.

The clinician should therefore ask why the medication is prescribed. The same compound can have different interpretive meaning when used for depression, panic, sleep, neuropathic pain, migraine, PMDD, or hot flashes. The QEEG does not reveal the indication. The intake form must.

6.11 Polypharmacy With Antidepressants

Antidepressants often appear in combinations: SSRI plus stimulant, SNRI plus gabapentinoid, antidepressant plus benzodiazepine, antidepressant plus antipsychotic augmentation, antidepressant plus sleep medication, antidepressant plus cannabis, or antidepressant plus caffeine. There is no reliable controlled within-subject pharmaco-EEG literature for most common psychotropic combinations. Combination interpretation is therefore usually a workflow heuristic.

Polypharmacy does not mean uninterpretable. It means the report should avoid single-cause language. If an SSRI-treated client also takes benzodiazepines, beta excess may be medication-shaped by the benzodiazepine even if the SSRI is the psychiatric anchor. If an SNRI-treated client also uses caffeine and bupropion, beta / arousal interpretation becomes more complex. If an antidepressant-treated client uses nightly cannabis for sleep, alpha and sleep-state interpretation require both chapters.

The report should state the competing contributors: "Alpha and beta findings are interpreted under SSRI exposure, sedating adjunct use, nightly cannabis, and poor sleep." That is more useful than assigning the map to "depression" alone.

6.12 Report Language Examples

Weak language: "FAA suggests SSRI response."

Better language: "FAA is present, but its antidepressant-response interpretation is sex-dependent and method-sensitive; confidence is adjusted for sex, reproductive hormone context, medication status, and recording pipeline."

Weak language: "The SSRI caused the beta excess."

Better language: "Beta excess is present under SSRI exposure with reported activation, caffeine use, and insomnia. Medication and state effects reduce confidence in interpreting beta as a stable endogenous hyperarousal phenotype."

Weak language: "The client is off antidepressants, so this is baseline."

Better language: "The recording occurred during recent SNRI taper with discontinuation symptoms. Findings should be interpreted as a discontinuation-state recording, not a pristine never-medicated baseline."

Weak language: "Antidepressant effects were considered."

Better language: "The recording was obtained under stable sertraline exposure, intermittent trazodone use, poor sleep, and perimenopausal symptoms; alpha and arousal interpretations are confidence-adjusted accordingly."

6.13 Choosing the Recording State

For antidepressant-treated clients, the usual clinical answer is to record the stable current state. Many clients will remain on antidepressants during neurofeedback. If the medication is stable, tolerated, and part of ordinary functioning, the current-state QEEG can be clinically useful. The report should say that interpretation is under stable antidepressant exposure.

Off-medication comparison is less straightforward than with short-acting stimulants (long adaptation, taper, discontinuation, relapse risk). When it is clinically justified, it belongs in a prescriber-coordinated plan, not a skip for QEEG convenience.

Recent dose changes deserve special caution. Starting an antidepressant, increasing an SNRI, tapering paroxetine, missing venlafaxine, adding trazodone, or stopping bupropion can all change sleep, arousal, mood, and cognition. A recording during this period is a real current-state recording, but it may be poor evidence for a durable phenotype.

The strongest antidepressant QEEG interpretation usually comes from stability: stable dose, stable sleep, stable mood state, documented side effects, documented hormone context, and no acute discontinuation. When stability is absent, the report should say so.

6.14 Practical Confidence Adjustments

For alpha and iAPF findings, reduce confidence when reproductive hormone context is unknown, when the client is perimenopausal, postpartum, on hormonal contraception, or recorded during an unusual cycle phase. This does not invalidate the finding. It limits trait interpretation.

For beta and arousal findings, reduce confidence when the client reports SSRI/SNRI activation, insomnia, caffeine escalation, stimulant co-treatment, akathisia-like restlessness, or recent dose increase. The beta may still be real, but the arousal explanation is less clean.

For theta or cordance-like findings, reduce confidence when the measure is being interpreted outside the method used in the source. Cordance literature should not be paraphrased as ordinary theta-power evidence. Raw QEEG maps and derived antidepressant-response biomarkers are related but not identical.

For discontinuation, reduce confidence broadly. A tapering or recently stopped antidepressant can alter mood, sleep, sensory symptoms, and autonomic state. Until the client is clinically stable, the recording should be treated as a transition-state measurement.

These confidence adjustments should be written in the report, not kept as private reasoning.

6.15 What Not to Claim

Five claims are not supportable from the antidepressant literature:

- Do not claim that an SSRI or SNRI produced a specific band-power magnitude unless the source directly reports it.

- Do not treat FAA as a universal antidepressant-response marker.
- Do not treat discontinuation as a clean unmedicated baseline.
- Do not assign alpha or iAPF changes to medication while ignoring sex, age, menstrual cycle, OCP use, pregnancy, postpartum state, perimenopause, or menopause.
- Do not use QEEG to recommend antidepressant start, stop, dose change, or switch; those decisions stay with the prescriber.

The more defensible claim is conditional: antidepressant exposure, clinical response, side effects, reproductive hormone context, sleep, and discontinuation state all change confidence in alpha, beta, arousal, and response-biomarker interpretation.

When the QEEG looks better after antidepressant treatment, the change may reflect medication effect, symptom remission, sleep improvement, reduced rumination, changed caffeine use, therapy response, time, or measurement differences. That is encouraging clinically, but causal attribution still requires careful comparison.

The same caution applies when the QEEG looks worse. A deteriorated map during antidepressant treatment may reflect side effects, relapse, sleep loss, pain, grief, substance use, discontinuation, or a new medical stressor. The map should prompt better questioning, not instant blame or a medication conclusion.

6.16 Interpretation traps

- **Using FAA as a universal SSRI biomarker.** FAA findings are sex-dependent and method-sensitive.
- **Confusing response prediction with drug effect.** Cordance or ML response predictors are not ordinary raw spectral signatures.
- **Ignoring reproductive hormone context.** Alpha and iAPF interpretation in women requires cycle, OCP, pregnancy, postpartum, and menopause context when relevant.
- **Treating discontinuation as clean baseline.** Tapering and withdrawal states can shape symptoms and EEG state.
- **Collapsing all antidepressants.** SSRIs, SNRIs, bupropion, mirtazapine, trazodone, TCAs, ketamine, and neurosteroids differ mechanistically.
- **Ignoring activation.** SSRI/SNRI activation or switching symptoms can alter arousal interpretation.

- **Ignoring CYP2D6 interactions with paroxetine.** Paroxetine is both a CYP2D6 substrate and a potent CYP2D6 inhibitor. Co-prescription with other CYP2D6 substrates (atomoxetine (Strattera), TCAs, some antipsychotics) can raise those drugs' levels. Codeine and tramadol (Ultram) are the reverse case: paroxetine raises the parent drug but blocks formation of the active metabolite (morphine, M1), so analgesia can fall while tramadol's seizure and serotonergic risks persist. A client whose QEEG looks "more medicated than the dose suggests" may be experiencing a paroxetine-driven 2D6 interaction.
- **Missing CYP2C19 PM risk with citalopram or escitalopram.** CYP2C19 poor metabolizers on citalopram or escitalopram are at increased QT-prolongation risk due to elevated drug exposure. This is a safety consideration, not a QEEG signature, but the QEEG clinician should document known pharmacogenomic status and communicate with the prescriber when relevant.
- **Overlooking fluvoxamine CYP3A4 inhibition.** Fluvoxamine is a potent CYP3A4 inhibitor. Clients on fluvoxamine plus a CYP3A4 substrate (certain benzodiazepines, quetiapine (Seroquel), some anticonvulsants) may have elevated exposure to the co-prescribed drug, which can alter the QEEG picture independently of the SSRI itself. Fluvoxamine is also the most potent CYP1A2 inhibitor among the SSRIs, which can raise caffeine exposure; a fluvoxamine client's caffeine history deserves extra weight when interpreting a recording, because the same intake produces higher caffeine exposure.

6.17 Intake questions

When antidepressants appear on the intake form, ask:

- **Which antidepressant, dose, and duration?** Record SSRI/SNRI/bupropion/trazodone/mirtazapine/TCA or other category.
- **Has the dose changed recently?** Mark start, increase, decrease, taper, missed doses, or discontinuation.
- **What side effects are present now?** Ask about activation, sedation, insomnia, emotional blunting, agitation, sexual side effects, and cognitive slowing.

- **What is the sleep context?** Insomnia, hypersomnia, sedating adjuncts, nightmares, and sleep apnea risk all matter.
- **For female clients, what is the reproductive-hormone context?** Document cycle phase if known, OCP use, pregnancy, postpartum, perimenopause, menopause, and hormone therapy.

6.18 Clinical recommendations

Interpret antidepressant-exposed QEEGs as current-state recordings unless a carefully planned comparison says otherwise. Stable antidepressant treatment can be the relevant clinical state for neurofeedback. The problem is not medication presence. The problem is undocumented medication, side effects, and discontinuation state.

Use constrained language for alpha and FAA. A report can say that FAA or alpha findings are present, but should not claim universal antidepressant-response prediction. If the client is female, document hormone context. If the client is tapering or recently changed dose, state that phenotype confidence is reduced by medication instability.

Do not recommend stopping antidepressants to obtain a cleaner QEEG. If a medication-state comparison is clinically useful, coordinate with the prescriber and justify it by safety, symptom stability, and treatment goals.

6.19 Evidence summary

- **Spectral effect:** Antidepressants can alter EEG/QEEG measures, but directions vary by compound, state, responder status, sex, method, and whether the claim concerns raw power, cordance, asymmetry, or connectivity. *Aperiodic caveat: cordance and FAA are the most replicated SSRI-response markers, but neither was validated with aperiodic-aware processing; the aperiodic contribution to apparent alpha and theta changes is unmeasured in most source studies.*
- **Phenotype inference:** SSRI/SNRI exposure, activation/sedation, reproductive hormone context, and discontinuation state can reduce confidence in alpha, FAA, beta, and arousal interpretations.
- **Workflow heuristic:** Treat antidepressant dose stability, side effects, sleep, tapering, and hormone context as required metadata for QEEG interpretation.

Ch 7: TCAs, MAOIs, and Atypical Antidepressants

7.1 Why this class matters in NFB practice

SSRIs and SNRIs are common enough to deserve their own chapter, but they do not exhaust antidepressant exposure. Many neurofeedback clients take tricyclic antidepressants, bupropion (Wellbutrin), trazodone (Desyrel), mirtazapine (Remeron), MAOIs, vortioxetine (Trintellix), vilazodone (Viibryd), agomelatine (Valdoxan) where available, or newer neurosteroid antidepressants. Some are prescribed for depression. Others are prescribed for sleep, pain, migraine, anxiety, smoking cessation, ADHD-adjacent symptoms, postpartum depression, or medically complex mood states.

Strongest evidence	Older TCA pharmaco-EEG literature supports EEG effects, but compound heterogeneity and sedating versus activating profiles limit class-wide claims.
Biggest interpretation trap	Treating antidepressant as a mechanism: TCAs, MAOIs, bupropion, trazodone, mirtazapine, vortioxetine, and neurosteroids differ.
Default clinical action	Treat non-SSRI antidepressants by mechanism, indication, timing, and side-effect state; label newer-agent claims as gaps unless direct QEEG evidence exists.

The QEEG problem is that "antidepressant" is an indication label, not an EEG mechanism. Amitriptyline (Elavil) for migraine, trazodone for sleep, bupropion for depression with low energy, and brexanolone for postpartum depression do not belong to one spectral category. This chapter therefore treats non-SSRI antidepressants as a set of mechanism groups rather than a single class.

These medications matter because they often carry anticholinergic, antihistaminergic, noradrenergic, dopaminergic, GABAergic, sleep, pain, and seizure-threshold implications. They can shape the same QEEG features clinicians use for arousal, slowing, attention, alpha organization, sleepiness, and safety decisions.

7.2 Mechanism (clinician-level pharmacology)

TCAs are pharmacologically broad. They can inhibit serotonin and norepinephrine reuptake, block histamine receptors, block muscarinic cholinergic receptors, affect alpha-adrenergic receptors, and influence cardiac conduction. The balance differs by compound. Amitriptyline and doxepin are often more sedating and anticholinergic. Nortriptyline (Pamelor) and desipramine can feel more activating. A TCA medication list therefore requires compound-specific interpretation.

MAOIs alter monoamine metabolism by inhibiting monoamine oxidase. They are less common in ordinary practice, but they are pharmacologically broad and interaction-heavy. Direct modern resting-QEEG evidence is sparse, so the book treats MAOIs as a gap category with strong clinical-medication documentation needs rather than a confident QEEG signature. Bupropion, a norepinephrine-dopamine reuptake inhibitor and nicotinic antagonist, is often clinically activating and is used for depression, ADHD-adjacent symptoms, and smoking cessation; its QEEG evidence base is discussed in the Bupropion section below.

Mirtazapine and trazodone often enter QEEG practice through sleep. Their antidepressant label may be less important than their sedating and sleep-architecture effects. Vortioxetine and vilazodone are serotonergic antidepressants with mechanisms that differ from classic SSRIs, but direct resting-QEEG evidence remains limited. Brexanolone and zuranolone are neurosteroid GABA-A positive allosteric modulators; their mechanism suggests GABAergic EEG relevance, but direct outpatient QEEG endpoints are sparse.

Compound	Primary QEEG Vectors	Claim type	Interaction Modes	Confidence
Tricyclic antidepressants	sedation anticholinergic context	heuristic	n/a	n/a
MAOIs	monoaminergic modulation	heuristic	n/a	n/a
Bupropion	seizure threshold context, activating profile	heuristic	n/a	n/a
Mirtazapine	sedation sleep context	heuristic	n/a	n/a
Trazodone	sleep eeg context	heuristic	n/a	n/a

Figure 7.1: TCA and other antidepressant confidence: compounds by QEEG vectors, claim type, and interaction modes.

7.3 Known spectral effects

The TCA pharmaco-EEG literature is older but important. Itil and colleagues' early pharmaco-EEG work on a single sedating tricyclic supports the broad point that sedating antidepressants can shift EEG measures in clinically visible ways (Itil et al., 1972). Armitage's later sleep-related work also supports the importance of separating waking QEEG from sleep-architecture effects (Armitage, 1996). The safest modern phrasing is that TCAs can alter EEG through a mixture of antidepressant, sedating, anticholinergic, and sleep effects, with compound-level heterogeneity.

TCAs should not be treated as uniform. Sedating and activating TCAs can differ. iAPF effects should be described as variable or possible decrease, not as a precise class-wide shift. Anticholinergic burden should be considered when slowing, cognitive inefficiency, or reduced reactivity appear in a client taking a TCA.

Bupropion spectral evidence is limited; the dedicated Bupropion section below covers the evidence base and clinical interpretation approach.

For newer agents such as vortioxetine, vilazodone, and many neurosteroid or melatonergic antidepressant strategies, direct resting-QEEG evidence is sparse. The chapter therefore uses gap language rather than inventing signatures.

7.4 Phenotype interaction effects

TCAs most often raise mimicry and exaggeration concerns. Sedating and anticholinergic agents can mimic underarousal, cognitive slowing, poor alpha reactivity, or diffuse slowing. In a client with chronic pain, migraine, insomnia, fibromyalgia, OSA, or aging-related slowing, the TCA may exaggerate a pattern already present. A frontal theta or slow-alpha interpretation should therefore be confidence-adjusted for anticholinergic load and sleep state.

Bupropion raises a different question. It may be clinically activating, may combine with stimulants or caffeine, and has seizure-threshold relevance. A beta/arousal or insomnia-related pattern under bupropion should be interpreted with side-effect and co-exposure context. The evidence does not support a clean bupropion resting-QEEG signature.

Trazodone and mirtazapine often transform the meaning of "antidepressant exposure." The clinical issue may be nighttime sedation, sleep architecture, morning hangover, or residual drowsiness, not mood treatment. A QEEG recorded after poor sleep or sedative hangover may show slowing that looks like underarousal or medication effect, but the correct exposure label is more specific: sleep-focused antidepressant use.

Neurosteroid antidepressants and newer serotonergic agents remain evidence-limited. Their mechanisms are meaningful, but the report should label interpretation as mechanistic extrapolation when direct QEEG endpoints are absent.

7.5 Tricyclic Antidepressants

TCAs are the most EEG-relevant group in this chapter because they combine antidepressant, sedating, anticholinergic, and sometimes analgesic properties. The same medication may be used at low dose for migraine or pain, at bedtime for sleep, or at higher dose for mood. The indication and dose context matter.

Anticholinergic burden is the main QEEG caution. Acetylcholine supports cortical activation, attention, sensory processing, and memory. Anticholinergic medications can therefore contribute to cognitive complaints, reduced vigilance, and slowing-like interpretations. In older adults, this concern becomes stronger because baseline slowing, cognitive vulnerability, polypharmacy, sleep disruption, and medical comorbidity already reduce interpretive specificity.

Sedation is the second caution. A nighttime TCA may improve sleep continuity and reduce pain, which could indirectly improve daytime EEG state. It may also produce morning hangover, drowsiness, or reduced reactivity. The direction is not guaranteed. The QEEG clinician should ask how the client feels on the medication.

Activating TCAs raise a different concern. Noradrenergic effects may shape arousal, insomnia, anxiety, or beta interpretation. A TCA label does not tell the clinician which side of this profile is dominant. The report should name the compound rather than writing "TCA effect" as if it were a unitary mechanism.

TCAs are CYP2D6 substrates, and CPIC provides genotype-informed dosing guidance for several tricyclics. CYP2D6 poor metabolizers have higher plasma levels at standard doses, leading to stronger sedation, anticholinergic burden, cognitive slowing, and potentially a more medication-shaped QEEG than the nominal dose would predict. When a client on a moderate TCA dose shows unexpectedly strong slowing or side effects, CYP2D6 status (if available) belongs in the interpretation context. The QEEG clinician does not manage genotype-guided dosing, but should document known pharmacogenomic results and flag exposure uncertainty.

TCAs also interact with cardiac and seizure-risk considerations. Those risks are medical and prescriber-managed, but they matter for neurofeedback context because aggressive arousal protocols, sleep deprivation, medication changes, and physiologic stress should not be considered in isolation from the broader safety picture.

7.6 MAOIs

MAOIs are uncommon but clinically important. They affect monoamine metabolism broadly and carry food, medication-interaction, and blood-pressure considerations. Direct modern resting-QEEG evidence is sparse. The correct QEEG stance is therefore not to invent a signature, but to document exposure and interaction context carefully.

MAOI-treated clients may have treatment-resistant depression histories, complex medication trials, dietary restrictions, stimulant or sympathomimetic contraindications, and prescriber-managed safety plans. The QEEG clinician should not treat MAOI exposure casually. If arousal, sleep, beta, autonomic symptoms, or medication interactions appear relevant, the report can note that MAOI exposure and interaction risk reduce confidence in simple phenotype attribution. Clinical documentation matters most.

7.7 Bupropion

Bupropion is one of the easiest medications to overinterpret. Clinically, it can feel activating, improve energy, help smoking cessation, and sometimes worsen anxiety or insomnia. Mechanistically, it differs from SSRIs and SNRIs. Practically, many clients combine it with caffeine, stimulants, nicotine replacement, SSRIs, or sleep medications.

No strong resting-QEEG bupropion signature has been identified. The clearest EEG-relevant anchor is seizure threshold, not band-power mapping (Kuate et al., 2004). This distinction is important. A clinician should not write that bupropion has a known beta, theta, or alpha pattern unless directly supported by evidence. The more defensible statement is that bupropion can affect arousal, sleep, activation, seizure-threshold context, and stimulant/caffeine interpretation, while direct resting-QEEG spectral evidence is limited.

In anxious depression, Papakostas and colleagues provide useful clinical context for bupropion versus SSRI outcomes (Papakostas et al., 2007). That helps the clinician understand why bupropion may appear in certain clinical profiles. It does not make bupropion a QEEG biomarker.

For QEEG reports, bupropion should trigger questions about dose, formulation, time of day, insomnia, anxiety, caffeine, stimulant co-treatment, seizure history, eating-disorder history, alcohol withdrawal, and nicotine use. Those variables may matter more than any proposed spectral signature.

7.8 Trazodone and Mirtazapine

Trazodone and mirtazapine are often antidepressants by label but sleep medications by use. This makes them common hidden confounders. A client may not volunteer trazodone when asked about "psychiatric meds" because they think of it as a sleep aid. A clinician may miss it when focusing only on antidepressant classes.

The QEEG question is usually state-related: did the medication improve sleep enough to improve daytime EEG stability, or did it produce morning sedation and reduced reactivity? Both are plausible. A well-rested trazodone user may produce a cleaner recording than an unmedicated insomniac. A sedated trazodone user may show slowing or reduced alpha reactivity. The medication cannot be interpreted apart from sleep quality.

Mirtazapine adds appetite, weight, sedation, sleep, and antihistaminergic questions. It may be used in depression with insomnia, anxiety, weight loss, or medically complex clients. Again, the QEEG issue is less a clean spectral fingerprint and more the combination of mood, sleep, sedation, metabolic state, and co-medications.

7.9 Newer and Gap Categories

Vortioxetine and vilazodone are clinically meaningful serotonergic antidepressants, but direct resting-QEEG literature is thin. Agomelatine is relevant where available because of circadian and melatonergic framing. Brexanolone and zuranolone are mechanistically important neurosteroid antidepressants that act through GABA-A modulation, especially in postpartum depression contexts. QEEG endpoints for these newer categories are sparse.

The book therefore treats these as gap or mechanism-extrapolation categories. A clinician may reasonably note that neurosteroid or circadian-active antidepressants could plausibly affect EEG through their respective mechanisms, but mechanism-based reasoning is not the same as having validated outpatient QEEG signatures.

Brexanolone (Zulresso) is a synthetic form of allopregnanolone, a neuroactive steroid that acts as a positive allosteric modulator of synaptic and extrasynaptic GABA-A receptors. FDA-approved in 2019 for postpartum depression, it is administered as a 60-hour continuous IV infusion in a certified healthcare facility. The mechanism differs from benzodiazepines: allopregnanolone modulates GABA-A receptors at sites distinct from the benzodiazepine binding site, with particular affinity for delta-subunit-containing extrasynaptic receptors that mediate tonic inhibition. The expected EEG effect is GABAergic: increased slow-wave activity and beta activity during infusion, with sedation as the main adverse effect (an FDA REMS program requires monitoring). However, no published resting-state QEEG studies in postpartum depression patients exist. The infusion context (60 hours in-facility, with monitoring) makes outpatient QEEG recording during treatment impractical. The clinically relevant question for QEEG is how long GABAergic spectral effects persist after the infusion ends. Given allopregnanolone's half-life of approximately 9 hours, pharmacokinetic clearance is expected within 2-3 days, but the antidepressant effect persists for weeks. Whether any spectral signature persists beyond pharmacokinetic clearance is unknown. A conservative recommendation is to wait at least one week after infusion completion before interpreting a resting-state QEEG as representative of the post-treatment state, and to document the infusion date and clinical response in the intake.

Zuranolone (Zurzuvae) is an oral neuroactive steroid GABA-A modulator FDA-approved in 2023 for postpartum depression, taken as 50 mg nightly for 14 days. Its mechanism parallels brexanolone (allopregnanolone pathway, extrasynaptic GABA-A modulation) but with oral bioavailability and outpatient use. Zuranolone has a half-life of approximately 16-23 hours. Sedation, dizziness, and somnolence are common during the 14-day treatment course. No published resting-state QEEG data exist for zuranolone. During the 14-day dosing window, the QEEG can be expected to show GABAergic features (increased slow activity, possible beta augmentation, sedation-related vigilance changes). After the 14-day course ends, pharmacokinetic clearance should occur within 3-5 days, but the antidepressant effect may persist. The clinical context (postpartum depression with sleep fragmentation, hormonal shifts, and infant care demands) adds marked state confounding. Document zuranolone exposure, course timing (day of 14, or days since completion), sedation, sleep quality, and postpartum month. Do not invent a spectral fingerprint; treat this as a time-limited GABAergic exposure with mechanism-based expectations and a pure evidence gap for resting-state outcomes.

Both neurosteroid antidepressants raise a broader interpretive point: they are designed to correct a peripartum allopregnanolone deficit, and their effect may partly restore a physiological state rather than adding a purely pharmacological overlay. That distinction matters for QEEG interpretation but cannot be resolved from a single recording.

7.10 Dextromethorphan-Bupropion (Auvelity): Evidence Gap

Auvelity (dextromethorphan 45 mg + bupropion 105 mg extended-release) was FDA-approved in 2022 for MDD. It carries zero direct resting-state QEEG evidence. The clinical trials did not incorporate EEG biomarkers. Limited dextromethorphan monotherapy data (TMS-EEG) suggest delta/theta reduction without alpha or gamma changes, but this has not been confirmed for the combination product at therapeutic doses. Mechanism-based extrapolation is a workflow heuristic only.

The main interpretive concern is pharmacokinetic: bupropion is a strong CYP2D6 inhibitor. A client on Auvelity plus a CYP2D6-dependent SSRI such as paroxetine or fluoxetine may show spectral features from elevated SSRI exposure (via 2D6 inhibition) rather than from any direct NMDA effect. Document Auvelity and all co-medications; do not claim a specific spectral signature.

For GLP-1 receptor agonists (semaglutide, tirzepatide), see Chapter 16.

7.11 Polypharmacy Patterns

Non-SSRI antidepressants often appear in combinations. Bupropion may be added to an SSRI. Trazodone may be added to an SNRI for sleep. A TCA may be used for pain alongside gabapentin (Neurontin), opioids, cannabis, or migraine medications. Mirtazapine may be combined with venlafaxine (Effexor). A neurosteroid antidepressant may appear in a postpartum medication and sleep context.

Combination interpretation is usually a workflow heuristic. The clinician should identify additive directions rather than assigning causality. Sedating antidepressant plus benzodiazepine plus cannabis plus OSA risk is a stronger slowing and vigilance concern than any one medication alone. Bupropion plus stimulant plus caffeine plus insomnia is a stronger activation and beta-context concern than bupropion alone.

The report should say that the QEEG is interpreted under combined exposure. It should not pretend that each drug can be subtracted cleanly from the map.

7.12 Report Language Examples

Weak language: "The client takes amitriptyline, so the slowing is medication-caused."
Better language: "Diffuse slowing is present under low-dose amitriptyline exposure, chronic pain, poor sleep, and intermittent antihistamine use. Anticholinergic and sedating exposures reduce confidence in interpreting the slowing as a stable endogenous underarousal phenotype."
Weak language: "Bupropion produces beta excess."
Better language: "Beta excess is present in a client taking bupropion with caffeine and poor sleep. Direct resting-QEEG evidence for a bupropion beta signature is limited, so interpretation should focus on arousal state, insomnia, stimulant / caffeine co-exposure, and artifact."
Weak language: "Trazodone is an antidepressant, so use the depression chapter."
Better language: "Trazodone is being used as a sleep medication; interpretation should document last dose, sleep quality, morning sedation, and alpha / reactivity effects."
Weak language: "Newer antidepressant effects are unknown, so ignore them."
Better language: "Direct resting-QEEG evidence for this newer antidepressant is limited. Mechanism and side-effect state are documented, and phenotype confidence is adjusted only where clinically plausible."

7.13 Choosing the Recording State

For TCAs and sleep-focused antidepressants, the ordinary treated state is often the most clinically relevant state. If the medication is taken nightly and the client will continue taking it during neurofeedback, the QEEG should usually be interpreted as a current-state recording under sedating or anticholinergic exposure. That can still guide training, especially if residual symptoms persist despite the medication.

Off-medication comparison is more complicated. Stopping a TCA, trazodone, mirtazapine, bupropion, or MAOI may change mood, sleep, pain, migraine control, seizure threshold, or withdrawal symptoms. A QEEG clinician should not ask for that change outside prescriber coordination. If the medication is being adjusted for clinical reasons, the recording should label the transition state.

For bupropion, the timing question often concerns activation, insomnia, caffeine, nicotine, stimulant co-treatment, and seizure-threshold context. For trazodone or mirtazapine, the timing question concerns last nighttime dose, sleep quality, and morning sedation. For TCAs, the timing question includes dose, compound, anticholinergic burden, pain indication, and age. For newer agents, the timing question may be less informative than documenting mechanism and side effects because direct QEEG evidence is thin.

7.14 What Not to Claim

Do not write that all TCAs slow the EEG in the same way. Do not write that bupropion has a known resting beta signature when the available literature covers seizure threshold rather than systematic QEEG mapping. Do not write that trazodone or mirtazapine are just antidepressants when they are being used as sleep medications. Do not invent signatures for vortioxetine, vilazodone, agomelatine, brexanolone, or zuranolone. Do not use QEEG to drive antidepressant or TCA prescribing; refer medication decisions to the prescriber.

The stronger clinical claim is narrower: non-SSRI antidepressants often alter QEEG interpretation through anticholinergic load, sedation, activation, sleep, pain, seizure-threshold context, and polypharmacy. Those are real clinical variables even when direct spectral evidence is incomplete, and documenting them makes the report safer and more useful for follow-up.

7.15 Case vignette

A fifty-eight-year-old client presents for neurofeedback because of brain fog, insomnia, chronic pain, and low mood. She takes low-dose amitriptyline at night for migraine and pain, bupropion in the morning for depression and low energy, and occasional diphenhydramine for sleep. The QEEG shows mild diffuse slowing, weak posterior alpha reactivity, and intermittent beta excess.

A simple report might call the slowing an underarousal phenotype and beta excess an anxiety marker. A better report recognizes competing mechanisms. Amitriptyline and diphenhydramine raise anticholinergic and sedating concerns. Chronic pain and poor sleep can also increase slowing. Bupropion, caffeine, anxiety, and muscle tension may contribute to beta. The map is clinically meaningful, but the phenotype labels are lower confidence unless medication timing, sleep, and raw-signal quality support them.

The defensible interpretation is: "Findings are interpreted under mixed antidepressant exposure, including anticholinergic/sedating nighttime medication and activating morning medication. Diffuse slowing and beta findings should be treated as current-state features with multiple plausible contributors."

7.16 Interpretation traps

- **Treating antidepressant as a mechanism.** TCAs, MAOIs, bupropion, trazodone, mirtazapine, vortioxetine, and neurosteroids differ.
- **Ignoring anticholinergic load.** Slowing and cognitive complaints under TCAs or OTC sleep aids need anticholinergic context.
- **Using bupropion seizure literature as a band-power signature.** Seizure-threshold evidence is not a resting-QEEG profile.
- **Missing sleep-focused prescribing.** Trazodone or mirtazapine may matter more as sleep-state modifiers than as antidepressants.
- **Inventing signatures for newer agents.** Pure gaps should be labeled as gaps.
- **Ignoring pain and migraine indications.** The treated condition can shape the QEEG independently of medication.

7.17 Intake questions

When non-SSRI antidepressants appear on the intake form, ask:

- **Why is the medication prescribed?** Depression, sleep, pain, migraine, smoking cessation, postpartum depression, or another indication changes interpretation.
- **Is the medication sedating, activating, or both?** Ask about morning hangover, insomnia, agitation, cognitive slowing, and daytime fatigue.

- **What is the anticholinergic burden?** Include TCAs, diphenhydramine, bladder medications, antipsychotics, and other OTC products.
- **Any seizure history, eating-disorder history, alcohol withdrawal, or high-dose bupropion exposure?** These are safety-context variables.
- **Any recent changes, additions, or switches?** New starts, dose changes, and sleep-medication substitution can destabilize interpretation.

7.18 Clinical recommendations

Interpret non-SSRI antidepressants by mechanism and indication. For TCAs, document sedating versus activating profile and anticholinergic load. For bupropion, document activation, insomnia, stimulant/caffeine combinations, and seizure-threshold context. For trazodone and mirtazapine, document sleep timing and next-day sedation. For newer agents with sparse QEEG evidence, label claims as mechanistic extrapolation or pure gap.

When the medication is prescribed for pain, migraine, sleep, or postpartum depression, the indication should appear in the QEEG interpretation because the treated condition can shape the recording as much as the drug, especially during symptom flares, unstable sleep, and recovery periods.

Do not recommend medication changes to clarify a QEEG. If anticholinergic load, seizure risk, or sedating polypharmacy appears clinically concerning, the neurofeedback clinician can recommend prescriber review, not medication discontinuation.

7.19 Evidence summary

- **Spectral effect:** Older TCA pharmaco-EEG literature supports EEG effects, but compound heterogeneity and sedating versus activating profiles limit class-wide claims.
- **Phenotype inference:** Anticholinergic burden, sedation, activation, sleep effects, pain indication, and seizure-threshold context can alter confidence in slowing, beta, alpha-reactivity, and arousal interpretations.

- **Workflow heuristic:** Treat non-SSRI antidepressants by mechanism, indication, timing, and side-effect state; label newer-agent claims as gaps unless direct QEEG evidence exists.

Ch 8: Benzodiazepines

8.1 Why this class matters in NFB practice

Benzodiazepines are among the most consequential medication classes for QEEG interpretation because they can produce a strong spectral signature while also changing cognition, anxiety, sleep, vigilance, and withdrawal risk. They are used for panic, generalized anxiety, insomnia, muscle spasm, seizure rescue, procedural anxiety, vertigo, alcohol withdrawal, and many off-label situations. A clinician may see alprazolam (Xanax), clonazepam (Klonopin), lorazepam (Ativan), diazepam (Valium), temazepam (Restoril), chlordiazepoxide (Librium), or intranasal rescue benzodiazepines on the intake form.

Strongest evidence	Benzodiazepines can increase beta activity and alter vigilance / reactivity; withdrawal is a distinct EEG-relevant state with safety implications.
Biggest interpretation trap	Reading benzodiazepine beta as ordinary activation: Beta can rise under sedation.
Default clinical action	Treat acute use, chronic use, tolerance, PRN dosing, tapering, withdrawal, paradoxical reactions, and sedative stacking as mandatory intake fields.

The main QEEG problem is that benzodiazepines can increase beta activity while also sedating the client. That combination makes simple band-language dangerous. Beta excess under benzodiazepine exposure does not mean the same thing as beta excess in an unmedicated anxious client. The surface map may look activated while the client's cognition, reactivity, or vigilance is blunted.

Benzodiazepines also make "baseline" language risky. A client who took clonazepam the night before, a client on long-term daily alprazolam, a client tapering diazepam, and a client in acute withdrawal are not in the same state. The medication state must be documented before beta, alpha reactivity, slowing, or arousal labels are interpreted.

8.2 Mechanism (clinician-level pharmacology)

Benzodiazepines are positive allosteric modulators at GABA-A receptors. They increase the effect of endogenous GABA at receptor subtypes to which they bind. Clinically, this can produce anxiolysis, sedation, anticonvulsant effects, muscle relaxation, impaired memory, slowed reaction time, and reduced arousal. The spectral signature is not a simple "more inhibition equals slower EEG" pattern. Benzodiazepines can produce prominent beta activity while also impairing performance and vigilance.

Pharmacokinetics matter. Alprazolam is shorter acting than diazepam. Diazepam has active metabolites and a long tail. Clonazepam is long acting and often used chronically. Lorazepam is common in medical settings. Intranasal diazepam or midazolam rescue medications produce acute exposure in a seizure or emergency context. The QEEG clinician should record compound, dose, timing, chronicity, and reason for use.

Tolerance and dependence matter as much as acute exposure. A one-time benzodiazepine dose in a healthy volunteer is not the same as years of nightly use. Long-term clients may have tolerance to sedative effects, persistent cognitive concerns, interdose withdrawal, or anxiety rebound. A QEEG can capture the current state, but should not be interpreted as if the client were benzodiazepine-naive.

8.3 Known spectral effects

Mandema and colleagues provide an important acute benzodiazepine EEG anchor (Mandema et al., 1992). The core clinical takeaway is that benzodiazepines can increase beta activity and alter vigilance-related EEG measures. The chapter does not quote unsupported magnitudes. It uses the directional claim: benzodiazepine exposure can create or amplify beta features relevant to QEEG phenotype interpretation.

Barker and colleagues are often tempting to cite because their meta-analysis documents cognitive effects of long-term benzodiazepine use (Barker et al., 2004). That source should not be used as an EEG-effects

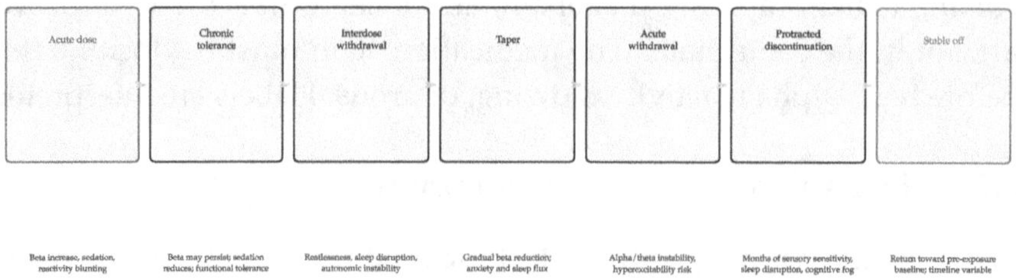

Figure 8.1: Benzodiazepine exposure-state map: acute dose through chronic tolerance, taper, withdrawal, protracted discontinuation, and stable off, with expected QEEG direction at each state.

citation. Its value in this chapter is clinical context: long-term benzodiazepine exposure can be associated with cognitive performance concerns, which means the QEEG clinician may see clients whose symptoms and spectral findings cannot be reduced to anxiety alone.

Withdrawal is its own EEG topic. Ashton observations and withdrawal literature describe acute and protracted benzodiazepine withdrawal states (Ashton, 2002). Acute withdrawal is a higher-risk period with possible beta rebound, epileptiform risk, and seizure concerns, especially after abrupt sedative changes. This is not a state in which phenotype interpretation should be casual.

Paradoxical responses are also real. Mancuso and colleagues review paradoxical reactions to benzodiazepines (Mancuso et al., 2004). A client who becomes disinhibited, agitated, activated, or behaviorally worse after benzodiazepine exposure should not be forced into the usual sedative model. The QEEG report should document the paradoxical history and lower confidence in population-average expectations.

8.4 Phenotype interaction effects

Benzodiazepines most often create mimicry and transformation. They can mimic beta excess while transforming the meaning of beta. A benzodiazepine-associated beta pattern may reflect pharmacological GABA-A modulation, not endogenous hyperarousal. The client may look spectrally fast while feeling sedated, foggy, or slowed.

They can also mask anxiety-related physiology. If a client takes alprazolam shortly before the recording, panic-related arousal may be reduced, while medication-related beta is increased. The current-state QEEG is still real, but it does not represent the client's unmedicated anxiety physiology. The benzodiazepine-associated beta and the endogenous anxiety-related beta can look identical on a topographic map. They do not mean the same thing. Treating them as interchangeable is the most common error in medicated-QEEG beta interpretation.

Exaggeration occurs when benzodiazepines combine with alcohol, opioids, sedating antidepressants, cannabis, antihistamines, OSA, chronic pain, or sleep deprivation. The resulting recording may show beta, slowing, poor reactivity, and vigilance instability. A single-cause explanation is rarely safe.

Withdrawal transforms the whole interpretation (see Withdrawal and Tapering, below).

8.5 Acute Exposure

Acute benzodiazepine exposure is the cleanest state to describe conceptually and the easiest to miss clinically. A client may take a PRN dose before the appointment because the QEEG itself is stressful. The technician may record the medication list but not the last-dose timing. The report then treats a peak or near-peak medication state as ordinary baseline.

Acute exposure can produce beta augmentation, altered vigilance, slowed reaction time, memory effects, reduced anxiety, and reduced reactivity. In QEEG terms, this means the map may show beta while the clinical state is calmer or more sedated. The report should not translate beta directly into endogenous hyperarousal.

PRN use is especially important. A client who uses alprazolam twice per month may be unexposed on most days and acutely exposed during the recording. A client who takes lorazepam before medical appointments may create a QEEG that is less anxious but more benzodiazepine-shaped than ordinary life. A client using intranasal benzodiazepine rescue medication is in an acute neurological context, not a routine outpatient baseline.

The intake phrase should be specific: "recorded two hours after PRN alprazolam" is far more useful than "takes alprazolam as needed."

8.6 Chronic Use and Tolerance

Chronic benzodiazepine use creates a different interpretation problem. The client may not feel sedated because tolerance has developed, but the EEG may still be shaped by long-term GABAergic exposure, sleep changes, cognitive effects, interdose withdrawal, or polypharmacy. A chronic user is not the same as an acute-dose volunteer.

Tolerance also separates subjective state from spectral state. A client may say, "It does not affect me anymore," while still showing medication-relevant timing, sleep, or withdrawal patterns. The clinician should respect the report but still document chronicity, dose stability, and missed-dose sensitivity.

Long half-life compounds complicate last-dose interpretation. Diazepam and metabolites may remain relevant long after the last pill. Clonazepam may create a steadier exposure profile than short-acting alprazolam. A same-day dose question is therefore insufficient. The clinician should record usual schedule, duration, dose changes, and whether the client experiences interdose symptoms.

Chronic use also intersects with age. Older adults may have higher fall risk, cognitive vulnerability, slower clearance, sleep apnea risk, and polypharmacy. Geriatric pharmaco-EEG data are sparse despite clinical importance, so the chapter uses clinical caution rather than compound-specific prediction.

8.7 Withdrawal and Tapering

Benzodiazepine withdrawal is a distinct physiological state with potential hyperexcitability, insomnia, autonomic symptoms, anxiety rebound, perceptual symptoms, and seizure risk, not a return to baseline. Acute withdrawal after abrupt changes can be medically dangerous. Protracted symptoms can persist after the most acute period.

From a QEEG standpoint, withdrawal creates several hazards. Beta rebound or hyperarousal features may be interpreted as trait anxiety. Sleep deprivation may create slow activity. Epileptiform risk may complicate interpretation and safety. Emotional distress may change artifact and muscle tension. The result can look like several phenotypes at once.

The Ashton materials are not a controlled QEEG trial, but they are clinically important for understanding benzodiazepine tapering and protracted withdrawal (Ashton, 2002). This book uses them as withdrawal-context guidance, not as a precise spectral model. The key point is that tapering state must be documented and phenotype interpretation should be conservative.

Abrupt sedative changes should usually trigger deferral rather than confident phenotyping. If the client recently stopped or sharply reduced benzodiazepines, the QEEG may still be useful as a current-state record, but it should not be used as the main basis for a stable neurofeedback phenotype. The report should say "recorded during benzodiazepine taper" or "recorded after missed doses" rather than "off benzodiazepines."

8.8 Paradoxical Reactions

Most benzodiazepine discussions emphasize sedation and anxiolysis. Some clients respond differently. Paradoxical reactions can include agitation, disinhibition, irritability, rage, impulsivity, activation, or worsened anxiety. Mancuso and colleagues review these reactions (Mancuso et al., 2004).

Paradoxical responders matter for QEEG because the expected drug-state model may be wrong. A client who becomes disinhibited after benzodiazepines is not a typical sedated benzodiazepine user. Their beta, muscle artifact, movement, and arousal signs may reflect activation under a drug expected to calm. The report should document the history rather than forcing the pattern into the average response.

Prevalence in the general adult population is low (under 1%), but rates are higher in children, older adults, individuals with TBI or brain injury, and those with personality disorders or impulse-control vulnerabilities. Developmental variants, substance use, neurocognitive vulnerability, and polypharmacy may all raise the importance of asking about paradoxical responses. The literature is not strong enough to create a QEEG paradoxical-responder signature. The clinical rule is simpler: ask, document, and reduce confidence in ordinary assumptions.

8.9 Sedative Stacking

Benzodiazepines rarely appear alone in complex clinical practice. They may be combined with alcohol, opioids, cannabis, gabapentinoids, sedating antidepressants, antipsychotics, antihistamines, melatonin, Z-drugs, muscle relaxants, or untreated OSA. This is both an interpretation problem and a safety problem.

Sedative stacking can create slowing, poor alpha reactivity, vigilance instability, memory complaints, and daytime fatigue. It can also increase respiratory and fall risk depending on the combination. The QEEG clinician should not manage these medications, but should notice when the recording occurs under stacked depressant exposure.

Polypharmacy also makes single-drug interpretation unreliable. If a client on clonazepam, trazodone (Desyrel), cannabis, and possible OSA shows slowing, the correct report is not "benzodiazepine slowing." It is "slowing under combined sedative exposure and sleep-disordered breathing risk." That phrasing is less tidy and more accurate.

8.10 Choosing the Recording State

The current-state recording is often appropriate if the client will continue benzodiazepines during neurofeedback. The map then represents treated functioning. That is useful when the clinical goal is to improve symptoms under ordinary medication exposure.

An off-benzodiazepine recording should not be requested casually. Benzodiazepine discontinuation can be medically risky (see Withdrawal and Tapering, above). If a prescriber-supervised taper is already underway, the QEEG can document the transition state with appropriate labeling.

If the question is whether beta excess is endogenous or benzodiazepine-associated, the answer may require repeated stable-state recordings, careful timing, symptom tracking, and prescriber involvement. A single recording cannot usually separate those sources.

8.11 Report Language Examples

Weak language: "The beta excess indicates anxiety."

Better language: "Beta excess is present under recent benzodiazepine exposure. Interpretation as endogenous anxiety-related hyperarousal is reduced because benzodiazepines can increase beta while also producing sedation."

Weak language: "The client stopped benzodiazepines, so this is baseline."

Better language: "The recording occurred during benzodiazepine taper with withdrawal symptoms. Findings should be interpreted as a withdrawal-state QEEG, not a pristine unmedicated baseline."

Weak language: "Benzodiazepine effects explain the whole map."

Better language: "Benzodiazepine exposure, alcohol use, possible OSA, poor sleep, and chronic anxiety all plausibly contribute to beta, slowing, and reactivity findings; confidence in a single phenotype explanation is reduced."

Weak language: "Hold the medication before repeat QEEG."

Better language: "Any medication-state comparison should be discussed with the prescriber because benzodiazepine interruption can produce withdrawal and seizure risk."

8.12 Practical Confidence Levels

High-confidence benzodiazepine interpretation is possible when the exposure state is clear, the recording is clean, and the finding matches known benzodiazepine effects. For example, beta excess recorded soon after a documented benzodiazepine dose should reduce confidence in endogenous hyperarousal interpretation.

Moderate-confidence interpretation is common when benzodiazepine exposure is chronic, stable, and part of ordinary functioning, but other factors such as sleep, anxiety, or comedication also contribute. The report can still guide training, but should avoid single-cause language.

Low-confidence interpretation applies when the client is tapering, missing doses, acutely withdrawing, stacking sedatives, intoxicated, severely sleep deprived, or medically unstable. In those cases, the QEEG may be useful for documenting current state, but phenotype selection should be cautious or deferred.

This confidence language belongs in the report. It prevents the clinician from treating a benzodiazepine-shaped map as a direct trait phenotype.

8.13 What Not to Claim

Six overclaims are not defensible with this drug class:

- Do not claim that benzodiazepine beta proves calm, anxiety, or hyperarousal.
- Do not claim that withdrawal is a clean baseline.
- Do not cite cognitive meta-analyses as if they measured QEEG.
- Do not tell clients to skip benzodiazepines for a recording.
- Do not ignore alcohol, opioids, antihistamines, cannabis, Z-drugs, OSA, or sleep deprivation as co-drivers of the pattern.
- QEEG is not a reason to hold, reduce, or stop benzodiazepines without prescriber management; withdrawal and seizure risk are real.

The stronger claim is conditional: benzodiazepine exposure and withdrawal state alter confidence in beta, alpha reactivity, slowing, vigilance, and arousal interpretations.

8.14 Case vignette

A client presents with anxiety, insomnia, and cognitive fog. She takes clonazepam nightly, uses alprazolam as needed, drinks wine several nights per week, and reports possible sleep apnea. She took alprazolam two hours before the QEEG because the appointment made her anxious. The QEEG shows beta excess, weak alpha reactivity, and intermittent slow activity.

A quick report might call this hyperarousal with underarousal features. A better report separates the layers. The beta excess may be benzodiazepine-associated, anxiety-related, caffeine-related, muscle-related, or mixed. Weak alpha reactivity may reflect sedative exposure, poor sleep, or drowsiness. Slow activity may reflect OSA risk, sedative stacking, sleep restriction, or artifact. The recording is clinically useful as a medicated anxious-state measurement, but confidence in an endogenous beta-excess phenotype is reduced.

The safest recommendation is documentation and prescriber coordination, not medication advice. If a comparison recording is clinically needed, it must be planned around safety, withdrawal risk, and the prescriber's judgment.

8.15 Interpretation traps

- **Reading benzodiazepine beta as ordinary activation.** Beta can rise under sedation.

- **Citing cognitive-effect literature as EEG evidence.** Barker is useful for cognitive context, not spectral claims.
- **Treating tapering as baseline.** Withdrawal is its own physiological state.
- **Ignoring alcohol, opioids, cannabis, OSA, and sleep medications.** Sedative stacking changes risk and interpretation.
- **Assuming paradoxical responders follow the usual sedative pattern.** Agitation or disinhibition after benzodiazepines should be documented.
- **Using QEEG to suggest discontinuation.** Benzodiazepine changes require prescriber management.
- **Missing stimulant interactions.** Clients tapering benzodiazepines may increase caffeine or have stimulant co-prescriptions that create mixed arousal states. See Chapter 5 for stimulant skipped-dose and caffeine interaction pitfalls.

8.16 Intake questions

When benzodiazepines appear on the intake form, ask:

- **Which benzodiazepine, dose, formulation, and timing?** Record last dose, usual schedule, PRN use, and long-acting metabolites.
- **How long has the client used it?** Separate acute, intermittent, chronic, tapering, and recently discontinued states.
- **Any withdrawal, interdose symptoms, missed doses, or dose reductions?** Treat these as major QEEG context.
- **Any alcohol, opioids, cannabis, antihistamines, sleep medications, or OSA risk?** Sedative combinations alter both safety and interpretation.
- **Any paradoxical reactions?** Ask about agitation, disinhibition, rage, activation, or worsened anxiety after benzodiazepines.

8.17 Clinical recommendations

Record benzodiazepine exposure precisely and interpret beta, alpha reactivity, slowing, and vigilance in that context. A benzodiazepine-exposed QEEG can guide current-state neurofeedback if the client will remain on the medication, but the report should not treat the map as an unmedicated trait baseline. Do not suggest skipping or tapering benzodiazepines to improve a recording; the prescriber must weigh withdrawal and seizure risk.

When withdrawal or recent dose reduction is present, label the recording as a withdrawal or transition-state QEEG. Phenotype interpretation should be reduced-confidence or deferred if the client is acutely unstable.

If the client is medically stable but symptomatically complex, the report can still be useful by naming the uncertainty: beta is present, sedation is present, withdrawal is absent or present, and confidence is adjusted accordingly.

Safety notice. Benzodiazepine withdrawal can cause seizures and is potentially fatal without medical supervision. Nothing in this chapter is a tapering protocol. Abrupt discontinuation or rapid taper of benzodiazepines requires physician management. If a client is considering reducing or stopping benzodiazepines, that conversation belongs with their prescribing clinician, not with the QEEG report.

8.18 Evidence summary

- **Spectral effect:** Benzodiazepines can increase beta activity and alter vigilance/reactivity; withdrawal is a distinct EEG-relevant state with safety implications. *Aperiodic caveat: the benzodiazepine-beta literature is among the most replicated in pharmaco-EEG, but was conducted with band-power methods; whether the beta increase reflects oscillatory spindles, aperiodic slope changes, or both is not resolved in the source studies.*
- **Phenotype inference:** Benzodiazepine exposure can mimic or transform beta-excess interpretation and reduce confidence in arousal, anxiety, and alpha-reactivity phenotypes.
- **Workflow heuristic:** Treat acute use, chronic use, tolerance, PRN dosing, tapering, withdrawal, paradoxical reactions, and sedative stacking as mandatory interpretation metadata.

Ch 9: Typical Antipsychotics

9.1 Why this class matters in NFB practice

Typical antipsychotics are less common than atypical antipsychotics in many outpatient neurofeedback referrals, but they remain clinically important. Clients may take haloperidol (Haldol), chlorpromazine (Thorazine), perphenazine, fluphenazine, thiothixene, or depot formulations for psychotic disorders, bipolar disorder, severe agitation, Tourette syndrome, nausea, or off-label behavioral control. Some may have current psychosis, residual negative symptoms, extrapyramidal symptoms, akathisia, sedation, or medication-induced cognitive slowing.

Strongest evidence	Typical antipsychotics are associated qualitatively with increased slow activity and alpha-profile changes, but clean percentage magnitudes are unreliable.
Biggest interpretation trap	Quoting fabricated percentages: Do not use Centorrino for continuous theta / delta magnitudes.
Default clinical action	Document route, last dose, LAI cycle position, EPS / akathisia, adjuncts, nicotine / cannabis, psychosis state, and sleep before assigning a phenotype.

For QEEG interpretation, typical antipsychotics raise two problems. First, they can shift the EEG toward slowing and alpha-profile changes that overlap with underarousal, frontal theta, encephalopathic, drowsiness, or medication-burden interpretations. Second, the treated condition itself can shape the recording. Psychosis state, sleep disruption, anticholinergic adjuncts, benzodiazepines, cannabis, nicotine, and hospitalization history may all appear in the same client.

This chapter focuses on first-generation antipsychotics. Atypical antipsychotics receive their own chapter because clozapine (Clozaril), olanzapine (Zyprexa), risperidone (Risperdal), quetiapine (Seroquel), aripiprazole (Abilify), and newer agents differ enough that combining them with typical antipsychotics would blur the evidence.

9.2 Mechanism (clinician-level pharmacology)

Typical antipsychotics are primarily dopamine D2 receptor antagonists, with additional receptor effects depending on the compound. High-potency agents such as haloperidol and fluphenazine tend to carry more extrapyramidal risk. Lower-potency agents such as chlorpromazine often carry more sedating, anticholinergic, antihistaminergic, and autonomic effects. These differences matter because QEEG features may reflect dopamine blockade, sedation, anticholinergic burden, motor restlessness, or adjunctive medications rather than one uniform "antipsychotic effect."

Medication route also matters. Oral daily use, short-acting IM use, emergency sedation, and depot/long-acting injectable exposure do not represent the same recording state. A depot cycle has timing: recent injection, mid-cycle plateau, or end-of-cycle trough. Direct QEEG data across depot cycles are sparse, so LAI timing is treated as mandatory metadata rather than as a validated spectral predictor.

Typical antipsychotics are also often paired with other medications (anticholinergics, benzodiazepines, mood stabilizers, and more), making most typical-antipsychotic QEEGs polypharmacy QEEGs (see Adjunctive Medication Context below).

9.3 Known spectral effects

The strongest defensible statement is qualitative. Computerized EEG profiles of haloperidol, chlorpromazine, and related antipsychotics support a pattern of increased slow activity, modest alpha slowing, and sometimes reduced faster activity, with differences by compound (Small et al., 1987). The chapter does not quote percentage changes because no clean, defensible class-wide band-power percentages exist in the literature.

Saletu's topography and tomography work supports the broader pharmaco-EEG idea that neuroleptic drug profiles can be described with topographic EEG methods (B. Saletu et al., 2002). The critical correction is that this paper does not report an explicit antipsychotic iAPF slowing magnitude in Hz. Any sentence giving a precise Hz shift should be removed. The safer wording is that sedative neuroleptics can shift alpha profiles toward slower, higher-amplitude activity, while explicit Hz magnitudes are not consistently reported.

Centorrino and colleagues are useful for categorical EEG abnormality rates during antipsychotic treatment, but not for continuous theta or delta percentage changes (Centorrino et al., 2002). Band-power magnitudes attributed to that paper are not in it. This chapter uses Centorrino only for categorical abnormality context, not for band-power quantification.

> **Typical antipsychotic spectral direction.** Expected changes under first-generation antipsychotic exposure: delta and theta increase (qualitative), alpha slowing and profile shift, possible beta decrease. Magnitude varies by compound, dose, route, and adjunctive medications. Clean percentage magnitudes are not defensible from the available sources. Interpret as directional guidance, not quantified prediction.

9.4 Phenotype interaction effects

Typical antipsychotics most often create mimicry and exaggeration. Slowing can mimic underarousal, frontal theta, drowsiness, medication burden, post-concussive effects, OSA, Long COVID, or encephalopathic patterns. If the client also has poor sleep, anticholinergic adjuncts, benzodiazepines, opioids, cannabis, or medical illness, the same direction of change may be exaggerated.

Transformation occurs when a QEEG feature has a different meaning under dopamine blockade and psychosis treatment. A frontal theta pattern in an unmedicated attention referral is not the same clinical object as frontal theta in a client taking haloperidol plus benztropine after recent hospitalization. The map may look similar, but the interpretive frame changes.

Masking is possible when antipsychotic treatment reduces agitation, psychotic arousal, insomnia, or substance-driven instability. A treated recording may look more stable than the acute untreated state. That can be useful for current-state neurofeedback planning, but it should not be described as the client's never-medicated baseline.

Akathisia can contaminate beta and arousal interpretation and should be flagged at intake; see Chapter 10 for the fuller akathisia-beta discussion.

9.5 Route, Depot Cycle, and Acute Use

For oral typical antipsychotics, last-dose timing, dose stability, and recent changes matter. A recent dose increase may produce sedation, extrapyramidal symptoms, or cognitive slowing that differs from stable treatment. A missed dose may produce rebound insomnia, agitation, or relapse risk.

Depot and long-acting injectable formulations add another timing layer. The report should document date of last injection, usual interval, and whether the client is near early-cycle peak, mid-cycle plateau, or end-of-cycle trough. The book does not claim a validated LAI-cycle QEEG curve. It treats cycle position as an exposure variable that may explain state differences across recordings.

Acute IM antipsychotic use, emergency sedation, or recent inpatient medication changes should be treated as a transition state. Phenotype interpretation is lower confidence when the client is recently hospitalized, acutely psychotic, heavily sedated, or medically unstable.

9.6 Adjunctive Medication Context

Typical antipsychotics often bring adjuncts. Benztropine, trihexyphenidyl, or other anticholinergic medications may be used for extrapyramidal symptoms. These can contribute to cognitive complaints, reduced activation, and possible slowing-like interpretation. Benzodiazepines may be used for agitation or anxiety and can add beta effects. Mood stabilizers may add slowing or other spectral effects. Nicotine use is common in psychosis populations and can alter arousal. Cannabis can complicate both psychosis and EEG interpretation.

The report should not treat the typical antipsychotic as the only active exposure. A better phrase is "interpreted under typical antipsychotic exposure with anticholinergic adjunct and benzodiazepine PRN use" than "antipsychotic effect."

9.7 Typical Versus Atypical Framing

The typical / atypical distinction is clinically useful but imperfect. Typical antipsychotics are often associated with stronger D2 blockade and higher extrapyramidal burden, while atypical agents vary widely across dopamine, serotonin, histamine, muscarinic, adrenergic, and metabolic profiles. From a QEEG standpoint, the distinction matters less than the actual compound, dose, route, adjuncts, and clinical state.

Haloperidol is not chlorpromazine. A high-potency medication with akathisia risk may produce a different recording context from a sedating low-potency medication with anticholinergic effects. A depot fluphenazine case differs from an oral chlorpromazine case. A medication used chronically for psychosis differs from a recent IM dose used for emergency agitation.

The chapter therefore uses typical antipsychotic as a starting category, not as a final explanation. If the recording shows slowing, the clinician should ask whether the likely contributors are D2 blockade, sedation, anticholinergic adjuncts, psychosis state, sleep disruption, hospitalization effects, nicotine / cannabis exposure, or medical illness. The answer is often several at once.

9.8 EPS, Akathisia, and Artifact

Extrapyramidal symptoms can affect both the client and the recording. Tremor, rigidity, restlessness, jaw tension, facial movement, and medication-induced parkinsonism can produce artifact or change vigilance. Akathisia can look like anxiety while arising from medication effect; a beta-heavy recording in a client with akathisia should not be treated as ordinary anxiety without qualification (see Chapter 10 for the fuller akathisia-beta discussion).

Anticholinergic treatment for EPS adds another layer. Benztropine or related medications may reduce movement symptoms while increasing cognitive and anticholinergic burden. If slowing or poor reactivity appears, the adjunct may be as relevant as the antipsychotic.

9.9 What Not to Claim

Do not give class-wide band-power percentages for typical antipsychotics unless a source directly reports them under the relevant conditions. Do not claim an explicit antipsychotic iAPF Hz shift from Saletu 2002. Do not use Centorrino as a continuous band-power source. Do not treat depot cycle timing as a validated QEEG curve. Do not equate akathisia with anxiety or ignore anticholinergic adjuncts. Do not use QEEG to recommend antipsychotic changes; relapse and safety sit with the prescriber.

The stronger claim is qualitative and conditional: typical antipsychotics can contribute to slowing and alpha-profile changes, and those effects reduce confidence in underarousal, frontal theta, slow-alpha, and arousal interpretations. The exact reading depends on compound, route, dose stability, adjuncts, psychosis state, sleep, and movement symptoms.

9.10 Report Language Examples

Weak language: "The antipsychotic caused the slowing."

Better language: "Diffuse slowing is present under haloperidol exposure with anticholinergic adjunct, poor sleep, and recent clinical instability. Typical antipsychotic exposure reduces confidence in interpreting the slowing as a stable endogenous underarousal phenotype."

Weak language: "The QEEG shows anxiety."

Better language: "Intermittent beta activity is present, but akathisia-like restlessness, nicotine use, and possible muscle artifact reduce confidence in interpreting beta as ordinary anxiety-related hyperarousal."

Weak language: "The client is stable because the map is improved."

Better language: "The recording appears more organized than the prior acute-state QEEG, but differences may reflect treatment stabilization, improved sleep, medication timing, artifact differences, or symptom improvement."

Weak language: "Depot antipsychotic effects are not relevant because the last pill was not today."

Better language: "The client receives a depot antipsychotic; the report should document injection date and cycle position because exposure may vary across the interval."

9.11 Choosing the Recording State

For most clients taking typical antipsychotics, the stable treated state is the clinically relevant state. Neurofeedback will usually occur while the medication remains in place, and the QEEG should be interpreted as a treated-state map that shows what physiology remains under ordinary treatment.

Off-medication comparison is usually inappropriate unless it is part of a prescriber-managed clinical plan. Antipsychotic interruption can carry relapse, agitation, insomnia, withdrawal, and safety risks.

When medication is changing for clinical reasons, the report should label the transition state. A client newly started on haloperidol, recently injected with a depot, or recovering from hospitalization is not at a stable baseline. The recording may still be useful, but phenotype confidence is lower.

9.12 Case vignette

A client with a history of schizophrenia is referred for QEEG-guided neurofeedback for cognitive fog, sleep disruption, and anxiety. He takes haloperidol, benztropine, and occasional lorazepam (Ativan), smokes nicotine daily, and recently reduced cannabis use. The QEEG shows frontal theta elevation, mild diffuse slowing, weak alpha organization, and intermittent beta activity.

A simple report might call the frontal theta an attention phenotype and the beta an anxiety marker. A better report is more cautious. The slowing and frontal theta overlap with typical antipsychotic exposure, anticholinergic adjunct, sleep disruption, psychosis history, and cannabis change. The beta may reflect lorazepam timing, anxiety, nicotine, muscle artifact, or akathisia-like restlessness. The recording is clinically useful as a treated-state map, but confidence in a simple endogenous attention phenotype is reduced.

The defensible interpretation is: "Findings are interpreted under typical antipsychotic exposure, anticholinergic adjunct, intermittent benzodiazepine use, nicotine exposure, and recent cannabis change. Slowing and theta findings should be treated as current-state features with multiple plausible contributors."

9.13 Interpretation traps

- **Quoting fabricated percentages.** Do not use Centorrino for continuous theta / delta magnitudes.
- **Quoting unsupported iAPF Hz shifts.** Saletu 2002 does not report an antipsychotic iAPF magnitude in Hz.
- **Ignoring anticholinergic adjuncts.** EPS medications can affect cognition and interpretation.
- **Interpreting akathisia as ordinary anxiety.** Restlessness can shape artifact and arousal features.
- **Ignoring depot timing.** LAI cycle position should be documented even if the evidence is limited to workflow heuristics.
- **Treating psychosis state as background.** Acute, residual, and stable treated states are different recordings.

9.14 Intake questions

When a typical antipsychotic appears on the intake form, ask:

- **Which antipsychotic, dose, route, and timing?** Record oral, IM, depot / LAI, recent dose changes, and last dose.
- **For depot/LAI use, where is the client in the injection cycle?** Record last injection date and usual interval.
- **Any extrapyramidal symptoms, akathisia, tremor, rigidity, or restlessness?** These alter artifact and arousal interpretation.
- **Any anticholinergic, benzodiazepine, mood stabilizer, sleep medication, nicotine, cannabis, or alcohol use?** Polypharmacy is common and clinically relevant.
- **What is the current psychosis and sleep state?** Recent hospitalization, relapse, insomnia, sedation, or instability changes confidence.

9.15 Clinical recommendations

Interpret typical-antipsychotic QEEGs as treated-state recordings unless a comparison initiated or explicitly designed by the treating prescriber is explicitly planned. Relapse, agitation, withdrawal, movement symptoms, and safety risks belong under prescriber management.

Use qualitative language for spectral effects. Say "slowing and alpha-profile changes may reduce confidence in underarousal or frontal-theta interpretations" rather than quoting unsupported magnitudes.

State depot cycle, adjunctive medications, EPS / akathisia symptoms, and current psychosis / sleep state in the report.

9.16 Evidence summary

- **Spectral effect:** Typical antipsychotics are associated qualitatively with increased slow activity and alpha-profile changes, but clean percentage magnitudes and explicit iAPF Hz shifts are not defensible from the available sources. *Aperiodic caveat: the antipsychotic slow-wave literature was analyzed with band-power methods; much of the reported delta/theta elevation may reflect aperiodic (1/f) background elevation as much as discrete oscillation increases.*
- **Phenotype inference:** Typical antipsychotic exposure can reduce confidence in frontal theta, diffuse slowing, slow-alpha, and arousal interpretations, especially with adjunctive anticholinergics or benzodiazepines.
- **Workflow heuristic:** Document route, last dose, LAI cycle position, EPS / akathisia, adjuncts, nicotine / cannabis, psychosis state, and sleep before assigning phenotype meaning.

Ch 10: Atypical Antipsychotics

10.1 Why this class matters in NFB practice

Atypical antipsychotics are common in neurofeedback referrals because they are prescribed across psychosis, bipolar disorder, depression augmentation, irritability, insomnia, autism-related behavioral indications, trauma-related agitation, and off-label sleep or anxiety use. The medication list may include clozapine (Clozaril), olanzapine (Zyprexa), risperidone (Risperdal), quetiapine (Seroquel), aripiprazole (Abilify), ziprasidone (Geodon), paliperidone (Invega), lurasidone (Latuda), lumateperone (Caplyta), brexpiprazole (Rexulti), pimavanserin (Nuplazid), cariprazine (Vraylar), or xanomeline-trospium (Cobenfy).

Strongest evidence	Clozapine, olanzapine, and risperidone support compound-specific EEG effects; aripiprazole has no single-dose spectral profile, only a qualitative epileptiform / abnormality grading, milder than clozapine, from a cross-sectional sample that cannot separate drug from diagnosis or dose; quetiapine and newer atypicals remain gaps.
Biggest interpretation trap	Treating atypicals as one EEG class: Clozapine, quetiapine, risperidone, and aripiprazole differ across EEG signatures.
Default clinical action	Document compound, route, LAI cycle position, indication, side effects, adjuncts, psychosis / mood state, and sleep before assigning a phenotype.

The class label hides large differences. Clozapine is not aripiprazole. Quetiapine at low dose for sleep is not risperidone in a first-episode psychosis study. A paliperidone long-acting injection is not the same exposure problem as an oral nightly quetiapine tablet. A clinician who writes "atypical antipsychotic effect" without compound, dose, indication, timing, side-effect state, and formulation is usually saying too little.

For QEEG interpretation, atypical antipsychotics matter because they can overlap with diffuse slowing, frontal theta, alpha-profile changes, beta / arousal findings, akathisia, sedation, seizure threshold, sleep disruption, metabolic burden, and condition effects. Some compounds have meaningful pharmaco-EEG evidence. Others remain pure or near-pure gaps.

10.2 Mechanism (clinician-level pharmacology)

Atypical antipsychotics generally combine dopamine and serotonin effects, but the details vary widely. Some are strong dopamine D2 antagonists. Some are dopamine partial agonists. Some have strong histaminergic, muscarinic, adrenergic, or serotonergic profiles. Those differences influence sedation, akathisia, metabolic burden, cognition, seizure risk, and EEG interpretation.

Clozapine is pharmacologically broad and clinically distinctive. It carries sedation, anticholinergic effects, seizure-threshold concerns, metabolic effects, and unique efficacy in treatment-resistant schizophrenia. Olanzapine shares some sedating and metabolic features but is not clozapine. Risperidone and paliperidone have stronger D2-related features and prolactin concerns. Quetiapine is often used at low doses for sleep, creating a different clinical context from antipsychotic-dose treatment. Aripiprazole, brexpiprazole, and cariprazine are dopamine partial agonist-spectrum agents. Lurasidone and lumateperone have newer profiles with limited direct QEEG evidence.

Route and formulation matter. Oral daily dosing differs from long-acting injectable paliperidone or aripiprazole. IM olanzapine for acute agitation differs from chronic oral olanzapine. LAI cycle position, recent dose changes, adherence, and missed doses should be documented.

10.3 Known spectral effects

Clozapine has one of the better-described atypical-antipsychotic QEEG profiles, with increases in slow activity and decreases in fast activity reported in healthy volunteers (Galderisi et al., 1996), and is discussed in detail under Compound-Specific Clinical Notes and Seizure Threshold and Clozapine below.

Olanzapine appears to produce less slow-wave enhancement than clozapine in a comparative EEG study of the two agents (Schuld et al., 2000). That does not make olanzapine EEG-neutral. It means olanzapine should be interpreted as a sedating atypical with a profile that may be milder than clozapine in available comparative data. The chapter uses qualitative direction, not percentage magnitudes.

Risperidone has a clean acute pharmaco-EEG reference. Lee and colleagues modeled risperidone effects on EEG in healthy volunteers and reported increased absolute delta and theta across leads after a single dose (Lee et al., 1999). This supports caution when interpreting frontal theta, diffuse slowing, and underarousal-like findings under risperidone exposure.

Aripiprazole has no clean acute reference of that kind. There is no single-dose spectral or coherence profile for aripiprazole that this book is willing to stand behind, and no alpha-frequency claim for it is supported. What does exist is qualitative. Dias Alves and colleagues graded routine EEG in 84 patients on strict atypical antipsychotic monotherapy and found modifications in about three-fifths of the sample (Dias Alves et al., 2018). Half the aripiprazole patients showed sharp or epileptiform activity, less than the nine in ten seen under clozapine, so aripiprazole should not be assumed to leave the record clean, though this design cannot separate drug from diagnosis, dose history, or selection. Across that sample, EEG modification tracked chlorpromazine-equivalent dose rather than the specific agent. The defensible claim is narrow. Do not assume aripiprazole leaves the record alone, and do not assume it slows the record the way a sedating neuroleptic does, because the spectral profile is not established in either direction.

Quetiapine is a major clinical gap; no reliable quantitative resting-QEEG support for strong theta / delta claims exists (see Low-Dose Quetiapine below for the full discussion).

Compound	Primary QEEG Vectors	Claim type	Interaction Modes	Confidence
Clozapine	delta theta increase, slow alpha increase, beta decrease	heuristic	transformation	reduced
Olanzapine	sedation slowing context	heuristic	n/a	n/a
Risperidone / paliperidone	delta theta increase	heuristic	n/a	n/a
Quetiapine	sedation context gap	heuristic	n/a	n/a
Aripiprazole	nonclassical profile, akathisia context	heuristic	n/a	n/a
Newer atypical antipsychotics	gap	heuristic	n/a	n/a

Figure 10.1: Atypical antipsychotic evidence-confidence matrix: compounds by QEEG vectors, claim type, and interaction modes.

For cariprazine, ziprasidone, lurasidone, lumateperone, brexpiprazole, pimavanserin, and xanomeline-trospium (Cobenfy), see Newer Agents and Pure Gaps below.

10.4 Phenotype interaction effects

Atypical antipsychotics can mimic underarousal, diffuse slowing, frontal theta, slow-alpha, or medication-burden phenotypes. Clozapine and olanzapine are especially relevant to slowing and vigilance. Risperidone can reduce confidence in theta and diffuse-slowing interpretations. Strong quetiapine QEEG claims need qualification (see Low-Dose Quetiapine).

They can also transform beta and arousal interpretation. Aripiprazole and other partial agonists may produce akathisia or activation in some clients. A beta-heavy or movement-contaminated recording under aripiprazole should not automatically be read as ordinary anxiety. Akathisia, restlessness, and medication tolerability belong in the QEEG context.

Exaggeration is common with polypharmacy. Antipsychotics are often combined with benzodiazepines, SSRIs/SNRIs, mood stabilizers, sleep medications, anticholinergics, cannabis, nicotine, and caffeine. The resulting QEEG may reflect medication stack, illness state, sleep, and side effects together. When a client on quetiapine plus an SSRI plus a sleep aid shows diffuse slowing, the clinician is not reading one drug's effect. The clinician is reading what three drugs, a diagnosis, and last night's sleep look like when they all show up in the same five minutes of eyes-closed data. A report that assigns the slowing to the antipsychotic has not made an error of fact. It has made an error of precision.

Masking can occur when antipsychotic treatment stabilizes psychosis, agitation, insomnia, or mood cycling. A treated-state recording may be calmer and more organized than an acute episode, which is clinically useful. It should not be mistaken for never-medicated trait physiology.

10.5 Compound-Specific Clinical Notes

Clozapine deserves the most caution. It has strong EEG relevance, seizure-threshold concerns, sedation, anticholinergic effects, metabolic burden, and treatment-resistant schizophrenia context. Slowing under clozapine should not be overread as a primary underarousal phenotype without medication context. Clozapine is also a CYP1A2 substrate: smoking induces CYP1A2 and lowers clozapine exposure, while smoking cessation reverses that induction and can raise plasma levels by 50% or more without a dose change. A client who recently quit smoking may show increased sedation, slowing, and side effects on the same clozapine dose, and the QEEG will look more medicated even though the prescription has not changed. Document smoking status and any recent changes at every recording.

Olanzapine can be sedating and metabolically burdensome. Its EEG effects appear less intense than clozapine in available comparative evidence, but it remains relevant to slowing, vigilance, sleep, and weight/metabolic context. Like clozapine, olanzapine is partially metabolized by CYP1A2, and smoking cessation can raise exposure. The effect is smaller than with clozapine but clinically relevant in heavy smokers.

Risperidone and paliperidone raise theta/delta and LAI-cycle questions. Paliperidone LAI timing should be documented, even though direct cycle-position QEEG curves are not validated.

Quetiapine at antipsychotic or low doses should be interpreted using the Low-Dose Quetiapine section below.

Aripiprazole should be treated as nonclassical. It may be activating or akathisia-producing in some clients and should not be described as a simple slowing agent. Direct evidence is limited and small-sample. Akathisia-related restlessness can produce muscle artifact and beta-range contamination that mimics anxiety-related beta excess (phenotype inference). The clinician should explicitly ask about inner restlessness, need to move, and inability to sit still, and should not interpret aripiprazole-associated beta as an anxiety phenotype without ruling out akathisia.

10.6 LAIs, Adherence, and Cycle Position

Long-acting injectable antipsychotics solve some adherence problems but create timing questions for QEEG. Paliperidone palmitate and aripiprazole LAI formulations can produce cycle-related exposure differences. The report should document last injection date, dosing interval, loading or maintenance phase, missed injections, and whether the recording occurred near early-cycle or end-cycle timing.

Direct QEEG evidence for LAI cycle effects is limited. The point is not to infer a precise spectral curve. The point is to avoid comparing two recordings as if medication exposure were identical when one occurred just after injection and another near the end of the interval.

10.7 Side-Effect States

Side effects often matter as much as the compound. Sedation can reduce vigilance, alter alpha reactivity, and make slow activity more likely. Akathisia can increase movement, muscle artifact, beta-range contamination, and anxiety-like symptoms. Tremor and rigidity can change recording quality. Metabolic changes can worsen sleep apnea risk, fatigue, inflammation, and daytime sleepiness. Anticholinergic effects can contribute to cognitive fog and reduced activation.

The same antipsychotic can therefore produce different QEEG contexts in different clients. A client tolerating olanzapine well on a stable dose is not the same as a client newly started on olanzapine with severe sedation and rapid weight gain. A client taking aripiprazole without akathisia is not the same as a client pacing in the chair during the recording. The report should describe the side-effect state directly.

Sedation should be separated from slowing. The client may feel sedated without dramatic slow activity, or show slowing from sleep deprivation, OSA, cannabis, benzodiazepines, or illness rather than the antipsychotic alone. Akathisia should be separated from anxiety. Both can feel distressing, but medication-induced restlessness changes the interpretation of beta and artifact.

10.8 Condition and Indication

Atypical antipsychotics are prescribed for different reasons. Clozapine for treatment-resistant schizophrenia, risperidone for irritability, quetiapine for sleep, aripiprazole for depression augmentation, olanzapine for bipolar mania, and pimavanserin for Parkinson-related psychosis represent different clinical contexts. The indication helps explain the recording.

Psychosis-spectrum clients may have illness-related EEG differences, high nicotine use, cannabis exposure, sleep disruption, cognitive symptoms, and anticholinergic adjuncts. Bipolar clients may have mood-state, sleep, stimulant, antidepressant, lithium, or anticonvulsant interactions. Depression-augmentation clients may have SSRI/SNRI exposure, residual depression, insomnia, and anxiety. Sleep-dose quetiapine clients may present primarily as insomnia or trauma cases rather than psychosis cases.

The QEEG should therefore not treat antipsychotic exposure as a single confound. The treated condition and the medication both shape the map.

10.9 Newer Agents and Pure Gaps

The newer-atypical category is where the book's gap discipline matters most. Ziprasidone, lurasidone, lumateperone, brexpiprazole, pimavanserin, and related agents have clinically important mechanisms, but no mature human resting-QEEG evidence base has been identified for most of them. The correct response is not to omit the medication or invent a signature. The correct response is to label the gap.

For a client taking lurasidone, the clinician can document dose, timing with food, akathisia, sleep, and mood/psychosis state. For lumateperone, document sedation, cognition, and indication. For brexpiprazole, document partial-agonist context and activation/akathisia. For pimavanserin, document Parkinsonian context, psychosis indication, and comorbid neurodegeneration. None of those documentation steps requires a fabricated band pattern.

Cariprazine has emerging evidence, including high-density EEG work (Czobor et al., 2026). Because that literature is new, it should be cited as emerging and not overgeneralized. A single emerging source does not make a routine clinical signature.

Gap language should sound like this: "Direct human resting-QEEG evidence for this compound is limited; interpretation is based on mechanism, side-effect state, indication, and class-adjacent evidence."

Xanomeline-trospium (Cobenfy) is a mechanism-boundary case. FDA-approved in September 2024 for schizophrenia in adults, it is first in class: a muscarinic agonist, not a dopamine blocker. Efficacy is attributed to xanomeline agonism at M1 and M4 muscarinic acetylcholine receptors in the CNS, reducing dopamine release in the associative striatum while sparing sensorimotor regions; the exact mechanism is not fully established. Trospium chloride is a peripheral muscarinic antagonist that does not appreciably cross the blood-brain barrier and is included to blunt xanomeline's peripheral cholinergic side effects (nausea, vomiting, sweating). No resting-QEEG data exist. The mechanism boundary matters for interpretation: cholinergic agonism in the CNS is pharmacologically opposite to the anticholinergic sedation that shapes the EEG discussion for most antipsychotics in this chapter, so a clinician reasoning from anticholinergic class effects would get the direction backwards. Until direct evidence appears, Cobenfy is a pure gap, and spectral claims in either direction are unsupported.

10.10 Low-Dose Quetiapine

Low-dose quetiapine is common enough to deserve special handling. It is often used for sleep, anxiety, trauma-related insomnia, bipolar sleep stabilization, or agitation rather than for psychosis at antipsychotic doses. Clinicians may assume it produces strong EEG slowing because it feels sedating. The available evidence does not support a strong quantified resting-QEEG claim.

That does not mean quetiapine is irrelevant. It means the mechanism of relevance may be sleep, sedation, next-day fatigue, antihistaminergic effect, anticholinergic burden, weight/metabolic effects, and co-medication context. A quetiapine user with poor sleep and morning fog may show slowing because of several interacting pathways.

The report should avoid saying "quetiapine caused diffuse slowing" unless evidence from timing, repeat recording, and clinical context supports that inference. Better language is: "Low-dose quetiapine use and sleep-state factors reduce confidence in interpreting slowing as a stable endogenous underarousal phenotype; direct resting-QEEG quantification for low-dose quetiapine is limited."

10.11 Seizure Threshold and Clozapine

Clozapine has special EEG and safety relevance because of seizure-threshold concerns. The QEEG clinician is not managing clozapine, but should recognize that clozapine cases often involve higher medical complexity, treatment resistance, sedation, anticholinergic effects, metabolic issues, and seizure-risk monitoring by the prescriber.

If paroxysmal activity, unusual slowing, or clinical seizure history appears, the report should recommend appropriate medical review rather than neurofeedback-only interpretation. QEEG findings should not be used to alter clozapine dosing. They can support communication with the prescriber when safety-relevant findings are present.

10.12 Report Language Examples

Weak language: "The atypical antipsychotic explains the slowing."

Better language: "Diffuse slowing is present under olanzapine exposure with poor sleep and metabolic/OSA risk. Atypical antipsychotic exposure reduces confidence in interpreting slowing as a stable endogenous underarousal phenotype."

Weak language: "Quetiapine produces heavy theta slowing."

Better language: "Low-dose quetiapine is clinically sedating, but direct resting-QEEG quantification is limited; interpretation should focus on sleep quality, next-day sedation, dose timing, and co-medications."

Weak language: "Aripiprazole is an antipsychotic, so it should slow the EEG."

Better language: "Aripiprazole has a nonclassical profile and may be associated with activation or akathisia in some clients; beta and movement findings should be interpreted with side-effect context."

Weak language: "No data means no concern."

Better language: "Direct resting-QEEG evidence for this newer atypical is limited. The report documents mechanism, side effects, indication, and co-medications, and avoids compound-specific spectral claims."

10.13 Choosing the Recording State

Stable treated-state recordings are usually appropriate. Most clients taking antipsychotics should not interrupt medication for QEEG interpretation. The current-state map can still guide neurofeedback if the client will continue the medication.

Recent starts, dose changes, LAI loading phases, missed injections, acute hospitalization, and medication switches should be labeled as transition states. Phenotype interpretation may be lower confidence during these periods.

If repeat QEEGs are used, medication state should be documented the same way each time. A change from oral to LAI, a dose increase, or a shift in injection-cycle timing can change the comparison.

10.14 Akathisia, Activation, and Beta

Akathisia is one of the easiest antipsychotic side effects to misread in QEEG practice. The client may describe anxiety, agitation, inability to sit still, inner restlessness, or panic-like distress. The clinician may see movement, jaw tension, muscle artifact, or beta-range contamination. If the report calls this hyperarousal without naming akathisia, it misses the medication context.

Aripiprazole and some other agents can be activating or akathisia-producing in susceptible clients. That does not mean every beta finding under aripiprazole is medication-caused. It means the report should document side effects before assigning beta to endogenous anxiety, trauma arousal, or cortical overactivation.

Akathisia can also drive nonadherence, sleep disruption, and substance use. A client may use cannabis, alcohol, benzodiazepines, or extra sleep medications to manage restlessness. The QEEG then reflects antipsychotic exposure plus compensatory exposures. The medication list alone may not reveal the behavioral response.

10.15 Metabolic and Sleep Confounds

Several atypical antipsychotics can contribute to weight gain, metabolic changes, sedation, and sleep-disordered breathing risk. Olanzapine and clozapine are especially important in this regard, but the clinical context matters for every compound. OSA, fragmented sleep, daytime fatigue, and circadian disruption can produce slowing and poor alpha reactivity that may be wrongly assigned to the medication or the psychiatric condition.

The QEEG clinician should therefore ask about snoring, witnessed apneas, morning headaches, daytime sleepiness, weight change, and sleep schedule. A slow or drowsy recording in a client taking olanzapine may reflect medication sedation, OSA, insufficient sleep, cannabis, benzodiazepines, metabolic burden, or psychosis recovery. The correct report keeps those possibilities visible.

Quetiapine adds similar concerns (see Low-Dose Quetiapine above).

10.16 Polypharmacy Patterns

Atypical antipsychotics often anchor a medication stack. Common pairings include antipsychotic plus SSRI/SNRI, antipsychotic plus mood stabilizer, antipsychotic plus benzodiazepine, antipsychotic plus stimulant, antipsychotic plus sleep medication, and antipsychotic plus cannabis or nicotine. Controlled pharmaco-EEG evidence for these combinations is limited, so interpretation is usually a workflow heuristic.

The practical task is to identify additive and competing directions. Clozapine plus benzodiazepine plus OSA risk points toward sedation and vigilance concerns. Aripiprazole plus stimulant plus caffeine points toward activation, akathisia, and beta/artifact concerns. Quetiapine plus cannabis plus trazodone (Desyrel) points toward sleep and sedation interpretation. Risperidone plus anticholinergic adjunct points toward theta/slowing plus cognitive-burden questions.

Polypharmacy language should be explicit. "The QEEG was recorded under olanzapine, valproate (Depakote), clonazepam (Klonopin), nicotine, and poor sleep" is more clinically useful than "antipsychotic effects may be present."

10.17 What Not to Claim

Do not treat atypical antipsychotics as a single spectral class. Do not claim low-dose quetiapine has a quantified resting-QEEG slowing signature. Do not convert Centorrino's categorical abnormality rates into continuous power changes. Do not present aripiprazole as a classical sedative-slowing agent. Do not invent signatures for newer agents with no direct resting-QEEG evidence. Do not ignore LAI cycle position or side effects. Do not use QEEG to recommend antipsychotic dose, hold, or switch; those decisions and their risks stay with the prescriber.

The stronger claim is conditional: atypical antipsychotics can shape QEEG interpretation through compound-specific spectral effects, sedation, akathisia, metabolic/sleep pathways, seizure threshold, route, adherence, and polypharmacy. The clinician's job is to make those conditions visible before assigning phenotype meaning.

10.18 Practical Confidence Levels

High-confidence interpretation is possible when the compound has direct evidence, exposure state is stable, side effects are documented, the recording is clean, and the finding matches the expected direction. Clozapine-associated slowing under stable dosing is a stronger inference than a band claim for a newer agent without QEEG data.

Moderate-confidence interpretation applies when the medication is stable but other factors point in the same direction. Olanzapine plus OSA risk, risperidone plus benzodiazepine use, or quetiapine plus poor sleep all lower specificity while preserving clinical usefulness.

Low-confidence interpretation applies during acute medication changes, hospitalization, severe akathisia, heavy sedative stacking, active intoxication or withdrawal, unstable sleep, or when the compound is a pure gap. In those cases, the recording may document the current state, but phenotype labels should be tentative or deferred.

This confidence language should be written into the report. A future clinician cannot reconstruct the medication logic if it remains only in the interpreter's head.

10.19 Case vignette

A client with bipolar disorder and psychotic features presents for neurofeedback because of cognitive fog, anxiety, and sleep disruption. She takes quetiapine at night, lamotrigine (Lamictal) in the morning, and occasional clonazepam. She recently stopped cannabis and reports restlessness since an aripiprazole trial was discontinued. The QEEG shows mild diffuse slowing, weak posterior alpha reactivity, and intermittent beta activity.

A simplistic report might describe underarousal with hyperarousal. A better report identifies competing contributors. Quetiapine may be clinically sedating, but strong resting-QEEG claims are not well quantified. Lamotrigine has its own anticonvulsant profile. Clonazepam can affect beta and reactivity. Cannabis discontinuation and sleep instability may shape both slowing and beta. Recent aripiprazole-related restlessness may complicate arousal interpretation.

The defensible report states that the recording is interpreted under atypical-antipsychotic exposure, mood-stabilizer exposure, intermittent benzodiazepine use, recent cannabis change, and sleep disruption. Slowing and beta findings are current-state features with reduced confidence as simple trait phenotypes.

10.20 Interpretation traps

- **Treating atypicals as one EEG class.** Clozapine, quetiapine, risperidone, and aripiprazole differ across EEG signatures.
- **Overclaiming quetiapine slowing.** Strong low-dose quetiapine QEEG claims are clinician lore unless quantified.
- **Using Centorrino for continuous band-power magnitudes.** It reports categorical abnormality rates, not continuous spectral percentages.
- **Mislabeling aripiprazole as classical slowing.** Its limited evidence suggests a nonclassical profile.
- **Inventing signatures for newer agents.** Lurasidone, lumateperone, brexpiprazole, pimavanserin, and similar drugs need gap labels when direct QEEG evidence is absent.
- **Ignoring LAI cycle position.** Injection timing should be documented for paliperidone and aripiprazole LAIs.

- **Treating end-of-cycle or missed LAI recordings as unmedicated baseline.** Injection timing and cycle position are part of exposure state. A recording near the end of a LAI cycle may show declining plasma levels and emerging symptoms, but it is not equivalent to a drug-free state.

10.21 Intake questions

When an atypical antipsychotic appears on the intake form, ask:

- **Which compound, dose, route, and indication?** Psychosis, bipolar disorder, depression augmentation, sleep, irritability, and agitation have different contexts.
- **Is the medication oral, IM, or LAI?** For LAIs, record last injection date, interval, and missed/loading doses.
- **What side effects are active?** Sedation, akathisia, tremor, rigidity, cognitive fog, weight/metabolic changes, and insomnia all matter.
- **What adjuncts are present?** Benzodiazepines, mood stabilizers, antidepressants, anticholinergics, sleep medications, cannabis, nicotine, and caffeine should be recorded.
- **What is the current clinical state?** Stable maintenance, recent hospitalization, acute psychosis, mood episode, taper, or medication switch.

10.22 Clinical recommendations

Interpret atypical-antipsychotic QEEGs compound by compound. Use stronger language for clozapine, olanzapine, and risperidone where direct evidence exists. Use constrained language for aripiprazole. Use gap language for quetiapine low-dose claims and newer agents where resting-QEEG evidence is absent or emerging.

Antipsychotic changes can destabilize mood, psychosis, sleep, safety, and withdrawal state. If a different medication state is clinically relevant, it must be prescriber-directed.

> **Scope of practice.** QEEG interpretation does not direct prescribing. Medication decisions, including discontinuation, dose changes, and substitution, rest with the prescriber.

Reports should explicitly state medication state: "recorded under stable clozapine exposure," "recorded near end of paliperidone LAI cycle," "recorded during quetiapine sleep-dose use," or "recorded after recent aripiprazole discontinuation." This makes later comparisons interpretable.

10.23 Evidence summary

- **Spectral effect:** Clozapine, olanzapine, and risperidone support compound-specific EEG effects; aripiprazole has no single-dose spectral profile, only a qualitative epileptiform / abnormality grading, milder than clozapine, from a cross-sectional sample that cannot separate drug from diagnosis or dose; quetiapine and newer atypicals have major evidence gaps. *Aperiodic caveat: the antipsychotic slow-wave literature was analyzed with band-power methods; much of the reported delta/theta elevation may reflect aperiodic (1/f) background elevation as much as discrete oscillation increases.*
- **Phenotype inference:** Atypical antipsychotics can reduce confidence in slowing, frontal theta, alpha, beta / arousal, and vigilance interpretations, with direction depending on compound and side-effect state.
- **Workflow heuristic:** Document compound, route, LAI cycle position, indication, side effects, adjuncts, psychosis / mood state, and sleep before assigning phenotype meaning.

Ch 11: Anticonvulsants and Mood Stabilizers

11.1 Why this class matters in NFB practice

Anticonvulsants and mood stabilizers are frequent in neurofeedback referrals because they are used for epilepsy, bipolar disorder, migraine, chronic pain, fibromyalgia, neuropathy, mood instability, aggression, sleep, and psychiatric augmentation. A medication list may include lithium, valproate (Depakote), carbamazepine (Tegretol), oxcarbazepine (Trileptal), lamotrigine (Lamictal), levetiracetam (Keppra), topiramate (Topamax), gabapentin (Neurontin), pregabalin (Lyrica), perampanel, brivaracetam, or related agents.

Strongest evidence	Lithium, lamotrigine, topiramate, and broader antiepileptic literature support compound-specific EEG effects, but directions differ and magnitudes vary.
Biggest interpretation trap	Repeating the lamotrigine error: Do not write that lamotrigine increases alpha power.
Default clinical action	Document indication, dose stability, missed doses, pregnancy / postpartum PK, seizure history, side effects, and comedications before assigning a phenotype.

This class matters because it sits at the intersection of QEEG interpretation and neurological safety. Some agents can contribute to slowing, cognitive fog, drowsiness, alpha-frequency shifts, or seizure-threshold changes. Some are prescribed because the client has epilepsy or paroxysmal risk. Some are used for pain or migraine, where the treated condition itself can shape the QEEG. A clinician cannot interpret these medications only as psychiatric drugs or only as neurological drugs.

The chapter's main rule is compound specificity. Lamotrigine differs from topiramate; lithium differs from valproate; gabapentin for fibromyalgia differs from carbamazepine for seizures. A broad "mood stabilizer" label is too vague for QEEG interpretation.

11.2 Mechanism (clinician-level pharmacology)

Mood stabilizers and anticonvulsants act through many mechanisms: sodium-channel modulation, calcium-channel effects, GABAergic effects, glutamatergic modulation, intracellular signaling, synaptic vesicle effects, and network-stability changes. These mechanisms can reduce seizure risk, stabilize mood, treat pain, or reduce migraine frequency, but they do not share one EEG signature.

Lithium has a distinctive clinical and pharmacokinetic profile, with narrow therapeutic monitoring and sensitivity to kidney function, hydration, drug interactions, and toxicity. Valproate is broad-spectrum and can be sedating or cognitively dulling for some clients. Carbamazepine and oxcarbazepine involve sodium-channel effects and drug interactions. Lamotrigine is often considered relatively cognitively sparing. Topiramate is notorious clinically for cognitive slowing in some clients. Gabapentin and pregabalin often enter through pain, sleep, anxiety, or fibromyalgia, where drowsiness and condition effects overlap.

That matters here because the EEG effect may reflect the drug, the treated condition, dose level, toxicity, sleep, comedications, or withdrawal state.

11.3 Known spectral effects

Lithium has a verified replacement anchor in Schulz and colleagues (Schulz et al., 2000), discussed in the Lithium subsection below.

Clemens and colleagues provide the key directional evidence for several antiepileptic drugs (Clemens et al., 2006). Lamotrigine is associated with reduced broad-band power while alpha mean frequency is preserved or slightly increased, not an alpha-power elevation. This makes lamotrigine relatively EEG-sparing compared with more sedating or slowing agents, but not irrelevant.

Compound	Primary QEEG Vectors	Claim type	Interaction Modes	Confidence
Anticonvulsants and mood stabilizers	compound specific	heuristic	exaggeration, transformation	reduced, substantially reduced
Lithium	slow activity, alpha iapf context	spectral	n/a	n/a
Lamotrigine	delta theta reduction, alpha frequency preserved	spectral	mimicry	reduced
Topiramate	slowing cognitive context	spectral	transformation	reduced

Figure 11.1: Anticonvulsant and mood-stabilizer evidence map: compounds by QEEG vectors, claim type, and interaction modes.

Topiramate has a verified replacement source in Wang and colleagues (W. W. Wang et al., 2003), discussed in the Topiramate subsection below.

Perucca and colleagues provide a broader review anchor for the adverse-effect and tolerability profile of antiepileptic drugs, including sedation and cognitive slowing (Perucca & Gilliam, 2012). This is useful for class-level orientation when individual compounds have sparse direct QEEG evidence, but it is not spectral evidence and should not be used to blur compound differences.

Gabapentinoids are best treated as drowsiness-mediated and condition-context medications rather than as a clean spectral fingerprint (see Gabapentin and Pregabalin below).

11.4 Phenotype interaction effects

Anticonvulsants and mood stabilizers most often create mimicry and exaggeration. Lithium, topiramate, valproate, carbamazepine, gabapentinoids, drowsiness, chronic pain, migraine, fibromyalgia, and epilepsy history can all overlap with slowing or frontal-theta interpretations. A diffuse-slowing map in a client on multiple mood stabilizers should not be treated as a pure underarousal phenotype.

Lamotrigine creates a different interpretive problem. Because it may reduce slow activity without shifting alpha mean frequency, a normal-looking QEEG under lamotrigine does not necessarily represent the unmedicated state. It may reflect treated stabilization. The clinician should avoid the opposite error of calling lamotrigine EEG-neutral in every context.

Topiramate can mimic cognitive-slowing phenotypes. A client taking topiramate for migraine who complains of word-finding problems and shows slow activity may be reflecting medication effect, migraine biology, sleep, or all three. The report should not assign causality from the map alone.

Gabapentinoids can exaggerate condition confounds by adding sedation to already fatigue-shaped recordings in fibromyalgia, chronic pain, or sleep disruption (see Gabapentin and Pregabalin below).

Withdrawal and missed doses transform interpretation. Anticonvulsant discontinuation can affect seizure risk, mood stability, sleep, and hyperexcitability. A tapering or recently missed-dose recording should be labeled as a transition state.

11.5 Compound-Specific Notes

Lithium should trigger questions about dose, serum level monitoring, kidney function, hydration, recent illness, NSAID/diuretic interactions, tremor, cognitive slowing, and toxicity symptoms. A QEEG suggesting unusual slowing in a lithium-treated client should be interpreted with medical context.

Valproate may appear in bipolar disorder, epilepsy, migraine, or aggression contexts. Sedation, weight gain, tremor, and comedications matter. Valproate withdrawal or nonadherence can carry seizure and mood risks.

Carbamazepine and oxcarbazepine raise sodium-channel, drug-interaction, and hyponatremia context questions. Drowsiness, slowing, and cognitive effects should be interpreted alongside dose and comedications.

Lamotrigine should be written with the corrected direction: reduced delta/theta power and preserved alpha mean frequency in the primary source, not alpha-power elevation. Pregnancy and postpartum pharmacokinetics are important because lamotrigine clearance through UGT1A4 glucuronidation can increase two- to threefold during pregnancy due to estrogen-mediated enzyme induction, then reverse rapidly postpartum, altering effective exposure even at the same dose. Valproate co-prescription roughly doubles lamotrigine levels by inhibiting the same UGT1A4 pathway. Hormonal contraceptives containing ethinyl estradiol can also induce UGT1A4 and lower lamotrigine exposure. See Appendix E for the full UGT1A4 pharmacogenomic discussion and Chapter 29 for pregnancy / postpartum timing context.

Topiramate is clinically important for migraine and weight contexts as well as epilepsy. Cognitive complaints, slowed processing, word-finding problems, and QEEG slowing should be interpreted together.

Gabapentin and pregabalin are often pain, sleep, and anxiety medications in practice. Their QEEG relevance is often drowsiness and condition overlap rather than a precise fingerprint.

Levetiracetam, brivaracetam, perampanel, eslicarbazepine, and newer agents should be handled with gap-aware language unless direct resting-QEEG evidence is available. Behavioral side effects, sleep, seizure history, and indication may outweigh any claimed band signature.

11.6 Lithium

Lithium is both a mood stabilizer and a medical-monitoring medication. QEEG interpretation should not separate the map from serum level, renal function, hydration, thyroid state, medication interactions, and toxicity symptoms. A client on stable lithium with good monitoring is different from a client who is dehydrated, acutely ill, taking NSAIDs, or experiencing tremor and cognitive slowing.

The replacement source supports qualitative lithium-related slowing and alpha / iAPF effects (Schulz et al., 2000). That does not permit invented magnitudes. It does justify lowering confidence when slow activity, reduced alpha organization, or cognitive-slowing complaints appear under lithium exposure.

Lithium also complicates mood-state interpretation. A QEEG recorded during mania recovery, depression, mixed state, or stable maintenance may differ because of mood state as well as medication. The report should state whether the client is stable, recently hospitalized, recently dose-adjusted, or symptomatic.

11.7 Valproate, Carbamazepine, and Oxcarbazepine

Valproate, carbamazepine, and oxcarbazepine often appear in epilepsy, bipolar disorder, migraine, aggression, and mood-instability cases. They can be sedating for some clients and are often combined with antipsychotics, antidepressants, benzodiazepines, or sleep medications. The QEEG effect may therefore reflect the medication, the treated condition, and the stack.

Valproate cases should document dose stability, sedation, tremor, weight/metabolic issues, menstrual/reproductive context, and liver or ammonia-related clinical concerns when relevant. The QEEG clinician is not managing labs, but should recognize that unusual slowing or cognitive change under valproate may warrant medical context.

Carbamazepine and oxcarbazepine raise interaction and sodium-context questions. Hyponatremia, drowsiness, drug interactions, and seizure/mood indication can all affect the clinical picture. If a client reports confusion, instability, or new cognitive symptoms, the QEEG report should not reduce the issue to phenotype language.

Carbamazepine and oxcarbazepine also carry a pharmacogenomic safety consideration that the QEEG clinician should be aware of. HLA-B*15:02, prevalent in Southeast and East Asian populations, is strongly associated with carbamazepine- and oxcarbazepine-induced Stevens-Johnson syndrome and toxic epidermal necrolysis; the FDA requires screening in at-risk ancestry groups before initiation. HLA-A*31:01, more common in European and Japanese populations, is associated with DRESS and broader hypersensitivity. These reactions typically emerge in the first one to three months of therapy. A client who develops rash, fever, or encephalopathic symptoms during early carbamazepine treatment and whose QEEG shows new diffuse slowing should be sent for same-day emergency evaluation, with the prescriber notified in parallel; drug discontinuation decisions and SJS/TEN/DRESS management are medical emergencies outside the scope of neurofeedback practice. Abrupt carbamazepine withdrawal in this context can lower seizure threshold, which should be noted when interpreting any subsequent QEEG. See Appendix E for HLA allele frequencies, CPIC guidance, and the broader anticonvulsant HLA table.

11.8 Topiramate

Topiramate deserves special caution because cognitive side effects are common enough in clinical practice to influence referral questions. Clients may report word-finding difficulty, slowed thinking, fog, fatigue, or academic/work impairment. The verified QEEG replacement source supports topiramate as a slowing-relevant medication (W. W. Wang et al., 2003), but the chapter does not quote unsupported magnitudes.

Topiramate is often used for migraine, seizures, weight-related indications, or mood stabilization. Migraine itself can affect posterior alpha and reactivity. Sleep disruption and pain can add slowing. If a topiramate-treated migraine client shows slowing, the correct interpretation is layered.

Reports should say: "Topiramate exposure and migraine history reduce confidence in interpreting slowing as a stable endogenous underarousal phenotype." That sentence is more defensible than saying the medication caused the entire pattern.

11.9 Gabapentin and Pregabalin

Gabapentin and pregabalin often enter through pain, fibromyalgia, neuropathy, anxiety, sleep, or seizure contexts. They can be sedating and may contribute to fatigue or drowsiness. Perucca's review provides broad context on antiepileptic adverse effects, sedation among them (Perucca & Gilliam, 2012), but gabapentinoid interpretation in ordinary neurofeedback practice is often more about drowsiness and condition overlap than a unique QEEG signature.

Fibromyalgia and chronic pain can already alter theta, alpha, connectivity, sleep, and arousal. Adding pregabalin or gabapentin may deepen fatigue or improve sleep. Either direction can change the recording. A current-state QEEG may still be clinically useful, but causal attribution is weak without repeat-state comparison.

The report should document dose timing, sedation, pain flare, sleep, opioid use, cannabis use, and whether the medication is new or stable.

11.10 Newer Antiseizure Medications

Levetiracetam, brivaracetam, perampanel, eslicarbazepine, lacosamide, zonisamide, and related agents should be handled with evidence-specific language. Some may have behavioral side effects, fatigue, sleep effects, or seizure-control implications. Direct resting-QEEG evidence may be limited or compound-specific.

Two newer agents deserve mention. **Cenobamate** (Xcopri), FDA-approved in 2019 for focal epilepsy, acts through dual sodium-channel inhibition and positive GABA-A modulation. It can be markedly sedating, especially during titration, and carries a titration-rate-dependent DRESS risk requiring slow titration. No resting-QEEG data exist; expect sedation-driven spectral effects during titration. **Ganaxolone** (Ztalmy), FDA-approved in 2022 for seizures associated with CDKL5 deficiency disorder, is a neuroactive steroid GABA-A modulator related to allopregnanolone. Its mechanism predicts GABAergic spectral effects (increased slow activity, possible beta), but that is a mechanistic expectation only, a workflow heuristic, and no ganaxolone EEG data exist in either direction. The primary clinical population (pediatric genetic epilepsy) and the absence of resting-QEEG studies make it a pure gap for routine neurofeedback interpretation.

If direct QEEG evidence is absent, document mechanism, indication, side effects, seizure history, and comedications.

11.11 Withdrawal, Missed Doses, and Seizure Safety

Anticonvulsant discontinuation is not a neutral recording condition. Missed doses, tapering, generic switching concerns, pregnancy-related clearance changes, and poor adherence can affect seizure risk, mood stability, sleep, and arousal. The QEEG clinician should not interpret a missed-dose recording as a clean baseline.

Withdrawal and dose instability should be labeled as transition states. For epilepsy clients, safety is primary. For bipolar clients, mood destabilization may be the central risk. For migraine and pain clients, symptom flare may shape the recording.

The report can recommend prescriber review when the medication history suggests safety concerns. It should not recommend dose changes.

11.12 Generic Switching and Exposure Changes

Generic switching concerns are common in epilepsy and mood-stabilizer populations. Lamotrigine bioequivalence literature exists, but there is no direct QEEG evidence for generic-switch effects. The QEEG stance is documentation, not alarm.

If a client reports new symptoms after a brand/generic or generic/generic switch, document the timing and symptoms.

Do not claim a QEEG signature of generic switching. If the client has seizure breakthrough, severe symptoms, or medication concerns, refer back to the prescriber.

11.13 Report Language Examples

Weak language: "Lamotrigine increased alpha."

Better language: "The established direction for lamotrigine is reduced delta/theta with preserved alpha mean frequency. The current alpha finding should not be attributed to lamotrigine without additional evidence."

Weak language: "The slowing is lithium toxicity."

Better language: "Diffuse slowing is present under lithium exposure. Interpretation should consider dose stability, serum-level monitoring, hydration, renal context, mood state, and clinical toxicity symptoms; QEEG alone does not diagnose lithium toxicity."

Weak language: "Topiramate caused the cognitive fog."

Better language: "Cognitive fog and slowing are present under topiramate exposure and migraine history. Topiramate is a plausible contributor, but migraine, sleep, pain, and comedications also reduce confidence in a single-cause interpretation."

Weak language: "Pregabalin has a specific QEEG signature."

Better language: "Pregabalin is interpreted mainly through drowsiness, pain, sleep, and condition-overlap context; direct compound-specific resting-QEEG claims should remain cautious."

Weak language: "The client missed medication, so this is baseline."

Better language: "The recording occurred after missed anticonvulsant doses and should be interpreted as a transition-state QEEG with safety and seizure-context caveats."

11.14 Choosing the Recording State

The stable current state is usually the safest and most clinically relevant recording state. Clients taking anticonvulsants for epilepsy should not skip medication for QEEG clarity. Clients taking mood stabilizers should not alter medication to produce an unmedicated map. For pain or migraine clients, stopping medication may create symptom flares that make the recording less interpretable.

If a prescriber-directed medication change is already underway, the QEEG can document that transition. The report should call it a transition-state recording and avoid treating it as a durable phenotype.

If a comparison is clinically justified, the two recordings should document indication, dose, last dose, adherence, sleep, symptom severity, seizure history, and side effects. Without that metadata, the comparison is fragile.

11.15 What Not to Claim

Do not collapse anticonvulsants into a single slowing category. Do not repeat the lamotrigine alpha-power error. Do not use topiramate claims from the rejected wrong-topic source. Do not treat gabapentinoid drowsiness as a precise fingerprint. Do not call missed-dose recordings baseline. Do not use QEEG to recommend anticonvulsant start, stop, dose change, or substitution; seizure and mood risk are for the prescriber to manage.

The stronger claim is conditional: anticonvulsants and mood stabilizers can shape QEEG interpretation through compound-specific spectral effects, seizure safety, mood state, pain and migraine context, drowsiness, pregnancy pharmacokinetics, and withdrawal or missed-dose states.

11.16 Practical Confidence Levels

High-confidence interpretation is possible when the compound has direct evidence, dosing is stable, side effects are documented, and the finding matches the expected direction. Topiramate-associated slowing under stable topiramate exposure is a stronger inference than a claim about a newer medication with sparse evidence.

Moderate confidence applies when medication and condition point in the same direction. A fibromyalgia client on pregabalin with poor sleep may show slowing, but the source cannot be separated cleanly.

Low confidence applies during missed doses, tapering, pregnancy-related exposure shifts, acute seizure instability, intoxication, severe sleep loss, or active symptom flare. In these cases, the QEEG may document current state but should not be treated as a stable phenotype.

11.17 Case vignette

Lamotrigine, topiramate, pregabalin, and occasional trazodone (Desyrel): four CNS-active prescriptions, three different indications. The client carries bipolar II, migraine, and fibromyalgia, and is here for brain fog and fatigue. The QEEG shows mild frontal theta elevation, reduced posterior alpha organization, and intermittent diffuse slowing.

A quick report might call this underarousal with attention-related theta. A better report is layered. Lamotrigine should not be blamed for alpha-power increase because that is not what the source supports. Topiramate can contribute to cognitive-slowing concerns. Pregabalin and fibromyalgia can both add drowsiness and slowing. Migraine and poor sleep may shape posterior alpha. Trazodone timing may affect reactivity.

The defensible report says: "Findings are interpreted under multiple anticonvulsant/mood-stabilizer exposures used for mood, migraine, and pain. Frontal theta and slowing are current-state features with reduced confidence as simple endogenous attention or underarousal phenotypes."

11.18 Interpretation traps

- **Repeating the lamotrigine error.** Do not write that lamotrigine increases alpha power.
- **Using the wrong topiramate citation.** Use the verified QEEG source or qualitative language.
- **Treating gabapentinoids as a clean fingerprint.** Drowsiness and condition overlap are often the main issue.
- **Ignoring indication.** Epilepsy, bipolar disorder, migraine, pain, and fibromyalgia create different QEEG contexts.
- **Treating missed doses as baseline.** Anticonvulsant discontinuation can be a safety and transition state.
- **Ignoring pregnancy and postpartum PK.** Lamotrigine exposure can shift even when dose appears unchanged.

11.19 Intake questions

When anticonvulsants or mood stabilizers appear on the intake form, ask:

- **What is the indication?** Epilepsy, bipolar disorder, migraine, pain, fibromyalgia, sleep, or augmentation changes interpretation.
- **Has the dose changed, been missed, or been tapered recently?** Treat transition states cautiously.
- **Any seizure history, aura, syncope, or paroxysmal events?** Safety context matters.
- **Any sedation, cognitive slowing, tremor, word-finding difficulty, or mood instability?** Side effects guide phenotype confidence.
- **For pregnancy/postpartum clients, has dosing or serum monitoring changed?** Especially important for lamotrigine.

11.20 Clinical recommendations

Interpret anticonvulsant and mood-stabilizer QEEGs by compound, indication, dose stability, and side-effect state. Do not collapse the class into one slowing signature. Use corrected lamotrigine language, qualitative lithium / topiramate language, and gap labels for newer agents when direct QEEG evidence is absent.

Anticonvulsant changes can alter seizure risk, mood stability, migraine control, pain, sleep, and withdrawal state. If medication-state comparison is clinically relevant, it must be prescriber-directed.

> **Scope of practice.** QEEG interpretation does not direct prescribing. Medication decisions, including discontinuation, dose changes, and substitution, rest with the prescriber.

When the client is tapering, postpartum, acutely ill, sleep deprived, or missing doses, label the recording as a transition-state QEEG and reduce phenotype confidence.

11.21 Evidence summary

- **Spectral effect:** Lithium, lamotrigine, topiramate, and broader antiepileptic literature support compound-specific EEG effects, but directions differ and magnitudes should not be invented. *Aperiodic caveat: the slow-wave effects of antipsychotics and mood stabilizers were documented with band-power methods; much of the reported delta/theta elevation may reflect aperiodic exponent shifts as much as discrete oscillation increases.*

- **Phenotype inference:** These medications can reduce confidence in slowing, frontal theta, alpha, cognitive-fog, and underarousal interpretations, especially when pain, migraine, epilepsy, or bipolar state is active.
- **Workflow heuristic:** Document indication, dose stability, missed doses, pregnancy / postpartum PK, seizure history, side effects, and comedications before assigning phenotype meaning.

Ch 12: Anesthetics and the Bispectral Index

12.1 Why this class matters in NFB practice

Anesthetics matter for QEEG practice for two reasons. First, anesthesia is the clearest clinical example of drugs changing the EEG in a dose-dependent, state-dependent way. The bispectral index (BIS) exists because EEG features can track anesthetic depth well enough to guide intraoperative monitoring (Glass et al., 1997; Sigl & Chamoun, 1994). Second, many neurofeedback clients have recent surgery, procedural sedation, endoscopy, dental anesthesia, outpatient ketamine, or emergency medication exposure. If the recording occurs too soon afterward, the clinician may be reading a recovery state rather than a stable baseline.

Strongest evidence	Anesthetic agents produce clear drug- and state-dependent EEG signatures (propofol slow / frontal-alpha, dexmedetomidine spindle-like, ketamine gamma / broadband).
Biggest interpretation trap	Treating anesthesia as ordinary sleep. General anesthesia is a drug-induced brain state, not natural sleep.
Default clinical action	For uncomplicated elective anesthesia, wait at least one week before stable phenotype interpretation; defer longer for postoperative cognitive change, delirium, ICU recovery, or older clients.

This chapter is not an anesthesia manual. It uses anesthetics as a teaching model for medication-QEEG interpretation. Propofol, sevoflurane, dexmedetomidine, ketamine, midazolam, opioids, and nitrous oxide all alter consciousness through different mechanisms and produce different EEG patterns. That makes anesthesia a useful worked example: drug mechanism, dose, state, timing, and recovery all matter.

For neurofeedback practice, the practical question is narrower: when should recent anesthesia or procedural sedation reduce confidence in QEEG phenotype interpretation? The answer is usually "document and wait until clinically recovered." For uncomplicated elective anesthesia, this book uses a conservative heuristic of waiting at least one week before QEEG interpretation; longer waits are reasonable when older age, cardiac surgery, complicated recovery, delirium, postoperative cognitive change, or ongoing symptoms are present.

12.2 Mechanism (clinician-level pharmacology)

General anesthesia is a drug-induced state involving hypnosis, amnesia, immobility, analgesia, autonomic control, and altered thalamocortical and cortical dynamics, not sleep. Brown, Lydic, and Schiff describe anesthesia as a systems neuroscience problem rather than a single switch (Brown et al., 2010). Different anesthetics reach that state through different receptor systems.

Propofol acts primarily through GABA-A potentiation and produces characteristic slow oscillations and frontal alpha at anesthetic doses. Sevoflurane and other volatile agents have overlapping but distinct patterns. Dexmedetomidine, an alpha-2 agonist, produces a sleep-spindle-like profile that resembles some non-REM sleep features more than propofol anesthesia. Ketamine, an NMDA antagonist, can produce dissociative anesthesia with gamma and broadband features rather than the same slow-alpha profile.

BIS and related monitors compress EEG information into a single index to estimate anesthetic depth (Rampil, 1998). That compression is clinically useful, but it is not magic. BIS values depend on signal quality, drug class, age, EMG artifact, burst suppression, and the algorithm's assumptions. This makes BIS a useful lesson for QEEG: a derived number can be helpful without being a direct measure of one brain state.

12.3 Known spectral effects

Propofol has one of the clearest anesthetic EEG signatures. Purdon and colleagues described propofol-induced frontal alpha and slow oscillations during loss of consciousness (Purdon et al., 2013). For QEEG clinicians, propofol illustrates that a drug can create a strong rhythm that is state-specific and dose-dependent. It should not be interpreted as a trait alpha phenotype.

Sevoflurane and propofol share some anesthetic-depth features but are not identical. Akeju and colleagues' sevoflurane/propofol work shows that anesthetic EEG signatures depend on agent and state (Akeju et al., 2014b). A post-anesthesia outpatient recording should therefore document the type of anesthesia when known, not merely "had surgery."

Dexmedetomidine differs from propofol. Akeju and colleagues showed different EEG signatures for propofol and dexmedetomidine, consistent with different mechanisms and states (Akeju et al., 2014a). This reinforces a central book theme: clinical sedation does not imply one EEG signature.

Ketamine is different again. Akeju and colleagues describe ketamine-related gamma and burst patterns during anesthesia (Akeju et al., 2016). Later outpatient ketamine and esketamine chapters handle sub-anesthetic psychiatric use separately. Here the point is that NMDA-antagonist anesthesia is not interchangeable with GABAergic anesthesia.

Burst suppression is a deep-anesthesia or severe-brain-state marker, not an ordinary outpatient QEEG phenotype. If a client has recent critical illness, ICU sedation, or complicated surgery, the post-anesthesia question becomes much broader than routine elective recovery.

Prolonged slowing belongs more to postoperative cognitive dysfunction, delirium risk, older age, complicated surgery, inflammation, or medical vulnerability than to a simple residual anesthetic effect.

12.4 Phenotype interaction effects

Recent anesthesia can mimic slowing, drowsiness, poor alpha reactivity, cognitive fog, or underarousal. In uncomplicated recovery, this effect is usually time-limited. In complicated recovery, older adults, cardiac surgery, delirium, postoperative cognitive dysfunction, ICU

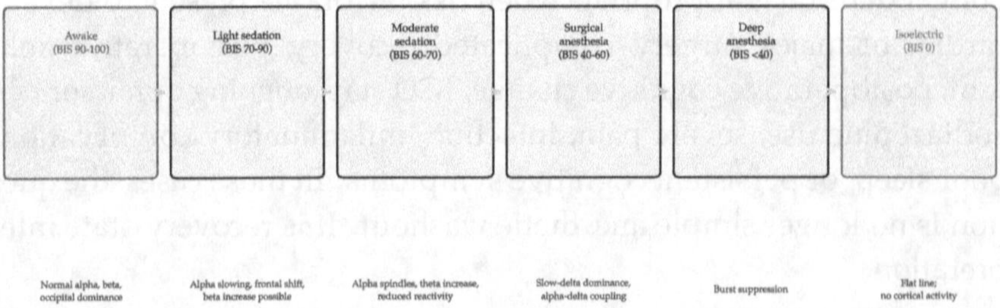

Figure 12.1: Anesthesia EEG state ladder: awake through sedation, surgical anesthesia, burst suppression, and isoelectric, with BIS index ranges.

exposure, or ongoing pain and sleep disruption, the QEEG may remain altered for longer.

Anesthesia can also transform interpretation. A slow QEEG two days after outpatient surgery does not mean the same thing as slow activity in a stable unmedicated baseline. It may reflect anesthetic recovery, sleep disruption, opioids, inflammation, pain, hospitalization, or postoperative fatigue. The finding is real but state-bound.

Exaggeration is common when anesthesia is paired with opioids, benzodiazepines, antihistamines, sleep medications, alcohol, cannabis, OSA, pain, or older age. The QEEG clinician should ask about the full perioperative medication stack, not only the anesthetic agent.

Masking can occur when surgery resolves pain or improves sleep over time. A later post-surgical QEEG may look better because the underlying pain state improved, not because medication washed out.

12.5 Post-Anesthesia Recovery Windows

No published study establishes how long uncomplicated anesthesia-related QEEG distortion takes to clear. This book's conservative heuristic is to avoid phenotype interpretation immediately after anesthesia or procedural sedation, and to wait at least one week after uncomplicated elective anesthesia when the goal is stable outpatient QEEG interpretation. The one-week buffer is not a measured washout time. It is room for sleep, pain, medication, and recovery stabilization.

Longer deferral is appropriate when risk factors are present: older age, cardiac or major surgery, complicated recovery, postoperative delirium, postoperative cognitive change, ICU stay, ongoing opioid or benzodiazepine use, severe pain, infection, inflammatory complications, poor sleep, or persistent cognitive symptoms. In those cases, the question is no longer simple anesthetic washout. It is recovery-state interpretation.

The report should document the type of procedure, anesthesia if known, date, complications, postoperative medications, sleep, pain, and cognitive recovery. "Had anesthesia recently" is too vague.

12.6 Case vignette

A sixty-eight-year-old client schedules QEEG-guided neurofeedback ten days after elective knee replacement. He had general anesthesia, postoperative opioids for several days, poor sleep, ongoing pain, and mild confusion for two days after surgery. The QEEG shows diffuse slowing, weak alpha reactivity, and fatigue-related drowsiness across the recording.

A simple report might call this underarousal or cognitive slowing. A better report treats it as a postoperative recovery-state recording. Anesthesia may no longer be the only driver. Pain, sleep disruption, opioids, age, inflammation, and recent confusion all reduce confidence in stable phenotype interpretation.

The defensible recommendation is to defer durable phenotype assignment until recovery stabilizes or to label the recording as current postoperative state. The QEEG may still document function during recovery, but it should not be treated as a pristine baseline.

12.7 Interpretation traps

- **Treating anesthesia as ordinary sleep.** General anesthesia is a drug-induced brain state, not natural sleep.
- **Using BIS as if it were a QEEG phenotype.** BIS is a derived anesthetic-depth index with context limits.
- **Ignoring the perioperative stack.** Opioids, benzodiazepines, antihistamines, pain, sleep loss, and inflammation matter.

- **Overextending uncomplicated recovery data.** Older age, delirium, cardiac surgery, ICU exposure, and complicated recovery require longer caution.
- **Failing to document procedure date.** Timing since anesthesia is mandatory metadata.
- **Confusing outpatient ketamine with anesthetic ketamine.** Dose, route, and clinical context differ.

12.8 Intake questions

When recent anesthesia or sedation appears on the intake form, ask:

- **What procedure occurred, and on what date?** Record days since anesthesia or sedation.
- **What type of anesthesia or sedation was used, if known?** Propofol, volatile anesthetic, dexmedetomidine, ketamine, midazolam, nitrous oxide, local only, or unknown.
- **Were there complications?** Delirium, prolonged confusion, ICU stay, infection, cardiac surgery, hypoxia, or difficult recovery.
- **What postoperative medications were used?** Opioids, benzodiazepines, sleep medications, antihistamines, antiemetics, steroids, cannabis, and alcohol matter.
- **How are sleep, pain, and cognition now?** Current recovery state determines interpretive confidence.

12.9 Clinical recommendations

The recovery-window heuristics above apply: wait at least one week after uncomplicated elective anesthesia; defer longer when risk factors are present. In complicated cases, the QEEG may document current state, but phenotype assignment should be reduced-confidence or deferred.

Do not use QEEG to guide postoperative or other medication decisions (dosing, holds, or substitutions). Coordinate with the prescriber or medical team.

12.10 Agent-Specific Notes

Propofol is the cleanest teaching example because its anesthetic EEG signature is well described. Frontal alpha and slow oscillations emerge with loss of consciousness and anesthetic depth. In outpatient QEEG, the relevance is not that propofol leaves a long-lasting alpha phenotype. The relevance is that a drug can create a strong, state-specific spectral pattern that would be meaningless if interpreted outside drug context.

Sevoflurane and other volatile agents create anesthetic EEG states that overlap with propofol in broad terms but differ in detail. For routine QEEG intake, the clinician rarely needs to reconstruct exact intraoperative spectra. The useful information is that the client had general anesthesia, the date, the recovery course, and whether complications or cognitive symptoms followed.

Dexmedetomidine is a good reminder that sedation mechanisms differ. Its EEG pattern can look more sleep-like than propofol, which matters for the book's broader argument: sedation is not one EEG state. If a client had ICU sedation or procedural dexmedetomidine, the recovery context may differ from a brief propofol case.

Ketamine is different from GABAergic anesthetics. At anesthetic doses, ketamine can produce broadband and gamma-related features, and at subanesthetic psychiatric doses it becomes a different chapter. The clinician should document whether ketamine was used as part of anesthesia, emergency sedation, pain treatment, or outpatient depression treatment.

Midazolam and other benzodiazepines are common in procedural sedation. Their EEG relevance overlaps with the benzodiazepine chapter: beta effects, sedation, amnesia, and withdrawal context in chronic users. A colonoscopy with midazolam and fentanyl is not the same exposure as general anesthesia, but it still belongs on the QEEG intake.

Opioids and nitrous oxide are often part of the perioperative or procedural context. Opioids can affect arousal, respiration, sleep, pain, and slowing. Nitrous oxide may be brief but should be documented when recent. The clinician should avoid focusing only on the named anesthetic while missing the perioperative stack.

12.11 Procedural Sedation and Outpatient Procedures

Many clients do not think of procedural sedation as anesthesia. They may report "just a colonoscopy," "just dental sedation," "just an injection," or "just a ketamine treatment." For QEEG interpretation, those details matter. A short sedated procedure can change sleep, pain, medications, anxiety, and recovery for several days.

Dental sedation, endoscopy, minor surgery, interventional pain procedures, imaging sedation, emergency sedation, and outpatient psychiatric ketamine should all be captured. The goal is to avoid interpreting a recovery state as stable phenotype physiology.

The same logic applies to local anesthesia with sedatives. A procedure may be "local" surgically but still include midazolam, fentanyl, propofol, or other centrally active medication. The intake question should ask about sedation, not only general anesthesia.

12.12 Raw EEG and Recovery-State Review

Post-anesthesia QEEGs require careful raw EEG review. Drowsiness, microsleeps, pain-related movement, medication tremor, opioid sedation, and poor sleep can all alter the spectrum. Automated maps may show slowing without revealing whether it was stable across alert epochs or driven by state drift.

Technician notes should document alertness, fatigue, pain behaviors, recent medication, and whether the client struggled to stay awake. If the recording contains late-session drowsiness, the report should say that vigilance instability limits trait interpretation.

Eyes-open data, alpha reactivity, and task engagement may be useful when available. A client who looks slow in eyes-closed rest but normalizes with eyes-open alertness may differ from a client with persistent slowing across states. Recovery-state interpretation should use more than one map when possible.

12.13 Report Language Examples

Weak language: "The QEEG shows underarousal."

Better language: "Diffuse slowing is present ten days after surgery with ongoing pain, poor sleep, and recent opioid exposure. Interpretation as a stable underarousal phenotype is reduced by postoperative recovery context."

Weak language: "The anesthesia should be gone by now, so ignore it."

Better language: "No published timeline for post-anesthesia QEEG normalization exists, but postoperative sleep, pain, medications, and cognitive symptoms are known confounds that remain relevant to QEEG interpretation regardless of how much time has passed."

Weak language: "Wait a long fixed interval after all anesthesia."

Better language: "For uncomplicated elective anesthesia, a one-week minimum buffer is a practical heuristic; longer deferral is based on recovery complexity and current symptoms."

Weak language: "Ketamine is ketamine."

Better language: "Anesthetic ketamine, outpatient subanesthetic ketamine, intranasal esketamine, and recreational ketamine differ by dose, route, context, and expected EEG state."

12.14 Practical Confidence Levels

High-confidence interpretation is possible when the procedure was uncomplicated, the client is fully recovered, sleep and pain have stabilized, postoperative centrally active medications have stopped, and the recording occurs after a reasonable buffer. In that case, recent anesthesia may still be documented but may not strongly reduce phenotype confidence.

Moderate confidence applies when the client is mostly recovered but still has pain, sleep disruption, mild fatigue, or recent medication changes. The QEEG can be useful, but slowing and alpha-reactivity findings should carry caveats.

Low confidence applies when the client has persistent confusion, delirium history, ICU stay, major surgery, ongoing opioids or benzodiazepines, severe pain, poor sleep, or active medical complications. In those cases, the recording is a recovery-state QEEG. It may have clinical value, but durable phenotype labels should usually wait.

12.15 What Not to Claim

Do not claim that all post-anesthesia QEEG abnormalities are direct residual anesthetic effects. Do not claim that all clients need long fixed delays after uncomplicated anesthesia. Do not ignore postoperative medications, pain, sleep, inflammation, delirium, or age. Do not treat BIS as a general outpatient phenotype metric. Do not collapse anesthetic ketamine and outpatient esketamine into one clinical context.

12.16 Documentation Standard

The minimum documentation standard is simple: procedure, date, anesthetic or sedative agents if known, complications, current pain, current sleep, current cognition, and postoperative medications. If the client cannot name the agents, the clinician can still document "unknown anesthesia type" and the recovery course.

For repeat QEEGs, document the same variables each time. A presurgery baseline, a two-week postoperative recovery recording, and a three-month follow-up can be clinically informative only if the perioperative context is visible. Otherwise, changes may be misattributed to neurofeedback, medication, or phenotype drift.

The chapter's practical stance is conservative but not alarmist. Recent uncomplicated anesthesia is usually a temporary state variable. Complicated recovery is a larger clinical context. Both should be documented before phenotype interpretation.

12.17 Evidence summary

- **Spectral effect:** Anesthetic agents produce clear drug- and state-dependent EEG signatures, including propofol slow / frontal-alpha patterns, dexmedetomidine sleep-like features, ketamine broadband / gamma features, and burst suppression at deep states.
- **Phenotype inference:** Recent anesthesia, procedural sedation, postoperative medications, sleep disruption, pain, delirium risk, and recovery state can reduce confidence in slowing, alpha-reactivity, vigilance, and underarousal interpretations.
- **Workflow heuristic:** For uncomplicated elective anesthesia, wait at least one week before stable phenotype interpretation; defer longer when postoperative cognitive or medical risk factors are present.

Ch 13: Outpatient Ketamine and Esketamine

13.1 Why this class matters in NFB practice

Outpatient ketamine and esketamine matter because many neurofeedback clients with treatment-resistant depression, trauma, chronic pain, suicidality history, or severe mood symptoms may have received IV ketamine, IM ketamine, intranasal esketamine, compounded ketamine, or ketamine-assisted psychotherapy. These treatments are not ordinary antidepressants, and they are not the same clinical context as anesthetic ketamine or recreational ketamine.

Strongest evidence	Ketamine / esketamine can acutely alter broadband power, aperiodic slope, gamma-related activity, and connectivity. Effects are timing- and dose-bound.
Biggest interpretation trap	Treating esketamine as a unique EEG fingerprint. Current evidence supports ketamine-family framing, not a separate esketamine signature.
Default clinical action	Document route, session timing, induction versus maintenance phase, dissociation, sleep, co-medications, and clinical goal before interpreting the recording.

The QEEG problem is timing. Ketamine and esketamine can produce acute oscillatory and aperiodic changes during or soon after dosing. A QEEG recorded during the treatment window, the same day, the next day, several days later, or between maintenance sessions answers different questions. A client may also be taking SSRIs / SNRIs, benzodiazepines, stimulants, antipsychotics, mood stabilizers, cannabis, or sleep medications.

This chapter treats esketamine and racemic ketamine as part of the same EEG family. There is no defensible evidence that intranasal esketamine has a unique resting-QEEG fingerprint separate from ketamine. Route, dose, supervision, and timing differ, but the core acute pattern belongs in the ketamine family.

13.2 Mechanism (clinician-level pharmacology)

Ketamine is a non-competitive NMDA receptor antagonist that blocks the ion channel in a use- and voltage-dependent manner rather than competing at the glutamate binding site. This mechanism produces complex downstream effects on glutamatergic signaling, disinhibition, plasticity, network dynamics, dissociation, and mood response. At anesthetic doses (typically 1–2 mg/kg IV) it can produce dissociative anesthesia. At subanesthetic outpatient doses (typically 0.5 mg/kg IV over ~40 minutes for depression protocols) it is used for treatment-resistant depression, suicidality, pain, and other off-label indications.

Esketamine is the S-enantiomer of ketamine and is FDA-approved as intranasal SPRAVATO (56 mg or 84 mg per session) under a REMS program. It has a clinic-session structure, observation period, and blood-pressure monitoring. In January 2025 the FDA approved esketamine as monotherapy for treatment-resistant depression in adults, the first monotherapy approved for that indication; the acute-suicidality indication remains adjunctive to an oral antidepressant. This changes the QEEG documentation problem: a clinician may now record a client on esketamine alone, with no oral antidepressant contributing to the spectral picture. Whether an antidepressant is co-prescribed should be captured rather than assumed, because the recording represents a different exposure state when esketamine is the only psychotropic on board.

The mechanism is not equivalent to classic stimulant activation or SSRI-style serotonergic treatment. Ketamine can alter broadband activity, gamma-related measures, aperiodic slope, and connectivity. A band-power-only interpretation can miss the most relevant part of the signal.

13.3 Known spectral effects

Guirguis and colleagues provide a key intranasal esketamine EEG anchor, reporting oscillatory and aperiodic changes consistent with network disinhibition during the monitored treatment window (Guirguis et al., 2025). The clinically important point is that acute esketamine can flatten the aperiodic spectrum and increase broadband power. Do not report this as a narrow single-band signature.

Lees and colleagues provide source-connectivity evidence in treatment-resistant depression after ketamine (Lees et al., 2026). These findings support the idea that ketamine can alter resting-state connectivity, not only spectral power. For QEEG practice, connectivity findings should be interpreted cautiously because source methods and pipelines matter.

Gilbert and Zarate reviewed the electrophysiology of ketamine in depression and in healthy controls, focusing on gamma oscillations and long-term potentiation as putative markers of synaptic potentiation, along with dynamic causal modeling of antidepressant response (Gilbert & Zarate, 2020). The review separates gamma's relationship to acute psychotomimetic drug effects from its relationship to delayed antidepressant response. This supports a timing-sensitive interpretation: the acute window differs from the post-acute window.

Soltanzadeh and colleagues compared S-ketamine and psilocybin in relation to aperiodic-spectrum effects, supporting the idea that S-ketamine alters the aperiodic component in a way that should not be collapsed into ordinary oscillatory band language (Soltanzadeh et al., 2025).

13.4 Phenotype interaction effects

Ketamine and esketamine can mimic or transform arousal, broadband, gamma, and connectivity interpretations. An acute post-dose QEEG is a treatment-state recording, not a stable trait baseline. Broadband increases and aperiodic flattening can make conventional band maps look shifted even when no narrow rhythm has changed in isolation.

They can also mask depression-related features if symptoms improve. A post-treatment QEEG may look more organized because mood, sleep, rumination, and network dynamics changed. That is clinically meaningful but not automatically a durable trait correction.

Exaggeration can occur when ketamine is combined with sleep deprivation, benzodiazepines, cannabis, stimulants, antipsychotics, chronic pain, or acute dissociation. Benzodiazepines are especially important because they may alter clinical response and EEG interpretation. The QEEG report should document co-medications on the day of treatment.

Transformation is central. A high-frequency or broadband finding during ketamine treatment does not carry the same meaning as beta / gamma findings in an ordinary unmedicated anxiety recording. Mechanism and timing change the interpretation.

13.5 Route and Treatment Context

IV ketamine, IM ketamine, intranasal esketamine, sublingual or oral compounded ketamine, and recreational ketamine are different clinical contexts. IV and IM treatment usually occur in clinic settings but protocols vary. Intranasal esketamine has a regulated monitoring model. Compounded troches or lozenges may have less standardized dosing and timing. Recreational use belongs in the substances chapter.

The intake form should ask route, dose if known, date and time of last session, number of sessions, maintenance frequency, acute side effects, dissociation, blood-pressure issues, nausea, sleep after treatment, and concurrent medications.

The QEEG clinician should avoid treating "ketamine history" as one variable. A client recorded two hours after intranasal esketamine differs from a client recorded two weeks after the last IV infusion.

13.6 Timing Windows

The acute treatment window is the lowest-confidence time for stable phenotype interpretation. It may be useful for research or treatment monitoring, but it should not be treated as a baseline.

Same-day recovery remains a transition state. Dissociation may have resolved behaviorally, but sleep, fatigue, nausea, blood pressure, and acute network effects may still matter.

The 24-72h window may be clinically interesting because antidepressant response can emerge quickly. It is not always a clean baseline, especially during induction series when treatments occur repeatedly. The report should say where in the dosing cycle the recording occurred.

Between maintenance sessions, QEEG may be more stable, but only if symptoms, sleep, and medications are stable. A client in an induction series should be treated differently from a client on monthly maintenance.

13.7 Case vignette

A client with treatment-resistant depression schedules QEEG-guided neurofeedback two days after intranasal esketamine. He takes an SSRI, uses clonazepam (Klonopin) occasionally, slept poorly after the session, and reports strong dissociation during treatment but mood improvement the next day. The QEEG shows flatter aperiodic slope, elevated broadband fast activity, and altered frontal connectivity measures.

A simplistic report might call the fast activity hyperarousal or the connectivity change a trait depression marker. A better report recognizes the treatment window. The recording occurred during a post-esketamine interval with poor sleep and benzodiazepine PRN context. Findings may reflect treatment-state physiology, symptom improvement, sleep disruption, medication stack, or pipeline sensitivity.

The defensible interpretation is: "QEEG was recorded two days after esketamine treatment during an active induction period. Oscillatory, aperiodic, and connectivity findings should be interpreted as post-treatment state markers, not stable trait phenotypes."

13.8 Interpretation traps

- **Treating esketamine as a unique EEG fingerprint.** Current evidence supports ketamine-family framing, not a separate esketamine signature.
- **Ignoring timing since session.** Acute, same-day, 24-72h, induction, and maintenance windows differ.
- **Collapsing aperiodic changes into band labels.** Broadband and slope effects can masquerade as band changes.
- **Confusing outpatient and anesthetic ketamine.** Dose, route, purpose, and EEG state differ.
- **Ignoring benzodiazepines and sleep.** Co-medications and post-treatment sleep can shape the map.
- **Treating response prediction as phenotype proof.** Symptom improvement does not prove a single QEEG mechanism.

13.9 Intake questions

When ketamine or esketamine appears on the intake form, ask:

- **Which route and protocol?** IV, IM, intranasal esketamine, compounded troche/lozenge, oral, or recreational.
- **When was the last session?** Record date, time, induction versus maintenance phase, and session number.
- **What happened during and after treatment?** Dissociation, nausea, blood pressure, sedation, anxiety, sleep, and next-day function.
- **What co-medications were used?** Benzodiazepines, antidepressants, stimulants, antipsychotics, cannabis, alcohol, sleep medications, and pain medications.
- **What is the clinical goal of the QEEG?** Baseline before treatment, treatment-state monitoring, or neurofeedback planning between sessions.

13.10 Clinical recommendations

Do not treat ketamine/esketamine recordings during acute or early post-dose windows as stable baseline QEEGs. Label them as treatment-state or post-treatment-state recordings. If the goal is durable neurofeedback phenotype selection, record at a stable point between sessions when sleep, mood, and co-medications are documented.

For active induction series, interpret QEEG cautiously because repeated treatments create a moving target. For maintenance treatment, document interval since last session and whether symptoms are stable.

Do not use QEEG to justify changes to ketamine, esketamine, benzodiazepines, antidepressants, or other medications. Coordinate with the prescribing clinic when timing, induction, or co-treatment questions affect interpretation.

13.11 Aperiodic Interpretation

Ketamine is one of the clearest reasons this book cannot rely only on classic frequency bands. A flattened aperiodic slope can change the apparent relationship among delta, theta, alpha, beta, and gamma without being a narrow oscillatory rhythm. If the pipeline does not separate oscillatory peaks from the aperiodic background, the clinician may mistake broad spectral tilt for a band-specific phenotype.

For ordinary neurofeedback reports, the practical answer is to add a caveat when ketamine or esketamine timing is close, not to overcomplicate every map: "Broadband and aperiodic effects may influence conventional band-power interpretation." If the software does not estimate aperiodic slope, the report should not pretend it does.

This matters most when the map shows broad fast activity, gamma-like elevation, or unusual beta / gamma features after a treatment session. The finding may reflect ketamine-family neurophysiology, muscle artifact, anxiety, sleep loss, or medication stack. Aperiodic-aware interpretation lowers overconfidence.

13.12 Route-Specific Caveats

Intranasal esketamine has a more standardized treatment environment than many compounded ketamine approaches. The REMS structure, observation period, and documented session schedule make the timing easier to record; whether an oral antidepressant is co-prescribed varies by indication and should be captured rather than assumed. Even then, QEEG interpretation depends on session timing, sleep, dissociation, and co-medications.

IV and IM ketamine protocols vary by clinic. Infusion length, dose, number of sessions, monitoring, psychotherapy pairing, and maintenance schedule may differ. A client may report "ketamine therapy" without knowing the dose or route. The QEEG clinician should record what is known and label unknowns.

Compounded troches, lozenges, and home-use models create larger documentation problems. Dose, absorption, timing, adherence, and supervision may be less clear. Direct QEEG evidence for these routes is limited, so interpretation should be conservative.

13.13 Recreational and Anesthetic Boundaries

This chapter covers outpatient therapeutic ketamine and esketamine. Recreational ketamine belongs in the recreational substances chapter because chronic heavy use, polysubstance context, bladder toxicity, dissociation patterns, and abstinence state raise different questions.

Anesthetic ketamine belongs in the anesthesia chapter because the dose and brain state are different.

The same molecule can therefore occupy three different clinical frames: anesthetic drug, psychiatric treatment, and recreational substance. QEEG interpretation must follow the frame, not just the molecule name.

13.14 Report Language Examples

Weak language: "The QEEG shows hyperarousal after ketamine."

Better language: "The recording occurred within the ketamine treatment interval; broadband fast activity and aperiodic flattening may reflect treatment-state physiology and should not be interpreted as ordinary hyperarousal without timing context."

Weak language: "Esketamine has a separate QEEG profile."

Better language: "Current evidence supports ketamine-family framing for esketamine; route and protocol differ, but a separate resting-QEEG fingerprint has not been established."

Weak language: "No effect remains after the session."

Better language: "Acute effects are strongest during and soon after dosing, while post-acute findings depend on timing, response, sleep, co-medications, and treatment phase."

Weak language: "This map predicts ketamine response."

Better language: "The QEEG may be useful as a within-client baseline or state marker, but response prediction requires protocol-specific evidence and should not be inferred from this clinical map alone."

13.15 Practical Confidence Levels

High confidence is possible when the client is outside the acute treatment window, the treatment schedule is stable, sleep has recovered, and co-medications are documented. Moderate confidence applies during stable maintenance treatment when the recording is close enough to a session that residual effects remain plausible; broadband, gamma, aperiodic, and connectivity findings should carry timing caveats. Low confidence applies during the acute session, same-day recovery, severe dissociation, active induction, unclear compounded dosing, heavy benzodiazepine use, intoxication, poor sleep, or major medication changes; durable phenotype assignment should wait.

13.16 What Not to Claim

Do not claim esketamine has a separate spectral identity from racemic ketamine. Do not treat acute broadband changes as a stable hyperarousal phenotype. Do not interpret aperiodic slope changes as a narrow band effect unless the pipeline supports that distinction. Do not use clinical QEEG alone to predict ketamine response. Do not merge anesthetic, therapeutic, and recreational ketamine contexts.

13.17 Co-Treatment Context

Most outpatient ketamine clients are not medication-free. They may be taking SSRIs, SNRIs, bupropion (Wellbutrin), lithium, lamotrigine (Lamictal), antipsychotics, benzodiazepines, stimulants, sleep medications, cannabis, or pain medications. Some are in psychotherapy on treatment days, tapering benzodiazepines, sleep deprived, or fasting before sessions.

The QEEG report should make co-treatment context visible. A broadband or connectivity shift after ketamine plus benzodiazepine PRN plus poor sleep should not be interpreted like ketamine alone. A stable maintenance client on unchanged antidepressant therapy is a different context from an induction client whose medications are being adjusted. For neurofeedback planning, ketamine timing is necessary but not sufficient. The medication stack, symptom response, sleep, and the client's ordinary treatment schedule all belong in the interpretive paragraph.

Safety notice. Intranasal esketamine (Spravato) is a REMS-restricted medication administered under clinical supervision because of dissociation and abuse potential. Intravenous ketamine infusion protocols vary by clinic and carry monitoring requirements. Ketamine use in clients with active suicidal ideation requires prescriber coordination; QEEG scheduling should follow the treating clinician's guidance on timing relative to the treatment schedule. Nothing in this chapter constitutes a dosing or monitoring protocol.

13.18 Evidence summary

- **Spectral effect:** Ketamine/esketamine can acutely alter broadband power, aperiodic slope, gamma-related activity, and connectivity; effects are timing- and method-dependent.
- **Phenotype inference:** Acute and early post-treatment recordings can reduce confidence in stable beta/gamma, arousal, connectivity, and depression-phenotype interpretations.
- **Workflow heuristic:** Document route, session timing, induction versus maintenance phase, dissociation, sleep, co-medications, and clinical goal before interpreting QEEG phenotype meaning.

Ch 14: Opioids

14.1 Why this class matters in NFB practice

Opioids appear in neurofeedback practice through chronic pain, postoperative recovery, cancer care, opioid use disorder treatment, medication-assisted treatment, emergency care, recreational exposure, and withdrawal. A medication list may include oxycodone, hydrocodone, morphine, fentanyl, tramadol (Ultram), methadone (Dolophine), buprenorphine (Subutex), buprenorphine/naloxone combination products (Suboxone), naltrexone (oral or Vivitrol depot), naloxone rescue history (Narcan), or kratom.

Strongest evidence	Methadone-maintenance data support qualitative theta and beta differences in that population; evidence is sparse for many other opioid compounds.
Biggest interpretation trap	Using rejected opioid citations: Do not cite wrong-topic sources for opioid claims.
Default clinical action	Document opioid type, indication, stability, last dose, withdrawal/intoxication state, pain severity, sleep/respiration, and co-medications before interpreting.

Opioids matter because they can alter arousal, respiration, sleep, pain, attention, mood, and withdrawal state. The QEEG map may reflect medication exposure, pain physiology, sleep-disordered breathing, benzodiazepine co-use, depression, trauma, opioid use disorder, or postoperative recovery. The same slowing pattern can mean different things in a stable buprenorphine-maintained client, an acute postoperative opioid user, and a client in withdrawal.

14.2 Mechanism (clinician-level pharmacology)

Most clinically used opioids act primarily through mu-opioid receptor agonism, with differences in potency, half-life, route, active metabolites, respiratory effects, and co-medication context. Methadone is long acting, has complex pharmacokinetics, and also interacts with NMDA and cardiac-risk considerations. Buprenorphine, a partial mu agonist with high receptor affinity, is often combined with naloxone for opioid use disorder treatment. Naltrexone blocks opioid receptors. Tramadol adds serotonergic and noradrenergic effects and has seizure-threshold considerations.

Opioids can produce sedation, analgesia, respiratory depression, sleep disruption, altered REM and slow-wave sleep, constipation, mood changes, and cognitive slowing. Withdrawal can produce the opposite direction clinically: agitation, insomnia, autonomic activation, pain sensitivity, anxiety, and restless sleep.

The QEEG question is therefore state-dependent. Is the client acutely dosed, stable on maintenance, in pain flare, tapering, intoxicated, withdrawing, recently postoperative, or combining opioids with benzodiazepines, alcohol, cannabis, gabapentinoids, or sleep medications?

14.3 Known spectral effects

Methadone-maintenance evidence supports qualitative theta and beta differences versus controls, without a defensible class-wide percentage magnitude. Wang and colleagues reported resting EEG changes in people receiving methadone treatment, supporting theta and beta directionality in that specific context (G. Y. Wang et al., 2015). The chapter does not quote an unsupported theta percentage.

Kerson's practitioner reference remains useful for class-level orientation across opioid and sedative effects, but it should be treated as a practice synthesis rather than a source for invented quantitative claims (Kerson, 2023).

Direct QEEG evidence for many outpatient opioid contexts is sparse. Acute postoperative opioids, chronic pain opioid therapy, buprenorphine maintenance, fentanyl patches, tramadol, naltrexone, and low-dose naltrexone all require gap-aware language unless a direct source is available. The clinician should not generalize methadone-maintenance findings to every opioid exposure.

Compound	Primary QEEG Vectors	Claim type	Interaction Modes	Confidence
Opioids	sedation slowing context, withdrawal hyperarousal	heuristic	exaggeration	substantially reduced

Figure 14.1: Opioid interpretation confidence: class-level QEEG vectors, claim type, and interaction modes.

Withdrawal is a distinct physiological state. It should not be treated as "off medication baseline." Opioid withdrawal can alter sleep, arousal, autonomic state, pain, and mood, making phenotype interpretation lower confidence.

14.4 Phenotype interaction effects

Opioids can mimic underarousal, diffuse slowing, drowsiness, poor vigilance, or cognitive-fog phenotypes. In chronic pain, the same features may also reflect pain, poor sleep, depression, fibromyalgia, OSA, gabapentinoids, cannabis, benzodiazepines, or inflammatory burden. The map is often composite.

Withdrawal can mimic hyperarousal, anxiety, insomnia, beta/artifact elevation, restlessness, and pain-related activation. It can also disrupt sleep enough to produce next-day slowing. This makes opioid withdrawal a transformation state, not a clean baseline.

Methadone and buprenorphine maintenance should be interpreted as stable treatment states when dose and timing are stable. The goal is not to remove the medication context. The goal is to understand the treated-state physiology under which neurofeedback will occur.

Tramadol needs special caution because it is both opioid-like and serotonergic/noradrenergic. It can interact with antidepressants and carries seizure-threshold concerns. A tramadol QEEG should not be interpreted as a simple opioid map.

14.5 Chronic Pain and Opioids

Chronic pain is not merely a reason for opioid exposure. Pain itself can shape attention, sleep, alpha rhythms, connectivity, mood, and arousal. A client with chronic back pain on oxycodone, pregabalin (Lyrica), duloxetine (Cymbalta), cannabis, and poor sleep is not a clean opioid case.

When pain is active during the recording, artifact, muscle tension, restlessness, fatigue, and state instability may all increase. If pain improves after surgery, injections, physical therapy, or medication changes, the QEEG may change because the pain state changed.

The report should name pain severity and timing. "Recorded during severe pain flare while taking hydrocodone and gabapentin (Neurontin)" is much more informative than "opioid exposure present."

14.6 Methadone and Buprenorphine

Methadone maintenance and buprenorphine treatment are common in opioid use disorder care. They should be treated respectfully as stabilizing treatments, not as merely confounds. A stable maintenance QEEG may be the clinically relevant state for neurofeedback.

Methadone has stronger QEEG evidence than many opioid contexts, but the claim remains qualitative. Buprenorphine evidence is thinner for routine resting QEEG, so the report should emphasize treatment stability, last dose, sleep, co-medications, withdrawal symptoms, and substance-use stability.

Dose timing matters. A trough state, missed dose, early induction, precipitated withdrawal, or recent relapse differs from stable maintenance. The report should label these states explicitly.

14.7 Antagonists and Low-Dose Naltrexone

Naltrexone and naloxone are not opioid agonists. Naltrexone may be used for opioid or alcohol use disorder, and low-dose naltrexone is used off-label in pain, autoimmune, and fatigue contexts. There is little direct resting-QEEG evidence for naltrexone or low-dose naltrexone.

The safest language is gap-aware: "No reliable resting-QEEG signature is established; interpretation should focus on indication, timing, symptoms, and comedications." For low-dose naltrexone in ME/CFS, fibromyalgia, or Long COVID contexts, the condition may be more QEEG-relevant than the medication evidence base.

14.8 Case vignette

Stable on buprenorphine/naloxone for opioid use disorder; pregabalin for neuropathic pain; chronic pain in the background; possible undiagnosed OSA; high daily caffeine to stay functional; sleeps poorly. That is the medication-and-state stack the client walks in with. The QEEG shows diffuse slowing, intermittent beta activity, and reduced alpha reactivity.

A simplistic report might call the slowing opioid-related and the beta anxiety-related. A better report treats the recording as a stable maintenance-state map shaped by pain, sleep, pregabalin, buprenorphine, caffeine, possible OSA, and mood. The beta may reflect caffeine, muscle tension, pain, or anxiety. The slowing may reflect sleep, pain, pregabalin, opioid state, or OSA.

The defensible report says: "Findings are interpreted under stable buprenorphine treatment with chronic pain, pregabalin exposure, poor sleep, and possible sleep-disordered breathing. Phenotype confidence is reduced for simple underarousal or hyperarousal labels." A client in opioid-use-disorder recovery is not a diagnostic puzzle to be solved by a map. The map is one frame of a person managing a chronic illness. Buprenorphine and naloxone should be treated respectfully as stabilizing treatments, not as confounds that make the QEEG less valid. The recording is valid. The interpretation has to carry more weight than usual.

14.9 Interpretation traps

- **Using rejected opioid citations.** Do not cite wrong-topic sources for opioid claims.
- **Quoting unsupported methadone magnitudes.** Use qualitative methadone directionality only.
- **Treating withdrawal as baseline.** Withdrawal is a distinct physiological state.
- **Ignoring respiratory sleep effects.** Opioids can worsen sleep-disordered breathing and daytime slowing.

- **Ignoring pain.** Chronic pain can shape QEEG independently of opioids.
- **Collapsing agonists and antagonists.** Methadone, buprenorphine, oxycodone, naltrexone, and naloxone are different contexts.

14.10 Intake questions

When opioid exposure appears on the intake form, ask:

- **Which opioid or antagonist, dose, route, and indication?** Pain, postoperative recovery, opioid use disorder, antagonist treatment, or off-label LDN.
- **When was the last dose and is dosing stable?** Trough, missed dose, induction, taper, or stable maintenance changes interpretation.
- **Any withdrawal, intoxication, craving, relapse, or recent overdose/naloxone history?** These are state variables and safety issues.
- **Any co-medications or substances?** Benzodiazepines, alcohol, cannabis, gabapentinoids, sleep medications, antidepressants, and caffeine are especially relevant.
- **How are pain, sleep, breathing, and daytime alertness?** OSA risk and pain flare can dominate the map.

14.11 Clinical recommendations

Interpret opioid QEEGs by exposure state: acute analgesia, chronic pain therapy, methadone maintenance, buprenorphine maintenance, antagonist treatment, postoperative recovery, taper, or withdrawal. Do not use one opioid signature for all contexts.

Use methadone QEEG evidence qualitatively. Label withdrawal and missed-dose recordings as transition states.

Do not recommend holding opioids, methadone, buprenorphine, naltrexone, or other analgesics for QEEG clarity. Do not use QEEG to justify discontinuation, dose changes, or substitution. Coordinate with the prescriber or treatment program when safety, withdrawal, or overdose concerns arise.

14.12 Acute, Chronic, and Trough States

Acute opioid exposure is not the same as stable chronic exposure. A client recorded after taking hydrocodone for a dental procedure may show sedation, pain relief, nausea, or sleepiness. A client on stable buprenorphine may show a treated maintenance state. A client nearing methadone trough may show emerging withdrawal, anxiety, pain, or autonomic arousal.

Last-dose timing is therefore mandatory. For short-acting opioids, same-day timing may matter. For long-acting opioids and maintenance medications, trough versus peak and missed-dose history matter. For transdermal fentanyl, patch timing, dose changes, fever, and heat exposure can matter clinically.

The QEEG report should not infer exposure from the medication list alone. A prescribed medication may not have been taken, an unreported medication may be present, or the recording may occur during withdrawal. Intake should ask directly and nonjudgmentally.

14.13 Respiratory and Sleep Effects

Opioids can affect respiration and sleep architecture. They may worsen sleep-disordered breathing or contribute to daytime sleepiness, especially when combined with benzodiazepines, alcohol, gabapentinoids, sedating antidepressants, or OSA risk. A slow QEEG in an opioid-treated client may be a sleep-breathing signal as much as a direct drug signal.

The clinician should ask about snoring, witnessed apneas, morning headaches, oxygen issues, CPAP use, sleep quality, and daytime sleepiness. If opioid and sedative stacking is present, respiratory safety belongs in the clinical context. QEEG cannot diagnose sleep apnea, but it can identify when sleep and respiration may be major confounders.

14.14 Codeine and CYP2D6 Prodrug Activation

Codeine is a CYP2D6-dependent prodrug: it requires CYP2D6-mediated O-demethylation to morphine for analgesic effect. CYP2D6 status is therefore clinically decisive here. Ultrarapid metabolizers convert codeine to morphine rapidly and at higher levels, with documented cases of respiratory depression, toxicity, and fatalities. The FDA added a boxed warning and a contraindication in children under 12. Poor metabolizers produce inadequate morphine and may experience minimal analgesia with preserved non-opioid side effects.

For QEEG interpretation, the implication is straightforward: two clients taking the same codeine dose can have dramatically different opioid brain exposure depending on CYP2D6 status. An ultrarapid metabolizer may show a more sedated, opioid-shaped recording than expected from the nominal dose. A poor metabolizer may show minimal opioid spectral contribution despite being "on an opioid." When a codeine-treated client's QEEG does not match the expected opioid picture, CYP2D6 status is a plausible explanation worth documenting.

14.15 Tramadol, CYP2D6, and Serotonergic Integration

Tramadol is often casually grouped with opioids, but it has a mixed mechanism that creates two distinct pharmacogenomic and interaction concerns. First, tramadol is a CYP2D6-dependent prodrug for its opioid activity: CYP2D6 converts tramadol to O-desmethyltramadol (M1), the metabolite responsible for mu-opioid receptor activation. Poor metabolizers produce less M1, leading to inadequate opioid analgesia, while ultrarapid metabolizers face higher opioid exposure and toxicity risk. CPIC provides genotype-based dosing recommendations.

Second, the parent tramadol compound retains serotonin and norepinephrine reuptake inhibition regardless of CYP2D6 status. This means a CYP2D6 poor metabolizer on tramadol gets less opioid effect but retains the full serotonergic load, creating a pharmacologic profile closer to an SNRI than to a traditional opioid. The serotonergic activity carries serotonin-syndrome risk when combined with SSRIs, SNRIs, MAOIs, triptans, or other serotonergic agents. Tramadol also lowers seizure threshold.

For QEEG interpretation, the critical point is that tramadol exposure cannot be treated as a simple opioid. The spectral picture may reflect opioid sedation, serotonergic modulation, noradrenergic effects, or all three, depending on CYP2D6 status and co-medications. A client on tramadol plus an SSRI presents a complex interpretive problem: the SSRI may also inhibit CYP2D6 (especially paroxetine (Paxil) and fluoxetine (Prozac)), further reducing opioid conversion while amplifying serotonergic burden. Document tramadol exposure, known CYP2D6 status, serotonergic co-medications, seizure-threshold context, and whether the client reports adequate analgesia.

14.16 Kratom and Grey-Zone Opioid Exposures

Kratom is not a prescription opioid, but it has opioid-receptor activity and appears in real-world intake. No high-quality chronic-user QEEG evidence has been identified. Withdrawal, dependence, stimulant-like reports at low doses, sedating reports at higher doses, and polysubstance context make interpretation difficult.

The QEEG clinician should ask about kratom specifically because clients may not list it as a medication. Document product, dose, timing, pattern, withdrawal symptoms, and other substances. Do not invent a kratom QEEG signature.

14.17 Xylazine Contamination

Xylazine is a veterinary alpha-2 adrenergic agonist increasingly found as an adulterant in illicit fentanyl and heroin, with high prevalence in the eastern United States. DEA estimates that xylazine was present in approximately 23% of fentanyl powder and 7% of fentanyl pills seized in 2022. It is not an opioid; naloxone does not reverse its effects. Clinically, xylazine produces profound sedation, bradycardia, hypotension, and respiratory depression that compound opioid effects and complicate overdose management. Because xylazine is almost always found with fentanyl or heroin, naloxone is still indicated in any suspected overdose to reverse the opioid component. Persistent sedation, bradycardia, and hypotension after naloxone are expected when xylazine is involved and do not mean naloxone has failed or should be withheld; call emergency services, support the airway, and continue monitoring.

No human resting-state EEG data exist for xylazine. Its mechanism (alpha-2 agonism) predicts EEG effects similar to clonidine or dexmedetomidine: increased slow-frequency power, reduced higher-frequency activity, and sedation-driven vigilance collapse. In combination with fentanyl, the expected spectral picture is additive or combined sedation.

The QEEG clinician cannot detect xylazine from the map, but should be aware that clients with illicit opioid exposure may be experiencing xylazine effects that amplify sedation beyond what opioid exposure alone would predict. If a client in opioid treatment shows unexpectedly deep slowing or fails to respond to naloxone, xylazine co-exposure is a possibility worth documenting. Incomplete naloxone response does not mean naloxone should be stopped. Suspected overdose in an adulterated supply still receives naloxone because an opioid component is usually present. Activate emergency services and support ventilation; the map is irrelevant until the client is stable.

14.18 Report Language Examples

Weak language: "The opioid caused theta."

Better language: "Theta/slowing findings are interpreted under opioid exposure, chronic pain, poor sleep, and possible sleep-disordered breathing. Current evidence does not support assigning a precise opioid-specific magnitude."

Weak language: "The client is off opioids, so this is baseline."

Better language: "The recording occurred during opioid taper/withdrawal and should be interpreted as a transition-state QEEG, not an unmedicated baseline."

Weak language: "Methadone produces a fixed theta increase."

Better language: "Methadone-maintenance evidence supports qualitative theta and beta differences in that population; individual interpretation should consider dose stability, last dose, withdrawal symptoms, and co-medications."

Weak language: "Buprenorphine invalidates the QEEG."

Better language: "Stable buprenorphine treatment is the client's current clinical state; the QEEG can guide neurofeedback under that treated-state condition with appropriate caveats."

14.19 Practical Confidence Levels

High confidence is possible when opioid exposure is stable, pain is stable, sleep is documented, and no withdrawal or intoxication is present. Moderate confidence applies when pain, sleep, or sedative co-medications are active but documented; phenotype labels should carry explicit caveats. Low confidence applies during intoxication, withdrawal, taper, missed doses, relapse, recent overdose, acute post-operative recovery, uncontrolled pain flare, heavy sedative stacking, or severe sleep disruption; durable phenotype assignment should wait.

14.20 What Not to Claim

Five specific overclaims apply to this drug class:

- Do not cite wrong-topic sources for opioid claims.
- Do not quote unsupported methadone percentages.
- Do not treat withdrawal as a clean baseline.
- Do not treat buprenorphine maintenance as invalidating a recording by default.
- Do not collapse agonists, partial agonists, antagonists, tramadol, and kratom into one spectral signature.

14.21 Documentation Standard

The minimum documentation standard is opioid or antagonist name, dose, route, indication, last dose, dose stability, withdrawal or intoxication symptoms, pain severity, sleep quality, respiratory risk, and co-medications. For maintenance treatment, record clinic stability, missed doses, recent induction, or tapering when known.

For repeat QEEGs, keep this documentation consistent. A baseline recorded during stable buprenorphine treatment and a follow-up recorded during taper are not directly comparable without the medication-state note. The same applies to pain flares, postoperative opioid use, or new gabapentinoid / benzodiazepine exposure. The chapter's stance is practical: opioids can matter, but the opioid label alone is never enough. The recording must be tied to state.

Safety notice. Opioid withdrawal can be severe and, in the context of xylazine-adulterated supply, is a medical emergency. Opioid discontinuation and taper require physician management. Clients who have recently reduced or stopped opioids are at elevated overdose risk on resumption because tolerance drops rapidly. Nothing in this chapter is a tapering protocol or a substitution recommendation. If a client reports opioid withdrawal symptoms or recent naloxone use, document and coordinate with their medical provider before proceeding with a non-emergency QEEG.

14.22 Evidence summary

- **Spectral effect:** Methadone-maintenance data support qualitative theta and beta differences in that population; evidence is sparse for many other opioid contexts.
- **Phenotype inference:** Opioids, pain, sleep-disordered breathing, gabapentinoids, benzodiazepines, and withdrawal can reduce confidence in slowing, vigilance, beta / arousal, and underarousal interpretations.
- **Workflow heuristic:** Document opioid type, indication, stability, last dose, withdrawal / intoxication state, pain severity, sleep / respiration, and co-medications before assigning phenotype meaning.

Ch 15: Z-drugs and Non-Benzo Sleep Medications

15.1 Why this class matters in NFB practice

Sleep medications are common in neurofeedback referrals because insomnia, trauma, anxiety, depression, chronic pain, ADHD, menopause, shift work, and medication side effects often disrupt sleep. A client may use zolpidem (Ambien), eszopiclone (Lunesta), zaleplon (Sonata), trazodone (Desyrel), low-dose doxepin, hydroxyzine, diphenhydramine, melatonin, ramelteon (Rozerem), suvorexant (Belsomra), lemborexant (Dayvigo), daridorexant (Quviviq), clonidine, cannabis, or several of these together.

Strongest evidence	Zolpidem and trazodone have sleep-EEG evidence, but waking resting-QEEG claims are much more limited; melatonin is mainly sleep / circadian evidence.
Biggest interpretation trap	Converting sleep EEG into waking claims: Sleep-stage effects are not automatically daytime resting-QEEG effects.
Default clinical action	Document last-night medications, sleep duration, sleep quality, OSA risk, next-day sedation, and recent medication changes before assigning a phenotype.

This chapter's central distinction is sleep EEG versus waking QEEG. A drug can change sleep architecture without having a strong next-day waking resting-QEEG signature. A drug can also leave morning sedation, drowsiness, poor reactivity, or rebound insomnia. The report must not convert nighttime sleep-stage effects into unsupported daytime phenotype claims.

The practical question is not "does this drug affect the EEG?" The better question is "what state was the client in during the recording?" A well-rested client after effective sleep treatment may look clearer than an untreated insomniac. A hungover or withdrawn hypnotic user may look slower or more unstable.

15.2 Mechanism (clinician-level pharmacology)

Z-drugs such as zolpidem, zaleplon, and eszopiclone act at benzodiazepine-site GABA-A receptors with preferential affinity for the $\alpha1$ subunit, which mediates sedation. Classical benzodiazepines, by contrast, bind non-selectively across $\alpha1$, $\alpha2$, $\alpha3$, and $\alpha5$ subtypes. This $\alpha1$ selectivity is the central pharmacological distinction: it produces hypnotic effects with less anxiolytic, anticonvulsant, and muscle-relaxant action. Half-lives differ across the class (zaleplon ~1 hour, zolpidem ~2.5 hours, eszopiclone ~6 hours), shaping next-day carryover risk. They are hypnotics, not daytime anxiolytics, though real-world use can drift.

Trazodone is an antidepressant often used at low doses for sleep, with serotonergic, antihistaminergic, and adrenergic effects. Low-dose doxepin is a histamine H1 antagonist at sleep doses. Diphenhydramine and hydroxyzine (both used off-label for sleep) are first-generation antihistamines with anticholinergic or sedating properties. Melatonin and ramelteon target melatonin signaling. Orexin antagonists reduce wake-promoting signaling.

These mechanisms differ, so "sleep medication" is not one EEG class. They share the clinical problem of recording-state contamination: next-day drowsiness, sleep debt, rebound insomnia, sleep architecture change, and untreated OSA can all shape the map.

15.3 Known spectral effects

Dijk and Czeisler's zolpidem work supports the important boundary condition that typical zolpidem sleep effects may be largely confined to the sleep period, with minimal next-day waking effects at the studied dose (Brunner et al., 1991). This does not mean every zolpidem user is next-day unaffected. It means the chapter should avoid assuming a strong waking-QEEG signature from sleep-use alone.

Saletu's trazodone work is primarily sleep EEG, not strong waking resting-QEEG evidence (Bemmel et al., 1992). Trazodone should therefore be described as sleep-relevant and potentially next-day-sedating in practice, while direct waking-QEEG claims remain limited.

Melatonin has cleaner sleep-onset and circadian relevance than many OTC sleep aids. Dijk and colleagues support melatonin-related sleep EEG context, reporting suppressed EEG low-frequency activity and enhanced spindle-frequency activity during daytime sleep (Dijk et al., 1995). The QEEG relevance is often timing, circadian alignment, and whether the client slept well, not a strong waking spectral fingerprint.

Orexin antagonists, ramelteon, low-dose doxepin, antihistamines, and adolescent sleep-medication use all need gap-aware language for waking resting QEEG unless direct evidence is present. Sleep EEG and medication mechanism can guide questions, but not precise QEEG band claims.

15.4 Phenotype interaction effects

Sleep medications can mimic underarousal, diffuse slowing, drowsiness, poor alpha reactivity, and reduced vigilance if the client is recorded during next-day sedation or inadequate sleep. They can also mask sleep-deprivation signatures by improving sleep.

Rebound insomnia and withdrawal can transform interpretation. A client who stopped zolpidem or trazodone abruptly and slept poorly before the QEEG is not in a clean baseline state. The map may reflect sleep debt, withdrawal arousal, anxiety, and poor recovery sleep.

Untreated OSA is a major confound. A client taking melatonin or trazodone who still has fragmented breathing may show severe slowing that is OSA-driven rather than medication-driven. The medication history and sleep history must be read together.

Antihistamines and anticholinergic burden can exaggerate cognitive fog and slowing, especially in older adults. Diphenhydramine used nightly should not be treated as a harmless supplement.

15.5 Compound-Specific Notes

Zolpidem, zaleplon, and eszopiclone should be interpreted through last dose, sleep duration, morning sedation, complex sleep behaviors, and withdrawal/rebound insomnia. Zaleplon has a shorter duration; eszopiclone may have more next-day concerns in some clients.

Trazodone should be treated as sleep-use antidepressant exposure with limited waking-QEEG evidence. Dose, morning grogginess, orthostasis, and co-medications matter.

Melatonin and ramelteon are primarily circadian/sleep-onset agents. The key questions are timing, dose, delayed sleep phase, adolescent use, and whether sleep improved.

Orexin antagonists may be clinically important but have limited direct waking-QEEG evidence for neurofeedback interpretation. Document dose, timing, next-day somnolence, nightmares, and sleep quality.

Antihistamines such as diphenhydramine and hydroxyzine can create sedation and anticholinergic burden. They are common because they are OTC or PRN, and clients may forget to list them.

15.6 Case vignette

A client with trauma-related insomnia takes trazodone most nights, diphenhydramine when sleep is severe, and melatonin irregularly. She schedules QEEG after four hours of sleep because she stopped trazodone the night before to "get a clean baseline." The map shows frontal theta, diffuse slowing, poor alpha reactivity, and intermittent beta from tension.

A simplistic report might call the slowing underarousal and the beta hyperarousal. A better report calls this a sleep-disrupted withdrawal/rebound state. The client is not medication-free in a useful sense. She is sleep deprived after changing a sleep medication pattern.

The defensible interpretation says: "QEEG was recorded after acute disruption of the client's usual sleep-medication pattern and short sleep. Findings are current-state features with reduced confidence for stable phenotype assignment."

15.7 Interpretation traps

- **Converting sleep EEG into waking claims.** Sleep-stage effects are not automatically daytime resting-QEEG effects.

- **Calling a skipped hypnotic night a baseline.** Rebound insomnia and sleep debt contaminate the map.
- **Ignoring OTC sleep aids.** Diphenhydramine, doxylamine, hydroxyzine, melatonin, and cannabis are often omitted.
- **Missing OSA.** Sleep medications can coexist with untreated sleep-disordered breathing.
- **Treating sleep improvement as drug artifact.** Better sleep can normalize a map.
- **Ignoring older-adult anticholinergic risk.** OTC antihistamines can be clinically meaningful.

15.8 Intake questions

When sleep medication appears on the intake form, ask:

- **What did you take last night and when?** Include prescriptions, OTC antihistamines, melatonin, cannabis, alcohol, and supplements.
- **How many hours did you sleep, and how rested are you now?** Current vigilance drives interpretation.
- **Did you skip, taper, or change a usual sleep medication?** Rebound insomnia is not baseline.
- **Any snoring, witnessed apneas, CPAP, morning headache, or daytime sleepiness?** Screen for OSA confounding.
- **Any next-day grogginess, memory gaps, or complex sleep behaviors?** These alter clinical confidence.

15.9 Clinical recommendations

Do not ask clients to stop sleep medication for QEEG clarity unless the prescriber has already directed that change. A skipped hypnotic may create a worse recording by producing rebound insomnia and sleep deprivation.

Record the client's usual sleep-medication state when the goal is neurofeedback planning under ordinary conditions. If the client is changing sleep medication, label the QEEG as a transition-state recording.

Separate sleep EEG evidence from waking-QEEG evidence. Use qualitative next-day sedation language when direct waking-QEEG data are thin.

15.10 Timing, Half-Life, and Morning State

Sleep medication timing matters because the QEEG is usually recorded during the day. A medication taken at 9 p.m. with eight hours of sleep is not the same state as a medication taken at 2 a.m. with four hours of sleep. A short-acting hypnotic may be mostly gone by morning, while sleep debt, rebound anxiety, or grogginess may remain.

The report should document time to bed, time of dose, time awake, total sleep time, awakenings, morning grogginess, caffeine rescue, and current alertness. This can be more useful than the medication name alone.

For clients who use PRN sleep medication, the QEEG date may not reflect their usual state. A map after a medicated night and a map after an unmedicated sleepless night can differ for reasons that have little to do with stable phenotype.

15.11 Withdrawal and Rebound

Withdrawal and rebound insomnia are distinct states. Stopping Z-drugs, trazodone, antihistamines, alcohol, cannabis, benzodiazepines, or melatonin routines can alter sleep and arousal. The client may believe the recording is "clean" because no pill was taken the night before. In reality, the recording may be dominated by acute sleep loss and autonomic arousal.

The QEEG clinician should ask whether the previous night was typical. If not, document why. If the QEEG is intended for stable phenotype selection, a typical sleep night is often more useful than an artificially medication-free night.

15.12 Adolescents and Emerging Adults

Melatonin, trazodone, hydroxyzine, clonidine, cannabis, and quetiapine (Seroquel) are common in adolescent sleep contexts. Adolescents also have developmental EEG features, delayed sleep phase, school-related sleep restriction, caffeine/energy drink use, ADHD medication, and anxiety. A slow or theta-heavy recording may reflect maturation, sleep debt, medication, circadian phase, or all of these.

The chapter does not treat adolescent sleep medication as adult sleep medication in smaller bodies. It calls for developmental context and documentation. If a teenager slept five hours after late-night screen use and melatonin, the QEEG should not be interpreted as a stable trait map without caveats.

15.13 Older Adults

Older adults are more vulnerable to anticholinergic burden, falls, cognitive side effects, residual sedation, OSA, pain, and polypharmacy. Diphenhydramine, doxylamine, hydroxyzine, low-dose doxepin, trazodone, benzodiazepines, alcohol, opioids, and gabapentinoids can stack.

In an older adult, slowing may reflect age, medication, sleep-disordered breathing, neurodegenerative vulnerability, pain, depression, or anticholinergic exposure. The QEEG should not reduce this to "sleep aid effect." OTC medications should be listed explicitly because clients may not consider them medications.

15.14 OSA and Sleep-Disordered Breathing

Sleep medications can worsen or obscure untreated sleep-disordered breathing in some clients, while insomnia treatment may improve sleep continuity in others. The QEEG cannot diagnose OSA, but waking slowing, fatigue, poor alpha reactivity, and drowsiness during the recording should prompt screening questions.

If the client uses CPAP, ask whether it was used the previous night and whether the mask fit, leak, or residual events were problematic. If CPAP was skipped, the QEEG should be labeled accordingly.

15.15 Report Language Examples

Weak language: "Melatonin caused the slowing."

Better language: "Slowing is present after short sleep with melatonin use and possible OSA symptoms. Medication, sleep duration, circadian timing, and sleep-disordered breathing all reduce confidence in a single-cause interpretation."

Weak language: "The client skipped zolpidem, so the recording is clean."

Better language: "The recording occurred after an atypical unmedicated night with reduced sleep; rebound insomnia and sleep debt reduce confidence in trait interpretation."

Weak language: "Trazodone has a waking QEEG signature."

Better language: "Trazodone has sleep-EEG evidence and clinical next-day sedation relevance, but strong waking resting-QEEG claims are limited."

Weak language: "OTC sleep aids do not matter."

Better language: "Nightly diphenhydramine or doxylamine can add sedation and anticholinergic burden, especially in older adults, and should be documented."

15.16 Practical Confidence Levels

High-confidence interpretation is possible when the client's sleep medication routine is stable, the previous night was typical, sleep duration is adequate, no rebound or withdrawal is present, and daytime alertness is stable.

Moderate confidence applies when sleep was mildly poor, the medication was used PRN, or next-day grogginess is present but documented. The map can still guide current-state training.

Low confidence applies after acute insomnia, skipped usual medication, rebound symptoms, intoxication, sedative stacking, untreated severe OSA symptoms, complex sleep behaviors, or major schedule disruption. In these cases, stable phenotype labels should usually wait.

15.17 What Not to Claim

Do not convert sleep-stage effects into waking resting-QEEG claims. Do not call a rebound insomnia night baseline. Do not ignore OTC antihistamines, cannabis, alcohol, or melatonin. Do not assign slowing to a sleep medication when untreated OSA or sleep deprivation is plausible.

15.18 Documentation Standard

The minimum documentation standard is sleep medication name, dose, timing, whether it was usual or atypical, total sleep time, sleep quality, awakenings, morning grogginess, caffeine rescue, alcohol/cannabis use, and OSA symptoms. For PRN medications, record how often the client uses them and whether the QEEG night matched the usual pattern.

For repeat QEEGs, use the same sleep questions each time. A baseline after an unmedicated sleepless night and a follow-up after a well-slept medicated night are not comparable without sleep-state notes. The same is true when CPAP adherence, bedtime, melatonin timing, or antihistamine use changes.

This chapter's practical stance is simple: sleep medications matter, but the previous night's sleep often matters more. The report should make both visible.

15.19 Multiple Sleep Aids

Clients often combine sleep aids without thinking of the combination as polypharmacy: melatonin plus diphenhydramine, trazodone plus cannabis, hydroxyzine plus alcohol, or a prescribed hypnotic plus an OTC antihistamine. The QEEG clinician should ask about combinations directly. Combination use can create next-day grogginess, unstable vigilance, and difficulty separating medication effects from sleep debt. It can also hide untreated insomnia when OSA, pain, nightmares, circadian delay, or restless legs remains unaddressed. The report should use stack language: "recorded after trazodone plus melatonin plus four hours of fragmented sleep" is more useful than "sleep medication present."

15.20 Evidence summary

- **Spectral effect:** Zolpidem and trazodone have sleep-EEG evidence, but waking resting-QEEG claims are much more limited; melatonin is mainly sleep/circadian relevant.
- **Phenotype inference:** Sleep medications, untreated insomnia, OSA, next-day sedation, and rebound insomnia can reduce confidence in slowing, theta, alpha-reactivity, and vigilance interpretations.
- **Workflow heuristic:** Document last-night medications, sleep duration, sleep quality, OSA risk, next-day sedation, and recent medication changes before assigning phenotype meaning.

Ch 16: OTC and Non-Psychotropic Medications

16.1 Why this class matters in NFB practice

OTC and non-psychotropic medications matter because clients often omit them. They may list antidepressants and stimulants but forget diphenhydramine, doxylamine, hydroxyzine, pseudoephedrine, cold medicine, PPIs, statins, beta-blockers, GLP-1 agonists, SGLT-2 inhibitors, PDE-5 inhibitors, steroids, antibiotics, or inhalers. Some of these are likely EEG-relevant. Many are pure gaps. Both facts matter.

Strongest evidence	Sedating first-generation antihistamines can produce drowsiness and slowing-like effects. Most other non-psychotropic categories have little direct resting-QEEG evidence.
Biggest interpretation trap	Ignoring OTC sleep aids. Diphenhydramine and doxylamine are common confounders that clients rarely report as "medications."
Default clinical action	Document all OTC, cold, allergy, sleep, and chronic non-psychotropic medications, and label pure-gap categories rather than inventing signatures.

This chapter is a triage chapter, not a catalog of every medication: which "non-psych" exposures should change QEEG confidence, which should be documented as gap categories, and which matter mainly through toxicity, deficiency, sleep, infection, hypoglycemia, or medical condition.

The biggest practical lesson is that OTC does not mean EEG-neutral. First-generation antihistamines can be sedating and anticholinergic.

Decongestants can be activating. Some antibiotics or medical toxicities can produce encephalopathic slowing. Do not invent QEEG signatures for statins, PPIs, or other chronic meds without direct evidence.

16.2 OTC Mechanism Families

Five mechanism families produce real (or possible) QEEG effects in OTC and non-psychotropic agents. Use these families to sort any OTC report quickly:

Family 1: Anticholinergic / sedating antihistaminergic. Diphenhydramine, doxylamine, hydroxyzine, promethazine (Phenergan), first-generation allergy and PM-pain products. Cross the blood-brain barrier; produce sedation, anticholinergic cognitive effects, drowsiness, and reduced alpha reactivity. Paradoxical excitation has been described in a small case series of CYP2D6 ultrarapid metabolizers. These are the OTC agents most likely to change the QEEG picture and least likely to be reported on intake forms (clients do not think of "Benadryl" as a medication).

Family 2: Sympathomimetic. Pseudoephedrine, phenylephrine. Increase arousal, anxiety, heart rate, and sleep disruption. May contribute to activation beta or fast-activity states.

Family 3: NSAID / acetaminophen / non-EEG direct. Most analgesics, PPIs, statins, GLP-1 agonists, SGLT-2 inhibitors, and PDE-5 inhibitors have little to no direct resting-QEEG evidence. Do not invent signatures. Document when present because metabolic, sleep, and medical contexts can create indirect effects (e.g., GLP-1 agents changing sleep; statins affecting rare patients with CNS side effects).

Family 4: Medical toxicity / encephalopathic context. Any medication, supplement, or medical state producing toxicity, infection, metabolic disruption, hypoglycemia, or acute illness can produce nonspecific EEG changes including diffuse slowing, focal changes, or paroxysmal activity. Theophylline, antibiotics with CNS penetration, and immune-mediated encephalopathy belong here.

Family 5: Dissociative. Dextromethorphan at high doses. It behaves as an NMDA-antagonist dissociative with sigma-1, serotonergic, and noradrenergic actions rather than as a decongestant-style sympathomimetic, so expect a dissociative picture, though tachycardia and agitation are common. Chapter 7 covers the same molecule in its Auvelity context.

16.3 Mechanism (clinician-level pharmacology)

First-generation antihistamines such as diphenhydramine and doxylamine cross the blood-brain barrier and can produce sedation, anticholinergic effects, cognitive fog, paradoxical excitation, and next-day impairment. Hydroxyzine is also sedating. Second-generation antihistamines such as loratadine, fexofenadine, and cetirizine are generally less sedating at therapeutic doses, though individual responses vary. The paradoxical-response literature for diphenhydramine includes CYP2D6 ultrarapid metabolism context (Leon & Nikoloff, 2008).

Steroids can affect mood and sleep, especially at high doses. Some antimicrobials can lower seizure threshold or contribute to encephalopathy in vulnerable medical contexts. Theophylline is stimulant-like. Insulin and sulfonylureas matter through hypoglycemia, not a direct EEG drug signature.

16.4 Known spectral effects

First-generation antihistamines have the most practical QEEG relevance in this chapter. The available evidence supports qualitative drowsiness/slowing and reduced reactivity framing for sedating antihistamines, without precise magnitudes. Diphenhydramine also has paradoxical-response literature, including CYP2D6 ultrarapid metabolism context (Leon & Nikoloff, 2008).

Second-generation antihistamines usually have minimal EEG impact at therapeutic doses. Individual clients can still be affected, but they should not be treated like diphenhydramine by default.

Statins, PPIs, GLP-1 agonists, SGLT-2 inhibitors, PDE-5 inhibitors, beta-blockers, naltrexone (Vivitrol)/LDN, and many routine non-psychotropic medications lack reliable human resting-QEEG signatures in the available literature. The correct clinical stance is gap labeling, not speculation.

Antimicrobials are mostly irrelevant to routine outpatient QEEG unless toxicity or encephalopathy is present. Cefepime, high-dose penicillins, fluoroquinolones, severe infection, renal impairment, and ICU

Compound	Primary QEEG Vectors	Claim type	Interaction Modes	Confidence
First-generation antihistamines	sedation slowing context, anticholinergic burden	heuristic	exaggeration, transformation	substantially reduced
Second-generation antihistamines	minimal expected effect	heuristic	n/a	n/a
OTC decongestants and cold medicines	activation sleep disruption context	heuristic	n/a	n/a

Figure 16.1: OTC/non-psychotropic triage: agents by QEEG vectors, claim type, and interaction modes.

states belong in medical red-flag territory, not ordinary phenotype interpretation.

16.5 Phenotype interaction effects

Sedating antihistamines can mimic drowsiness, underarousal, diffuse slowing, frontal theta, reduced alpha reactivity, and cognitive fog. Anticholinergic burden can exaggerate age-related or medication-related cognitive concerns, especially in older adults.

Paradoxical excitation can transform interpretation. A child, developmental-variant client, or CYP2D6 ultrarapid metabolizer may respond to diphenhydramine with activation rather than sedation. The QEEG cannot diagnose the mechanism, but the history should flag paradoxical response.

Decongestants can mimic activation, anxiety, tremor, insomnia, or beta/artifact findings. They can also worsen sleep, creating next-day slowing.

Gap-category drugs can mislead if the clinician invents effects. A statin or PPI should not be blamed for a QEEG pattern without evidence. However, B12 deficiency, hypoglycemia, infection, steroid psychosis, or drug toxicity can be relevant through indirect pathways.

16.6 Category Notes

First-generation antihistamines include diphenhydramine and doxylamine. Ask about sleep use, allergy use, cold medicine, PM pain medications, and paradoxical reactions.

Second-generation antihistamines include loratadine, fexofenadine, and cetirizine. Treat as usually minimal but document sedation if reported.

Decongestants and cold medicines often combine multiple ingredients. Pseudoephedrine, phenylephrine, dextromethorphan, antihistamines, acetaminophen, alcohol-containing syrups, and caffeine-like ingredients may appear together.

Statins, PPIs, GLP-1 agonists, SGLT-2 inhibitors, PDE-5 inhibitors, and beta-blockers are gap-labeled for routine resting QEEG. Do not invent signatures. Document them because medical context and indirect pathways may matter.

Steroids and antimicrobials matter mainly when mood, sleep, psychosis, seizure threshold, encephalopathy, infection, renal impairment, or toxicity are present.

16.7 Case vignette

A client with insomnia and allergies arrives for QEEG after taking diphenhydramine for sleep and pseudoephedrine for congestion the night before. She slept poorly, feels foggy, and had an extra coffee. The QEEG shows diffuse slowing, intermittent beta, and weak alpha reactivity.

A simplistic report might call the slowing underarousal and the beta anxiety. A better report identifies a mixed OTC state: sedating antihistamine, activating decongestant, poor sleep, caffeine compensation, and illness / allergy context.

The defensible report says: "QEEG was recorded after sedating and sympathomimetic OTC medication exposure with poor sleep and caffeine compensation; phenotype confidence is reduced for stable underarousal or hyperarousal labels."

16.8 Interpretation traps

- **Ignoring OTC sleep aids.** Diphenhydramine and doxylamine are common confounders.
- **Inventing statin or PPI signatures.** These are gap categories for routine resting QEEG.
- **Missing combination cold medicines.** Multiple active ingredients may be present.

- **Treating second-generation antihistamines like diphenhydramine.** Sedation risk differs.
- **Ignoring paradoxical reactions.** Antihistamines can activate some clients.
- **Missing medical toxicity.** Encephalopathy, hypoglycemia, infection, and renal impairment change the problem.

16.9 Intake questions

When OTC or non-psychotropic medications appear on the intake form, ask:

- **Any allergy, sleep, cold, pain, or PM medications in the last 48 hours?** Ask specifically about diphenhydramine, doxylamine, hydroxyzine, pseudoephedrine, dextromethorphan.
- **Any paradoxical reactions to antihistamines?** Activation, agitation, insomnia, or "Benadryl makes me wired."
- **Any chronic non-psychotropic prescriptions?** Statins, PPIs, beta-blockers, GLP-1 agonists, SGLT-2 inhibitors, PDE-5 inhibitors, steroids, antibiotics.
- **Any current infection, fever, steroid burst, hypoglycemia, or medication toxicity concern?** These may dominate the map.
- **Any OTC combination products?** Clients may not know every ingredient.

16.10 Clinical recommendations

Document OTC and non-psychotropic medications explicitly. Do not assume they are irrelevant because they are common or non-psychiatric.

Use qualitative caution for first-generation antihistamines and decongestants. Use gap labels for statins, PPIs, GLP-1 agonists, SGLT-2 inhibitors, PDE-5 inhibitors, beta-blockers, and LDN/naltrexone when no direct resting-QEEG evidence exists.

If encephalopathy, hypoglycemia, infection, steroid psychosis, seizure-risk, or medication toxicity is plausible, medical evaluation takes priority over phenotype interpretation.

16.11 Indirect Pathways

Non-psychotropic medications often matter indirectly. PPIs may matter through B12 deficiency in long-term use, not through a direct PPI rhythm. Diabetes medications may matter through hypoglycemia, not a direct drug signature. Beta-blockers may matter through fatigue, sleep, or exercise tolerance. GLP-1 agonists may matter through weight loss, nausea, appetite change, sleep apnea improvement, or metabolic change rather than direct resting EEG.

Statins may matter if a client reports muscle pain, sleep change, or cognitive complaints, but the QEEG should not assign a statin signature. PDE-5 inhibitors may matter through vascular, sleep, headache, or timing context, not a known resting-QEEG pattern.

This indirect-pathway framing keeps the chapter clinically useful without overstating evidence.

16.12 GLP-1 Receptor Agonists (Semaglutide, Tirzepatide)

Semaglutide (Ozempic, Wegovy) and tirzepatide (Mounjaro, Zepbound) are now among the most commonly prescribed medications in adults with obesity and type 2 diabetes, and many neurofeedback referrals will be taking one.

Mechanism. GLP-1 agonists work primarily through incretin-mediated glucose regulation, appetite suppression via hypothalamic and brainstem satiety circuits, and delayed gastric emptying. Tirzepatide adds GIP receptor agonism. CNS effects are plausible because GLP-1 receptors are expressed in hypothalamus, brainstem, hippocampus, and cortex, and emerging trials are investigating semaglutide for alcohol use disorder, binge eating, and substance-related cravings.

Known spectral effects. No published resting-state QEEG study of GLP-1 agonists exists. There is no validated spectral signature and no mechanistic reason to expect a large direct cortical effect at therapeutic doses. The indirect pathways that could matter for QEEG are weight loss (which can improve OSA, metabolic health, and daytime alertness), nausea and GI distress (which can worsen recording state), appetite suppression (which can change caffeine patterns and energy), and improved mood or energy as a secondary consequence of weight loss. None of these constitute a GLP-1 QEEG signature.

Interaction with psychiatric medications. GLP-1 agonists delay gastric emptying, which can theoretically alter absorption kinetics of co-prescribed oral medications. This is a prescriber concern, not a QEEG concern, but the clinician should be aware that a client who recently started semaglutide may be experiencing nausea, caloric restriction, changed caffeine intake, sleep changes, or medication absorption shifts that could show up in the recording.

This is a pure gap category: workflow heuristic only, no spectral claims. Document GLP-1 agonist exposure, recent start or dose escalation, nausea, weight loss, changed eating or caffeine patterns, and any relevant mood or energy changes. Do not invent a GLP-1 QEEG signature.

16.13 Anticholinergic Burden

Anticholinergic burden is especially relevant in older adults, clients with cognitive complaints, and clients taking multiple medications. Diphenhydramine, doxylamine, some bladder medications, some tricyclics, some antipsychotics, and other anticholinergic agents can stack.

A QEEG with slowing or poor reactivity in an older adult taking nightly diphenhydramine plus a TCA should not be interpreted as a simple neurodegenerative or underarousal pattern. Medication burden belongs in the paragraph.

Paradoxical reactions complicate the picture. Some clients report that diphenhydramine or hydroxyzine makes them agitated, wired, or unable to sleep. The clinician should believe and document that history rather than forcing the expected sedative model.

16.14 Steroids, Infection, and Encephalopathy

Corticosteroids can affect mood, sleep, anxiety, and psychosis risk in susceptible clients. A short steroid burst for asthma, autoimmune flare, or pain may change sleep and arousal enough to matter for QEEG even if no routine steroid signature exists.

Infection and antibiotics create a different safety context. Most outpatient antibiotics are not QEEG confounds by themselves. But severe infection, fever, renal impairment, cefepime, high-dose penicillins, fluoroquinolones, or delirium symptoms can shift the question toward encephalopathy or seizure threshold.

When confusion, acute cognitive change, fever, severe illness, or neurological symptoms are present, QEEG phenotype interpretation should pause.

16.15 Report Language Examples

Weak language: "The statin caused the slowing."

Better language: "No direct resting-QEEG signature is established for statins in the available evidence. Slowing should be interpreted with sleep, medical illness, medication burden, and symptom context."

Weak language: "Benadryl is just OTC."

Better language: "Diphenhydramine is a sedating first-generation antihistamine with anticholinergic effects; recent use reduces confidence in drowsiness, slowing, and underarousal interpretations."

Weak language: "The PPI is irrelevant."

Better language: "PPIs lack a direct QEEG signature in the available evidence, but long-term medical context such as B12 deficiency may be relevant if symptoms suggest it."

Weak language: "Beta-blockers reduce beta on QEEG."

Better language: "Beta-blocker resting-QEEG evidence is limited; interpret through fatigue, indication, dose timing, and comorbid cardiovascular/anxiety context rather than a presumed beta-band effect."

16.16 Training Implications

Non-psychotropic medications rarely dictate neurofeedback targets on their own. They change confidence and differential diagnosis. If a client took diphenhydramine last night, a slowing map may be rescheduled or labeled. If a client is on a statin, no special EEG adjustment is needed unless symptoms or medical context suggest an indirect pathway.

For clients with many OTC and chronic medications, the main intervention is documentation. A clean medication list can prevent overinterpretation and can identify safety referrals when acute illness, toxicity, hypoglycemia, or confusion is present.

Outcome tracking should note changes in sedating OTC use, steroid bursts, acute infections, cold medicines, GLP-1-related weight or sleep changes, and new beta-blockers. These may explain QEEG changes without implying direct signatures.

16.17 Practical Confidence Levels

High-confidence interpretation is possible when OTC sedatives, decongestants, acute illness, and toxicity concerns are absent or stable, and chronic non-psychotropic medications are documented.

Moderate confidence applies when a first-generation antihistamine, decongestant, steroid burst, acute allergy / cold symptoms, or mild sleep disruption is present but documented.

Low confidence applies during acute confusion, suspected encephalopathy, severe infection, hypoglycemia, medication toxicity, paradoxical OTC reaction, heavy anticholinergic burden, or recent sedating OTC use with marked drowsiness.

16.18 Documentation Standard

Minimum documentation includes all OTC sleep / allergy / cold products, chronic non-psychotropic prescriptions, last-dose timing for sedating or activating OTC agents, current illness, steroid bursts, antibiotics, hypoglycemia history, paradoxical reactions, and anticholinergic burden when relevant.

Ask clients to bring product names or photos when possible. Combination products are easy to misremember, and ingredient lists matter.

16.19 What Not to Claim

Do not invent signatures for statins, PPIs, GLP-1 agonists, SGLT-2 inhibitors, PDE-5 inhibitors, beta-blockers, LDN / naltrexone, or routine chronic medical drugs. Do not ignore diphenhydramine because it is OTC. Do not treat medical toxicity or encephalopathy as a neurofeedback phenotype.

16.20 When to Defer

Defer stable phenotype interpretation when the client is acutely ill, febrile, confused, hypoglycemic, heavily sedated, recently started a steroid burst with severe insomnia, or taking a new medication with strong side effects. The QEEG may document current state, but it is not a stable baseline.

Defer or refer when encephalopathy, delirium, seizure, medication toxicity, or acute neurological change is plausible. These are medical questions before they are neurofeedback questions.

If the medication is a pure-gap chronic drug and the client is otherwise stable, do not defer solely because it appears on the list. Document it and proceed with appropriate caveat.

16.21 Evidence summary

- **Spectral effect:** Sedating first-generation antihistamines can produce drowsiness / slowing-like effects; most other non-psychotropic categories have little direct resting-QEEG evidence.
- **Phenotype inference:** OTC sedatives, decongestants, sleep disruption, anticholinergic burden, toxicity, and medical illness can reduce confidence in underarousal, beta / arousal, slowing, and cognitive-fog interpretations.
- **Workflow heuristic:** Document all OTC, cold, allergy, sleep, and chronic non-psychotropic medications, and label pure-gap categories rather than inventing signatures.

Ch 17: Nutraceuticals and Herbal Preparations

17.1 Why this class matters in NFB practice

Nutraceuticals and herbal preparations are common in neurofeedback clients because they feel safer than prescription medications and are often used without clinician oversight. Clients may take L-theanine, melatonin, magnesium, omega-3 fatty acids, ashwagandha, rhodiola, bacopa, lion's mane, valerian, kava, NAC, ALCAR, racetams, kratom, phenibut, tianeptine, methylene blue, or multi-ingredient "brain" blends.

Strongest evidence	L-theanine and melatonin have specific task/sleep-context evidence. Most nutraceuticals lack reliable waking resting-QEEG signatures.
Biggest interpretation trap	Overstating L-theanine. Alpha effects are task- and state-dependent, not a simple resting-alpha claim.
Default clinical action	Document supplement names, blends, dose, timing, purpose, withdrawal risk, product uncertainty, and prescription interactions before assigning a phenotype.

The main QEEG problem is evidence mismatch. Some supplements have limited EEG data in specific tasks or sleep contexts. Many popular products have no rigorous waking resting-QEEG evidence. Product quality, dose accuracy, contaminants, interactions, and undisclosed use further complicate interpretation.

This chapter's rule is simple: document supplements like drugs, but do not grant them drug-like evidence when evidence is absent.

17.2 The Four-Bucket Framework

The clinician does not need to become a supplement pharmacologist to use this chapter. The practical task is to sort every supplement exposure into one of four buckets. This sorting step prevents the two most common errors: treating a popular supplement as invisible, or treating it as fully interpretable.

Bucket 1: Specific EEG evidence. Products with at least one controlled study measuring resting or task EEG in humans. *Examples:* L-theanine (alpha dynamics in task-dependent ways; Nobre et al., 2008; Gomez-Ramirez et al., 2009), melatonin (sleep EEG and sleep-onset timing), caffeine-theanine combinations.

Bucket 2: Sleep or arousal indirect effects. Products that influence sleep architecture, arousal, or cortisol, and therefore change what the QEEG captures, but without direct resting-QEEG data. *Examples:* magnesium glycinate, valerian, passionflower, ashwagandha, rhodiola, omega-3 fatty acids, adaptogenic blends.

Bucket 3: No usable QEEG evidence. Products where no direct resting-QEEG evidence exists and mechanism-extrapolation is too thin for even cautious inference. *Examples:* most vitamin supplements, most probiotic blends, most anti-inflammatory nutraceuticals (resveratrol, curcumin, quercetin). Document but do not assign QEEG significance.

Bucket 4: Safety and withdrawal concerns. Products with abuse potential, withdrawal risk, or significant drug interactions despite "supplement" or "natural" labeling. *Examples:* kratom (opioidergic, withdrawal-positive), phenibut (GABA-B agonist, withdrawal seizure risk), tianeptine (opioid-like at high doses), kava (sedative, hepatotoxicity at high doses), yohimbine (alpha-2 antagonist, cardiovascular effects). These belong in the same documentation category as scheduled medications.

17.3 Mechanism (clinician-level pharmacology)

Nutraceuticals span many mechanisms and highly variable regulatory oversight. A capsule may contain more, less, or different active ingredient than the label suggests. Multi-ingredient products can include caffeine, sedatives, stimulants, cannabinoids, or undisclosed compounds. Client language can also mislead: "I only take vitamins" may describe a multivitamin or it may describe magnesium glycinate, melatonin, ashwagandha, mushroom blends, green-tea extract, a pre-workout powder, CBD gummies, and an imported nootropic. The intake form should give the client enough examples to disclose what they use. Asking for product photos is often the most efficient approach.

17.4 Known spectral effects

L-theanine is the best example of why detail matters. Nobre and colleagues support alpha-related attention findings (Nobre et al., 2008), while Gomez-Ramirez and colleagues found reduced tonic alpha during a visuospatial task, with no measurable change in cue-related anticipatory alpha (Gomez-Ramirez et al., 2009). The corrected claim is not that L-theanine raises resting alpha. It can affect alpha dynamics in task/state-dependent ways.

Caffeine plus L-theanine combinations have behavioral and attention evidence, including Owen and colleagues (Owen et al., 2008). For QEEG, the combination should be documented as both caffeine exposure and theanine exposure, not treated as tea in a generic sense.

Melatonin has the cleanest sleep-onset and sleep EEG relevance (Dijk et al., 1995). The waking QEEG issue is usually sleep timing, sleep quality, circadian phase, and next-day state rather than a strong resting spectral signature.

Omega-3 fatty acids, ashwagandha, rhodiola, bacopa, lion's mane, NAC, ALCAR, magnesium forms, kava, valerian, racetams, and many nootropic blends have sparse, underpowered, or absent waking resting-QEEG evidence. They should be gap-labeled unless a specific source supports a specific claim.

This does not mean these products have no biological effect. A supplement may change sleep, anxiety, pain, or alertness, and those clinical changes may alter the recording state. But the book cannot translate that into a reliable resting spectral signature.

The highest-risk interpretive errors usually occur with broad labels. "Nootropic" is not a mechanism. "Adaptogen" is not an EEG category. "Sleep support" may include melatonin, valerian, magnesium, GABA, antihistamine-like ingredients, cannabinoids, or undisclosed

Compound	Primary QEEG Vectors	Claim type	Interaction Modes	Confidence
Caffeine plus L-theanine	attention alpha modulation context, caffeine context	heuristic	n/a	n/a
L-theanine	task alpha modulation, tonic alpha correction	heuristic	n/a	n/a
Melatonin	sleep onset context, circadian timing context, next day state	heuristic	n/a	n/a
Calming supplements and herbal sedatives	sedation context, sleep context, gap	heuristic	n/a	n/a
Adaptogens and wellness nootropics	gap, product quality uncertainty	heuristic	n/a	n/a

Figure 17.1: Nutraceutical/herbal evidence triage: agents by QEEG vectors, claim type, and interaction modes.

sedatives. The QEEG report should name the product and its timing rather than convert marketing language into neurophysiology.

17.5 Phenotype interaction effects

Supplements can mimic sedation, activation, sleep improvement, withdrawal, anxiety relief, or stimulant effects depending on product and dose. More often, they complicate attribution. A client taking melatonin, magnesium, ashwagandha, CBD, caffeine, and L-theanine may show changes driven by sleep, caffeine, product interactions, or expectation.

Grey-market substances can transform interpretation. Kratom may act partly through opioid pathways. Phenibut has GABA-B-like concerns and withdrawal risk. Tianeptine has opioid-like abuse potential. These should not be treated as harmless wellness products.

Product uncertainty is a phenotype confound. If the clinician cannot know what was in a blend, the report should state that uncertainty.

17.6 Product-Specific Notes

L-theanine belongs in a task/state category. If taken with caffeine, the caffeine exposure is usually the more familiar QEEG confound, while the theanine component may affect attention and alpha dynamics. The report should avoid a generic "tea raises alpha" explanation. It should say that caffeine-theanine exposure was present and that task-related alpha findings may not generalize to resting-QEEG interpretation.

Melatonin belongs in a circadian and sleep-onset category. Morning recordings after late or irregular melatonin use should be interpreted with attention to sleep duration, sleep quality, grogginess, dream intensity, and schedule drift. For many clients, the relevant question is whether the recording captured a rested state, a residual sleepiness state, or a shifted circadian state, not whether melatonin directly changed beta or theta.

Kava, valerian, magnesium, glycine, GABA-branded products, and similar calming supplements should be treated as sedative-adjacent exposures unless evidence proves otherwise. The QEEG effect may be absent, mild, or indirect. Still, they matter for drowsiness, blink rate, vigilance, and symptom-state interpretation.

Omega-3 fatty acids, NAC, ALCAR, bacopa, lion's mane, rhodiola, ashwagandha, and similar wellness products should usually be documented as gap exposures for QEEG purposes. They may be clinically relevant to the client, but the clinician should not infer a specific z-score pattern from their use.

Kratom, phenibut, tianeptine, and grey-market nootropics require a different level of caution. They are not ordinary wellness products in a QEEG intake. They can involve dependence, withdrawal, intoxication, sedation, agitation, sleep disruption, or interaction with psychiatric and pain medications. If use is active or recently changed, the recording may be less useful as a stable baseline.

17.7 Case vignette

"No psychiatric medications" reads the intake form. The supplement section, in smaller print, lists L-theanine with morning coffee, magnesium at night, melatonin irregularly, ashwagandha daily, and a "focus blend" before work. Anxiety and insomnia are the presenting concerns. The QEEG shows intermittent beta, weak alpha reactivity, and drowsiness late in the recording.

A simplistic report might call this anxiety plus underarousal. A better report documents caffeine-theanine timing, irregular melatonin and sleep, unknown focus-blend ingredients, and supplement polypharmacy. The QEEG remains usable, but supplement exposure reduces confidence in simple trait labels.

The defensible report says: "Findings are interpreted under nutraceutical polypharmacy, caffeine-theanine exposure, irregular melatonin use, and unknown focus-blend ingredients; phenotype labels should be cautious."

17.8 Report Language Examples

Use language that preserves uncertainty without sounding dismissive:

- "The recording was obtained under ongoing supplement use, including melatonin and magnesium for sleep and caffeine-theanine exposure before the session."
- "L-theanine has task/state-dependent EEG evidence; the present resting-QEEG findings should not be interpreted as a direct marker of theanine response."
- "The client reports a multi-ingredient nootropic blend of uncertain composition; this limits confidence in simple arousal-state attribution."
- "Kratom/phenibut/tianeptine exposure is clinically relevant and should be documented separately from routine vitamin or mineral supplementation."
- "The supplement list is treated as a potential recording-state confound, not as a basis for QEEG-guided supplement advice."

Avoid language that implies certainty:

- "The alpha pattern proves the theanine is working."
- "Low beta reflects magnesium deficiency."
- "Ashwagandha caused the client's theta pattern."
- "This QEEG indicates which supplements should be stopped."

The report can be useful without being overconfident. It can say that supplement exposure is present, identify the most plausible interpretive pathways, and recommend consistent documentation across follow-up recordings.

17.9 Interpretation traps

- **Overstating L-theanine.** Alpha effects are task/state-dependent, not a simple resting-alpha claim.
- **Ignoring supplement blends.** Multi-ingredient nootropics may contain stimulants or sedatives.
- **Treating "natural" as irrelevant.** Kratom, phenibut, and tianeptine can have serious effects.
- **Inventing adaptogen signatures.** Ashwagandha, rhodiola, lion's mane, and similar products are mostly gaps for QEEG.
- **Ignoring sleep pathway.** Melatonin and magnesium may matter through sleep, not direct waking EEG.
- **Ignoring product quality.** Label accuracy and contamination are real issues.

17.10 IV Infusion Therapies

Clients increasingly present for QEEG after receiving IV infusion therapies from longevity clinics, biohacking centers, addiction-recovery programs, naturopathic offices, and IV drip bars. These are rarely captured on standard medication intake forms because clients do not think of them as medications. The QEEG clinician should ask about them directly.

The most common IV therapies encountered in practice include NAD+ infusions, glutathione, Myers' cocktails (magnesium, calcium, B-complex, vitamin C), high-dose IV vitamin C, alpha-lipoic acid, phosphatidylcholine, amino acid infusions, and chelation therapy (EDTA, DMSA). IV ketamine is covered separately in Chapter 13.

Evidence base: effectively zero. As of 2026, there are no peer-reviewed human studies reporting resting-state EEG or QEEG changes during or after any of these IV nutrient/cofactor therapies. This includes NAD+ (despite a growing addiction-recovery literature), glutathione (despite off-label Parkinson's use), Myers' cocktails, and high-dose vitamin C (despite extensive oncology safety data). The addiction-recovery NAD+ protocol literature (BR+NAD, Springfield Wellness) describes clinical outcomes but provides no quantitative electrophysiology. A single older megadose vitamin C study reported EEG changes with non-modern methods and has not been replicated.

Mechanistic plausibility. The strongest case for acute EEG relevance is IV magnesium at high doses, given magnesium's role as an NMDA receptor antagonist and GABA-A modulator. However, eclampsia-level IV magnesium dosing (used with continuous EEG monitoring in ICU settings) is far above the 1–2 g doses in a typical Myers' cocktail. At wellness doses, any acute EEG effect would likely be subtle and indistinguishable from nonspecific relaxation. IV NAD+ infusions can produce intense autonomic side effects (chest tightness, nausea, anxiety, a "wired-tired" feeling) that could transiently alter arousal and sleep, but these are nonspecific state effects, not a NAD+ spectral signature.

Pre-recording timing. Given the absence of direct evidence, a conservative approach is reasonable:

- Defer a baseline recording while the client still reports effects of a recent infusion: sleep disruption, anxiety, flushing, headache, or any felt change. Symptom resolution is the signal, not a clock, because there is no evidence establishing a clearance interval.
- Where a recording is obtained close to an infusion, document the product, dose, route, and time since, and read it as a current-state map rather than a stable baseline.

Intake documentation. Add an "IV / injection therapies" block to the intake form:

- Have you received any IV or injection therapies in the past 4 weeks (for wellness, longevity, recovery, or detox)?
- What was infused, when, dose / duration, provider, and frequency?
- Any effects noticed during or after (anxiety, fog, insomnia, sedation, headache)?

If a client arrives having recently received an IV therapy and rescheduling is impractical, document the infusion in the recording metadata and add a standard caveat: "Baseline obtained within [time] of [IV therapy]; acute EEG effects have not been characterized in the literature, so findings may reflect transient state factors."

This is a pure gap category. Do not invent an IV nutrient EEG signature. The value of documenting these exposures is completeness: a recording state that includes a same-day NAD+ infusion, poor sleep from the infusion, and elevated caffeine to compensate is a different state from the client's usual day, and the report should say so.

17.11 Polypharmacy and Interaction Context

Supplement polypharmacy often clusters with medication polypharmacy. A client taking an SSRI may also take L-theanine, magnesium, melatonin, NAC, omega-3, cannabis, and a sleep tea. A client taking stimulants may also use caffeine-theanine stacks and pre-workout products. A client with chronic pain may use magnesium, CBD, kratom, and sedating antihistamines. These combinations make single-cause QEEG interpretation weak.

The useful question is not "Which one caused the map?" The useful question is "What state was recorded, and is that state stable enough to guide training?" If the answer is yes, the map may still guide neurofeedback cautiously. If the answer is no, repeat recording under a more stable state may be better than overreading the first map.

Interactions also affect adverse events. Kava, valerian, phenibut, alcohol, benzodiazepines, opioids, Z-drugs, sedating antihistamines, and cannabis can cluster around sleep and anxiety. Stimulants, caffeine, pre-workout products, thyroid medication, and activating antidepressants can cluster around alertness and insomnia. QEEG interpretation should follow the cluster, not the most familiar item.

17.12 Intake questions

When supplements or herbals appear on the intake form, ask:

- **What supplements, blends, powders, teas, or nootropics do you use?** Ask for product photos if possible.
- **Dose and timing?** Especially caffeine-theanine, melatonin, kava, valerian, magnesium, kratom, phenibut.
- **Any withdrawal or dependence concerns?** Kratom, phenibut, tianeptine, and sedative herbals need screening.
- **Any sleep, anxiety, or stimulant purpose?** Indication helps interpret the QEEG.
- **Any prescription interactions?** SSRIs, sedatives, stimulants, opioids, antipsychotics, and anticoagulants may matter.

17.13 Clinical recommendations

Treat supplements as exposure variables. Document them, but do not invent signatures for products without evidence. Use the strongest available claim: task-specific, sleep-context, gap, or safety concern.

If a supplement is part of the client's ordinary state and will continue during neurofeedback, recording under that stable state may be reasonable. If the client recently started, stopped, or stacked supplements, label the QEEG as a transition state.

Kratom, phenibut, tianeptine, severe sedative stacking, or withdrawal symptoms should prompt safety and medical context, not casual wellness framing.

Where possible, repeat measures should standardize supplement state. A follow-up QEEG after starting neurofeedback should record the same caffeine, melatonin, and supplement timing as the baseline unless the clinical question is specifically about a change. Inconsistent supplement timing can create apparent treatment effects that are state effects.

Clinicians should avoid giving supplement instructions outside their scope. It is reasonable to ask for documentation, recommend consistency for recording purposes, and coordinate with medical providers when safety concerns appear. It is not appropriate to use QEEG to prescribe, stop, or endorse supplement regimens, or to justify changes to prescription medications, as if the map were a pharmacologic decision tool.

Safety notice. High-dose IV infusions (NAD+, high-dose magnesium, chelation agents) carry medical risks including cardiac arrhythmia, acute hypotension, and electrolyte imbalance. These are medical procedures, not wellness services, and should be supervised by a licensed provider. A QEEG clinician who notices that a client has recently received an unusual IV infusion should document it as a potential confound and coordinate with the administering provider when there is any clinical uncertainty.

17.14 Evidence summary

- **Spectral effect:** L-theanine and melatonin have specific task / sleep-context evidence; most nutraceuticals lack reliable waking resting-QEEG signatures.
- **Phenotype inference:** Supplements can alter confidence in arousal, sleep, alpha, sedation, and withdrawal interpretations mainly through timing, sleep, caffeine pairing, and product uncertainty.
- **Workflow heuristic:** Document supplement names, blends, dose, timing, purpose, withdrawal risk, product uncertainty, and prescription interactions before assigning phenotype meaning.

Ch 18: Patterns Across Substances

If you remember nothing else from this chapter: The receptor system points to a spectral direction, not to a magnitude and not to an individual client. GABAergic enhancement points toward beta. Catecholaminergic drive points toward suppressed slow activity. Histaminergic and anticholinergic load points toward diffuse slowing. Withdrawal often runs against the acute picture, though the EEG evidence for that is thin outside the benzodiazepines. The families are built on anchor compounds that have actually been studied. Learn them and you can predict the direction for a drug you have never seen. You cannot predict its magnitude, its effect in one client, or what the recording will show once state and indication are in the mix.

18.1 Receptor-Family Quick Reference

The table below summarizes the eight mechanism families covered in this chapter. It is a starting point, not a complete map.

Receptor family	Representative drugs	Spectral direction (acute)	Phenotype confusion risk
GABAergic enhancement	Benzodiazepines, Z-drugs, barbiturates, alcohol, neurosteroids	Beta increase; sedation; reduced alpha reactivity	Drug beta misread as endogenous anxiety beta
Catecholaminergic (stimulant)	Methylphenidate, amphetamines, modafinil, caffeine	Slow-activity suppression; some beta increase	Medicated "normalization" misread as clean phenotype

Receptor family	Representative drugs	Spectral direction (acute)	Phenotype confusion risk
Sedative-histaminergic	Antihistamines, tricyclics, atypicals, quetiapine	Diffuse slowing; low-voltage; vigilance instability	Medication slowing misread as underarousal phenotype
Serotonergic	SSRIs, SNRIs, trazodone	Modest alpha shifts; FAA changes; variable	FAA and alpha misread as stable trait markers
Glutamatergic / NMDA antagonism	Ketamine, esketamine, memantine, dextromethorphan	Broadband and aperiodic shifts; gamma increase; no single-band fit	Aperiodic background change forced into standard band labels
Opioidergic	Opioids, buprenorphine	Theta and delta increase; pain confounds	Opioid slowing conflated with pain-state slowing
Cannabinoid	THC, CBD, synthetic cannabinoids	Frontal theta / alpha increase; slow iAPF in chronic use	Cannabis slowing misread as ADHD or depression phenotype
Anticonvulsant	Valproate, topiramate, lamotrigine, levetiracetam, lithium	Heterogeneous; no single pattern (slowing, beta, both, or neither)	"Anticonvulsant effect" read as one signature

Gabapentinoids are deliberately absent from the GABAergic row. They sit next to that family clinically because they sedate, but not mechanistically; see the anticonvulsant section below.

For worked differential examples across these families, see Chapter 25 (When It's Not the Drug).

18.2 The repeating patterns

The previous chapters covered medications one class at a time. That is the right way to learn the details: dose curves, formulation timing, withdrawal risk, and the specific evidence anchors differ enough that no shortcut replaces compound-level knowledge. But if you stop there, you are memorizing a medication list instead of building a framework.

This chapter is the framework. It is the heart of the perturbation engine: the level of abstraction at which individual drugs collapse back into the receptor-system families that generate their spectral signatures. A small number of receptor-system families account for most of the spectral patterns you will see in medicated clients. GABAergic drugs produce one family of changes. Catecholaminergic drugs produce another. Sedative-histaminergic and anticholinergic loads produce a third. Serotonergic, glutamatergic, opioidergic, and cannabinoid systems each contribute their own spectral tendencies. Most of these families have a recognizable spectral direction, a tolerance story, and a withdrawal signature; the anticonvulsants are the exception, and the table above gives them no shared direction because the literature does not support one. If you learn these mechanism-to-spectrum relationships, you can predict the approximate EEG signature of a drug you have never seen before, based on its receptor profile. You will not predict the magnitude or the individual response. You will predict the direction. That is enough to ask the right intake questions and to know which phenotype labels need confidence adjustments before the recording even starts.

The families are not only a teaching device. The largest pharmaco-EEG dataset yet assembled has now looked for them at scale: over 24,000 clinical EEG recordings, roughly 6000 hours, spanning a wide range of psychiatric diagnoses and medication regimens, compared across more than 75,000 spectral, connectivity, and nonlinear features (Szponar et al., 2026). The class-specific signatures that survived dimensionality reduction point the same way this chapter does. Benzodiazepines showed increased beta with reduced theta-alpha power. Antipsychotics and anticonvulsants both showed marked slow-wave amplification and reductions in signal complexity. SSRIs showed enhanced gamma-band coherence, a newer signal that has not yet reached the routine clinical vocabulary and that conventional band-power reporting is not built to see. The results are public through an interactive resource called BrainwavesRX, so a clinician can look at the class-level picture without waiting for it to be summarized.

Read the design before you read the findings. This is a cross-sectional observational study of naturalistic prescribing, not a controlled dose-response experiment. Nobody was randomized to anything. The drug and the reason for the drug arrive together, and the design does not address that: some share of the antipsychotic slowing in a dataset like this belongs to the conditions that get treated with antipsychotics. What the study earns is a spectral-effect claim about direction at the group level, supported by convergence rather than by control. What it does not earn is an individual-level inference. It tells you that a class-level association holds across 24,000 records under real-world conditions. It does not tell you what your client's beta means.

18.3 GABAergic enhancement: beta increase and rebound

Benzodiazepines, barbiturates, Z-drugs, alcohol, and neurosteroids share a common thread: positive modulation at GABA-A receptor sites. The shared spectral consequence is faster rhythmic activity, especially in the beta range (Mandema et al., 1992). This beta increase often coexists with sedation, reduced alpha reactivity, and vigilance instability. The client may look spectrally fast while feeling cognitively slow. That combination is the central interpretive trap for this family.

Gabapentinoids do not belong on that list, and it is worth saying why before the family logic gets applied to them. Gabapentin and pregabalin bind the alpha-2-delta subunit of voltage-gated calcium channels; the current gabapentin label states that the drug has no effect on GABA binding, uptake, or degradation. They are shelved near this family because they sedate and because they are used for overlapping indications, not because they share its mechanism, and they do not produce the beta augmentation the rest of the family produces. Treat them as their own category, described later in this chapter.

The beta does not mean activation. It means pharmacological inhibition organized into a faster cortical rhythm. A benzodiazepine-associated beta pattern and an endogenous anxiety-related beta pattern can look similar on a topographic map. They do not mean the same thing. Treating them as interchangeable is the most common error in medicated QEEG interpretation.

Tolerance develops with chronic exposure. A client on long-term clonazepam (Klonopin) may no longer feel sedated but may still carry a medication-shaped spectral profile. Interdose withdrawal can create its own signature: restlessness, sleep disruption, and autonomic instability between doses.

Full withdrawal inverts the story. Abrupt benzodiazepine discontinuation or rapid taper can produce alpha and theta instability, hyperexcitability, sleep disruption, and in serious cases paroxysmal abnormality risk (Ashton, 2002). Z-drug rebound is often described as following a similar logic at the sleep-wake boundary, but the direct evidence is thin: a single zolpidem dose in healthy volunteers left no residual sleep or EEG effect on the following drug-free night (Brunner et al., 1991). Gabapentinoid withdrawal can produce anxiety rebound and sleep disruption, though the EEG literature is thinner than for benzodiazepines. Alcohol withdrawal overlaps with benzodiazepine withdrawal because the mechanism overlaps: both are GABA-A states, and cross-tolerance is clinically real.

The clinical rule: when you see beta excess in a client taking any GABA-A positive modulator, do not call it activation until you have ruled out the medication as the source. And when a client recently stopped one of these drugs, do not call the recording a baseline. It is a withdrawal-state recording.

18.4 Stimulant and catecholaminergic: suppression of slow activity

Methylphenidate, amphetamines, atomoxetine (Strattera), modafinil (Provigil), and caffeine all increase catecholaminergic tone, though through different mechanisms. The shared spectral direction is a reduction in slow activity, especially theta, and sometimes an increase in beta or SMR-range power. In pediatric ADHD samples, a six-month stimulant trial shifted the EEG toward the normative range, and the shift sat mainly in theta and beta (Clarke, Barry, Bond, et al., 2002). That finding anchors the clinical concern: stimulant exposure can mask or reduce the theta features clinicians use to identify attention phenotypes.

The masking problem is the core issue. A client recorded near peak extended-release stimulant coverage may show a more normalized theta profile than their unmedicated state would produce. That recording is not wrong. It answers a question about treated functioning. It does not answer a question about endogenous physiology. The clinician who confuses the two will underestimate the attention phenotype.

Atomoxetine is a norepinephrine reuptake inhibitor (Barry et al., 2009) with slower onset and CYP2D6-dependent exposure, not a classic stimulant. Modafinil is a wake-promoting agent that acts primarily on vigilance systems rather than producing a methylphenidate-like theta-beta shift (Bodenmann & Landolt, 2010; Linton et al., 2022; D. Wang et al., 2015). Both can change the EEG, but they should not be collapsed into one stimulant signature.

Chronic stimulant use produces tolerance in some clients. Withdrawal and rebound can show theta increases, fatigue, and what looks like a return of the pre-treatment phenotype. A skipped-dose recording is a withdrawal-state recording, not a clean unmedicated baseline, especially if the client also slept poorly or increased caffeine to compensate. The clinician should also remember that caffeine and nicotine act through different pharmacology but push the same clinical confound: alertness, muscle tension, and beta-range shifts that overlap with arousal and TBR language.

18.5 Sedative, histaminergic, and anticholinergic: diffuse slowing and vigilance drop

First-generation antihistamines, sedating antidepressants (trazodone (Desyrel), mirtazapine (Remeron), doxepin), sedating antipsychotics at lower doses (quetiapine (Seroquel), olanzapine (Zyprexa)), and drugs with anticholinergic burden push the EEG toward delta and theta increases, alpha slowing, drowsiness intrusion, and reduced reactivity. The mechanisms differ. Histamine H1 blockade, muscarinic antagonism, and alpha-1 adrenergic blockade can all produce sedation and slowing, but the shared clinical consequence is the same spectral direction.

Not all antipsychotic slowing evidence is equally strong. Clozapine (Clozaril) produces the clearest slowing signal in the class, supported by spectral work in healthy volunteers showing delta and theta increases alongside reductions in fast activity (Galderisi et al., 1996). Olanzapine shows dose-dependent sedation and slowing in pharmaco-EEG work, though with less dramatic delta increases than clozapine (Schuld et al., 2000). Risperidone (Risperdal) shows acute delta and theta increases in early controlled work (Lee et al., 1999). For quetiapine, aripiprazole (Abilify), and newer atypical agents, the direct resting-QEEG evidence base is thinner; clinical expectations of slowing are often extrapolated from side-effect profiles and class membership rather than from controlled spectral studies. The clinician should not treat all antipsychotic slowing as equivalently evidenced; clozapine-level claims do not automatically transfer to aripiprazole. An early pharmaco-EEG study of a single sedating tricyclic showed that antimuscarinic load can produce sedation-shaped maps mimicking underarousal or cognitive decline (Itil et al., 1972); Chapter 7 discusses the broader TCA class evidence and compound heterogeneity. Diphenhydramine is easy to miss on an intake form because clients do not think of it as a psychiatric medication, but it can produce sedation, paradoxical activation in some clients, and day-after impairment that contaminates a recording (Leon & Nikoloff, 2008).

The clinical risk: these patterns mimic underarousal phenotypes, TBI residua, or early cognitive decline. A slow, drowsy map in a client on quetiapine, trazodone, and a PM antihistamine shows stacked sedation, not an endogenous slowing phenotype. The report should name the exposures before assigning a phenotype label. And the intake should specifically ask about OTC sleep aids, cold medications, and allergy products, because clients rarely think of these as psychiatric drugs even when they are shaping the recording.

18.6 Serotonergic modulation: subtle alpha and theta shifts

SSRIs, SNRIs, trazodone (which straddles this category and the sedative family), and serotonergic psychedelics all modulate 5-HT pathways. The spectral effects are compound-specific and often subtle at clinical QEEG resolution. This is the family where you are least likely to see a single recognizable signature and most likely to be misled by individual variation.

Older pharmaco-EEG mapping confirms that antidepressants produce measurable EEG changes, but not a single class fingerprint (B. Saletu et al., 1986; B. Saletu et al., 2006). Alpha frequency shifts, theta changes, and frontal alpha asymmetry modulation are all reported, but none is reliable enough to serve as a standalone biomarker. FAA in particular requires three qualifications: it is sex-dependent (male and female response patterns differ), method-sensitive (reference choice and asymmetry computation alter results), and the strongest SSRI-related FAA findings come from response-prediction designs rather than direct spectral-effect studies (Bruder et al., 2008). A medicated-client report should not treat FAA as a simple serotonergic biomarker without documenting sex, reproductive hormone context, and processing pipeline.

Response-prediction work is clinically interesting but operates at a different level than direct spectral effects. Theta cordance changes may predict treatment response (Bares et al., 2007; Bares et al., 2008), but cordance is a derived measure that combines absolute and relative power; it is not raw theta power. Confusing cordance with direct theta change is one of the more common interpretive errors in serotonergic QEEG discussion. A map that shows theta change under SSRI exposure is not the same as a cordance-based response prediction, and the two should not be cited interchangeably.

SNRIs add a noradrenergic activation component that can overlap with insomnia, blood pressure changes, and tremor. These side effects can shape the recording state without producing a private SNRI spectral code. The clinician should ask about the side-effect profile, not just the drug name.

Discontinuation produces its own signature. SSRI and SNRI withdrawal can alter sleep, arousal, and emotional reactivity in ways that spill into the waking EEG. A recording obtained shortly after antidepressant discontinuation is a withdrawal-state record, not a return to a pre-treatment baseline. Reproductive hormone context also matters here: menstrual cycle phase and OCP use can shift alpha independently of the antidepressant, most clearly the center frequency of the band rather than the individual alpha peak (Brötzner et al., 2014). Perimenopause and postpartum state belong in the same interpretive frame on clinical grounds, though that work does not test them. In serotonergic interpretation, context is everything and a single recording is rarely enough to separate drug from state.

18.7 Glutamatergic and NMDA antagonism: broadband and aperiodic effects

Ketamine, esketamine, memantine, dextromethorphan, and some psychedelics (partially) act through NMDA antagonism or glutamatergic modulation. These drugs produce spectral changes that do not fit neatly into single-band descriptions. Aperiodic slope flattening, broadband power shifts, and gamma-range activity increases can all appear (Gilbert & Zarate, 2020; Guirguis et al., 2025). If you try to force these changes into standard band-power labels, you will misread the map.

This matters because conventional QEEG software reports theta, alpha, beta, and sometimes gamma as discrete bands. A drug that changes the aperiodic background shifts apparent power in every band without producing a discrete oscillatory change in any of them. Separating periodic from aperiodic components is what the question actually requires when an NMDA-active compound is on board. Most clinical platforms will not do it, and specparam output is itself sensitive to fitting range, peak settings, line-noise handling, and data quality, so the fallback rule matters more here than the ideal one. When decomposition is unavailable, or available but not validated in your own pipeline, do not claim a narrow oscillatory mechanism from a broadband band-power shift. Report the finding as an unresolved periodic-versus-aperiodic change and name what you could not separate. Ketamine and psilocybin comparisons illustrate why (Soltanzadeh et al., 2025).

Timing is critical. A recording obtained hours after a ketamine infusion or esketamine session captures a treatment window, not a stable trait. The same client recorded a week later will look different. Session timing, co-administered benzodiazepines (common in ketamine clinics), and sleep state all matter.

These are among the hardest medication effects to interpret with conventional band-power QEEG. When the broadband picture does not match a simple phenotype story, consider whether an NMDA-active exposure is in play. Memantine in dementia care and dextromethorphan in combination products add milder NMDA-modulatory context that rarely dominates a recording but can contribute to a mixed picture, especially in polypharmacy.

18.8 Opioidergic: slow activity with pain-state confounding

Mu-opioid agonists (morphine, oxycodone, hydrocodone, fentanyl, methadone (Dolophine), buprenorphine (Subutex), kratom at higher doses) produce slowing in many acute and chronic contexts. Alpha reactivity may be reduced. Sedation and respiratory effects interact with the spectral picture, especially when opioids are combined with benzodiazepines, gabapentinoids, or other depressants.

Chronic opioid use produces tolerance, so the spectral signature in a stable methadone maintenance client is different from an acute post-operative opioid exposure (G. Y. Wang et al., 2015). A client rotating between short-acting opioids with unstable pain control presents yet another state.

The biggest interpretive problem with opioids is often the pain, not the drug alone. Chronic pain itself changes EEG features: attention, sleep architecture, arousal, alpha reactivity, and muscle tension all shift. A slow, fatigued map in a chronic-pain client on opioids cannot be cleanly separated into drug effect and pain effect from a single recording. The honest report says both are plausible contributors and does not pretend to resolve the ratio.

Withdrawal creates its own hazard. Missed doses, rapid taper, or transition to an antagonist can produce autonomic instability, sleep disruption, and arousal changes. Those states are not baselines. Tramadol (Ultram) deserves a separate note: it is a mixed serotonergic and opioid agent with drug-drug interaction context that does not fit the pure mu-agonist model (Kerson, 2023).

18.9 Cannabinoid: acute and chronic dissociation

THC, CBD, and synthetic cannabinoids produce different spectral effects. Acute THC can increase theta, alter alpha organization, and produce state-dependent changes that vary with dose, route, product, and tolerance. Chronic cannabis users may show different resting patterns than acute users: elevated frontal alpha in long-term users, and beta/gamma differences that do not replicate cleanly across cohorts, illustrate why a single "cannabis look" fails (Prashad et al., 2018; Prashad et al., 2026; Struve et al., 1999).

CBD effects are subtle and poorly characterized at clinical QEEG resolution. Most wellness-dose CBD products lack a defensible resting signature separate from their indication context. Even clinical CBD trials that collected EEG alongside symptom and cognitive outcomes have reported the clinical measures without a resting QEEG signature (Solowij et al., 2018).

The main clinical problem with cannabinoids is uncertainty. You rarely know the exact THC-to-CBD ratio, the dose, the route, the timing, or the tolerance state. A client who uses cannabis nightly may show attenuated spectral changes on a use day and instability on an abstinence day. Neither is a clean trait measurement.

I tell clinicians to document product, route, last use, and whether the recording day matched the client's usual pattern. A cannabis checkbox is not enough.

18.10 Anticonvulsant heterogeneity: no single pattern

Valproate (Depakote), carbamazepine (Tegretol), lamotrigine (Lamictal), topiramate (Topamax), levetiracetam (Keppra), and gabapentinoids are grouped by clinical indication, not by mechanism. Their spectral effects reflect this heterogeneity. Topiramate produces documented slowing (W. W. Wang et al., 2003). Valproate can increase slow activity and shows dose-dependent effects. Lithium can reduce alpha organization and increase slow-band prominence (Schulz et al., 2000). Lamotrigine acts differently, and the limited evidence suggests it may not produce the same slowing profile as valproate or topiramate (Clemens et al., 2006).

The shared pattern is the absence of a shared pattern. Each anticonvulsant must be evaluated by its own receptor and channel profile. Grouping them as "anticonvulsants" on a QEEG report is about as useful as grouping all clients as "medicated." The label tells you the clinical indication. It does not tell you the spectral direction.

Gabapentinoids (gabapentin (Neurontin), pregabalin (Lyrica)) belong partly here and partly in the GABAergic family. Their sedation and drowsiness are clinically real and sit inside the antiepileptic tolerability picture (Perucca & Gilliam, 2012), but they do not produce the same sharp beta augmentation as benzodiazepines. They are their own interpretive category. The practical point: when you see "anticonvulsant" on an intake form, your next question should be which one. The answer determines whether you expect slowing, beta, both, or neither.

18.11 What this framework gives you

You now have a receptor-to-spectrum mental model. When a new drug appears on a client's medication list, the first question is: what receptor system does it primarily affect? A GABAergic drug points toward beta and vigilance changes. A catecholaminergic drug points toward theta suppression. A sedative-histaminergic or anticholinergic drug points toward slowing. A serotonergic drug points toward subtle alpha and theta shifts. An NMDA antagonist points toward broadband and aperiodic changes. An opioid points toward slowing with pain confounding. A cannabinoid points toward dose-dependent and state-dependent uncertainty. An anticonvulsant points toward no single direction; the answer depends on which compound, so ask which one before predicting slowing, beta, both, or neither.

That directional prediction tells you which phenotype labels to question and which intake questions to ask first. It does not tell you the magnitude of the effect, the individual response, or the interaction with other exposures, conditions, and developmental factors. Those are what the rest of this book handles. The framework is a routing tool. It gets you to the right chapter, the right questions, and the right confidence adjustments faster than memorizing a list of brand names.

Mixed states are the default. Most adults in clinical practice carry more than one exposure. When two pattern families overlap in the same recording, write that down. A mixed-state label with documented exposures is more honest and more useful than a forced single-phenotype call. The later chapters on polypharmacy, condition confounders, and special populations add the next layer. The receptor-to-spectrum families stay the same. The stacking gets more complex, but the vocabulary you need to describe it starts here.

18.12 Evidence summary

- **Spectral effect:** Mechanism-family spectral directions are supported by controlled pharmaco-EEG evidence for the anchor compounds in each group: benzodiazepine beta augmentation (Mandema et al., 1992), stimulant theta reduction in ADHD samples (Clarke, Barry, Bond, et al., 2002), antipsychotic slowing profiles (Galderisi et al., 1996; Lee et al., 1999; Schuld et al., 2000), ketamine/esketamine broadband and aperiodic effects (Guirguis et al., 2025), and anticonvulsant-specific directions (Clemens et al., 2006; Schulz et al., 2000; W. W. Wang et al., 2003).

- **Spectral effect, observational convergence:** The largest pharmaco-EEG dataset in existence independently reproduces two of those directions at scale, benzodiazepine beta increase with reduced theta-alpha power and antipsychotic and anticonvulsant slow-wave amplification with reduced signal complexity, across more than 24,000 clinical recordings (Szponar et al., 2026). The design is cross-sectional and observational, so it corroborates direction at the group level under naturalistic prescribing without controlling for confounding by indication, and it licenses no individual-level inference.

- **Phenotype inference:** Cross-substance pattern families plausibly explain a large share of phenotype mimicry, masking, and transformation in medicated QEEG recordings. The translation from spectral direction to phenotype-misclassification risk has not been directly tested but follows from the spectral evidence and the four interaction modes (Chapter 1).

- **Workflow heuristic:** The receptor-to-spectrum routing model (identify mechanism family first, then narrow by compound, dose, timing, and state) is a clinical practice recommendation without controlled validation. In the author's clinical experience, this framework reduces the rate of premature phenotype labeling in medicated clients, but that observation has not been formally tested.

Cross-reference. The differential question, 'What else besides this drug could produce this pattern?', is the subject of Chapter 25 (When It's Not the Drug). That chapter applies the mechanism families described here to non-drug confounders: TBI, post-viral illness, obstructive sleep apnea, and sleep deprivation. The two chapters are designed to be read together. Chapter 18 builds the vocabulary. Chapter 25 tests it against the hardest clinical cases.

Part III

Phenotype Patterns

Ch 19: The Inverse Question and Its Limits

19.1 Why the Inverse Direction Is Harder

This book is the perturbation engine in a three-part clinical QEEG system. The forward direction (Parts I, II, IV, V, VI) asks what drugs do to the EEG. Part III asks the question that goes the other direction: what does the EEG say about which drugs will work? That is the inverse direction, and it is where the perturbation engine's logic reaches furthest from its empirical base. The limits in this chapter are the load-bearing architecture that keeps Part III from becoming overreach, not a disclaimer appended for form.

The preceding parts of this book address a forward question: given a medication, what happens to the EEG? Part III reverses the arrow.

Here the question becomes: given an EEG phenotype already present in the recording, what does the published literature say about how individuals carrying that pattern tend to respond to particular medication classes? This is the inverse direction, and it is the question that clients and prescribers ask most often.

19.2 Two Directions, One Dataset

Both directions use the same underlying data, but the inferential weight they can bear is not equivalent. When we ask "what does an SSRI do to the EEG?" we can draw on randomized controlled trials with pre-post spectral analysis, head-to-head comparisons, and dose-response curves. The causal direction is relatively clean: the drug is the intervention, the EEG change is the outcome.

When we invert the question, the logic shifts. Now we are asking whether a baseline EEG feature carries predictive information about clinical outcome under a given treatment. The evidence base for this question relies on prediction studies, pharmaco-EEG responder analyses, and retrospective phenotype-outcome correlations. The designs are observational or quasi-experimental. Sample sizes are often small. Replication is inconsistent.

The forward direction answers "what does the drug do to brain electrical activity?" The inverse direction attempts to answer "does this brain electrical pattern tell us something about who benefits from which drug?" The second question is harder, and the evidence supporting it is thinner.

19.3 The Group-to-Individual Translation Gap

The central caveat governs everything that follows: most of the prediction evidence reviewed in Part III comes from group-level studies. A study may demonstrate that patients with elevated frontal theta at baseline respond to a stimulant at higher rates than those without that feature. That finding describes a statistical tendency across a sample. Applying it to the individual client sitting in front of you is the step where confidence drops sharply.

Every framework in Chapter 20 and Chapter 21 was built and tested as a group exercise. Within-group spread routinely swamps between-group separation. Effect sizes in the best work stay small to moderate. The phenotype explains a slice of outcome variance; the rest sits in comorbidity, polypharmacy, sleep, substances, genetics, and factors the original study modeled partially or not at all.

When that finding meets the individual client, the screening math disappears. Your client was not run through inclusion criteria. Their stack of diagnoses and medications does not mirror the training sample. Spectral artifacts from their real-world pharmacology were not in the model. The gap between cohort association and bedside prediction is not a sample-size problem waiting for a bigger *n*; it is what happens when population tools meet single cases. Printing the map on letterhead does not convert cohort statistics into personal odds.

19.4 What Part III Is Not

Part III is not a prescribing guide. It does not tell the clinician which medication to recommend. QEEG findings should not be used to recommend medication discontinuation, dose changes, or pharmacologic substitution; those decisions rest with the prescriber. Every entry in Chapter 21 is hypothesis-generating; none constitutes a treatment directive.

What Part III provides is context. When a clinician identifies a phenotype and wonders whether the literature contains any signal about likely treatment response, Chapter 21 assembles that signal in one place, states its strength honestly, and leaves the clinical decision where it belongs: with the treating team.

19.5 Replication Issues Across Major Frameworks

The five major prediction frameworks underlying Chapter 21 each carry specific replication concerns. These should be read before relying on any individual entry.

Theta/beta ratio. TBR has the longest ADHD-related prediction history and the most forensic literature. The 2026 Strzelczyk multiverse analysis showed directly that defensible analytic choices (epoch selection, band boundaries, artifact handling) can create or erase apparent TBR effects from the same raw data (Strzelczyk et al., 2026). Boxum et al.'s (2024) EEG-subtyping work found no association between EEG subtype and behavioral traits, with small and non-significant effect sizes (Boxum et al., 2024). TBR retains some group-level signal; individual-level prediction is not supported by the current evidence base.

Frontal alpha asymmetry. A 2025 meta-analysis of resting FAA in depression found a small pooled effect for the standard F4-F3 measure (mean difference −0.03, 95% CI −0.05 to −0.01) with high heterogeneity across studies (Luo et al., 2025). Reference scheme changes the numbers: average, linked-ears, and Laplacian transforms can disagree on the same recording. Resting FAA is now better understood as a group-level association that survives pooling but is far too small to carry an individual prediction: a marker with strong theoretical backing whose effect size does not reach clinical usefulness.

Cordance. Cook and Leuchter's cordance metric was an early EEG response predictor. Uptake outside the originating labs was thin; a 2024 independent prospective trial in Indian MDD found early theta cordance shifts did not predict SSRI outcomes (Singh et al., 2024). The framework remains hypothesis-generating.

Brainmarker-I. Brainmarker-I (the iSPOT-D composite) is the most rigorously assembled SSRI-response predictor in major depressive disorder so far. Independent work has validated individual alpha peak frequency for TMS response (Baradits et al., 2026), but the pharmacotherapy claim (iAPF stratifies sertraline vs. placebo) still waits for an out-of-sample drug trial. Treat the sertraline finding as single-study until replication lands.

Suffin and Emory classification. This system has not received independent large-scale replication. The original studies were conducted by the system's developers. Until independent groups reproduce the predictive accuracy in adequately powered samples, the framework remains hypothesis-generating.

19.6 Known Failure Modes

Specific clinical scenarios reliably degrade prediction accuracy, and they are the scenarios most clinicians encounter daily.

Polypharmacy. When a client is taking multiple psychotropic medications, the recorded EEG phenotype reflects the combined spectral effects of all active compounds. The prediction frameworks were typically developed in medication-free or single-medication samples. Whether prediction retains any validity under polypharmacy is, for most frameworks, unknown.

State confounds. Sleep deprivation elevates theta and can shift TBR values into ADHD-mimic ranges. Recent caffeine changes arousal and is a live confound for alpha and asymmetry readings, though the literature does not fix a direction for either. Drowsiness during recording produces frontal theta that may be misidentified as a trait feature. Each of these state confounds can push a phenotype across a classification boundary without reflecting any stable trait relevant to medication response.

Pipeline variability. Reference scheme, artifact-rejection algorithm, normative database, epoch length, and frequency-band definitions all influence whether a phenotype is detected. The field lacks a standardized processing pipeline, and until one exists, phenotype detection will remain partially arbitrary.

Comorbidity. A client with comorbid ADHD, anxiety, and insomnia presents a spectral profile shaped by all three conditions. The prediction framework trained on isolated ADHD samples may misclassify or provide contradictory predictions when applied to a composite phenotype.

19.7 What Better Evidence Would Look Like

For the prediction frameworks in Part III to mature from hypothesis-generating associations into clinically actionable tools, the field needs: pre-registered multi-site replications powered to detect the modest observed effect sizes; within-subject longitudinal designs that track EEG phenotype stability and medication response; polypharmacy-inclusive samples; population-diverse samples; standardized processing pipelines; individual-level prediction accuracy reporting (not just group-level AUC); aperiodic-aware reanalysis of the key prediction datasets (most were conducted with band-power methods that do not separate periodic from aperiodic contributions); and cost-effectiveness trial data demonstrating that QEEG-guided treatment selection outperforms standard care. None of these standards is exotic. The field has not yet invested in them at the required scale.

19.8 Scope and Position

The associations described in Chapter 21 represent the best available signal from a literature whose evidence base has, if anything, weakened under recent scrutiny. No QEEG biomarker currently achieves the reliability required for standalone treatment decisions. Some clinical lore carries genuine signal even when the formal evidence base is thin.

The best use of inverse-direction inference is to ask better questions in the prescriber conversation, not to provide premature answers. The appropriate framing is: "The literature suggests this pattern is associated with differential response to this drug class, though the evidence has not been replicated consistently enough for clinical certainty. Does that inform your treatment planning?" That is a question, not a directive.

Chapter 20 picks up the lineages these signals came from. Chapter 21 presents the 45 entries themselves. The limits stated in this chapter apply to all of them.

For the clinical evidence trail on TBR as a prediction marker, see the companion Field Guide *Ch 6, Phenotype Atlas,* tbr_elevated *entry. For the developmental and age-graded normative work that defines "stable trait" against which medicated-state recordings are compared, see* Dynamic Brain *(the baseline engine in this trilogy).*

Ch 20: Pharmaco-EEG Prediction Lineages: From Suffin & Emory to Brainmarker-I

The premise of pharmaco-EEG is straightforward: if different brains respond differently to the same medication, and if EEG captures some of that difference before treatment begins, then a baseline recording should carry information about who will respond and who will not. Several research groups have pursued this idea across three decades. Each has produced real findings. None has delivered a tool that reliably predicts outcomes for a single patient sitting in a clinic. Understanding why requires tracing each lineage on its own terms.

20.1 Suffin & Emory: Neurometric Subgroups (1995)

The first serious attempt to use quantitative EEG for medication guidance came from Suffin and Emory, who applied John's neurometric framework to classify patients with attentional and affective disorders into EEG-defined subgroups (Suffin & Emory, 1995). The core claim was that these subgroups, defined by deviations from age-normed EEG databases, predicted differential treatment response with 80–85% accuracy, independent of the DSM diagnosis the patient carried.

The logic was appealing: DSM categories lump together patients with heterogeneous neurophysiology, so a physiologically grounded classification should outperform symptom checklists at matching patients to drugs. And the accuracy numbers looked strong. But several caveats limit what we can conclude. The samples were small. Independent replication at scale never materialized. The method was tied to a specific normative database (the NYU/E. Roy John database), meaning adoption required that exact infrastructure. Other labs working with different normative references could not straightforwardly reproduce the classification scheme.

Suffin and Emory's contribution was conceptual as much as empirical: the idea that EEG phenotypes might cut across diagnostic boundaries and predict pharmacological response became a guiding hypothesis for everything that followed. The evidence base for that specific classification system, however, remains thin.

No 2024-2026 work has changed this assessment. Reviews of EEG biomarkers cite the original study as historical and then note the absence of independent validation. The commercially derived rEEG/PEER Online platform, which descends from this lineage, has not produced independently run post-2014 RCTs demonstrating superior clinical outcomes over standard care. Commercial adoption has outpaced scientific validation, and clinicians should be aware that marketing claims for QEEG-guided prescribing in this tradition are not supported by peer-reviewed outcome data at the standard required for clinical recommendation.

20.2 Theta Cordance: Perfusion Proxies and Early Change (Leuchter, Bares)

Cordance is a derived EEG measure that combines absolute and relative power in a way that correlates with regional cerebral perfusion, as Leuchter and colleagues demonstrated in the mid-1990s (Leuchter et al., 1994). The measure gained clinical interest when subsequent work showed that early changes in prefrontal theta cordance, specifically reductions during the first one to two weeks of antidepressant treatment, predicted eventual treatment response.

Bares and colleagues provided key replication data. A 2007 study showed that prefrontal cordance at week one separated eventual responders from nonresponders to antidepressants (Bares et al., 2007), and a 2008 follow-up found the same week-one prefrontal cordance separation in treatment-resistant inpatients receiving venlafaxine (Bares et al., 2008). The timing specificity was the strongest feature of this work: the biomarker operated at a clinically useful window, potentially allowing clinicians to switch medications weeks before conventional symptom-based assessment would reveal nonresponse.

The BRITE-MD study, a randomized trial led by Leuchter's group, tested cordance prospectively as a biomarker for SSRI response (Leuchter et al., 2009). The results supported the association at the group level. But individual-level classification accuracy remained modest, and the method turned out to be sensitive to recording parameters, reference schemes, and analysis pipelines. Theta cordance has been replicated across multiple independent groups, which distinguishes it from some other pharmaco-EEG markers. Yet clinical adoption has been minimal. The gap between a statistically significant group-level predictor and a decision-grade clinical tool proved wider than the early enthusiasm suggested.

Subsequent work has reinforced these concerns. A 2024 prospective trial in an Indian MDD sample tested early frontal theta cordance changes as a predictor of SSRI response and found no significant predictive value ($p = 0.37$) (Singh et al., 2024). A 2024 meta-analysis of QEEG changes with antidepressant treatment found that cordance and related markers show reliable group-level change during treatment ($d \approx 0.8$), supporting the measure as a treatment-tracking marker, but emphasized that this does not translate into reliable individual-level prediction before treatment begins (Srivastava et al., 2024). The distinction matters: a marker that changes when treatment works is not the same as a marker that predicts who will respond before treatment starts. Cordance has earned its place as a historically important lineage, but its clinical utility as a prospective predictor remains unestablished.

20.3 Frontal Alpha Asymmetry: Approach, Withdrawal, and Sex Differences (Davidson, Bruder)

Davidson's approach-withdrawal model, first proposed in the early 1980s (Davidson & Fox, 1982) and refined over subsequent decades (Davidson, 2004), provided a theoretical scaffold for linking frontal alpha asymmetry (FAA) to affective processing. The model holds that relatively greater left frontal activity indexes approach motivation, while rightward asymmetry indexes withdrawal. Depression, in this framework, involves a deficit in approach-related left frontal engagement.

A convention note applies throughout this chapter and Chapter 21: alpha power and cortical activation run in opposite directions at a given scalp site. More alpha power means less cortical activation. When the text says "greater right-sided frontal alpha," it means higher alpha amplitude on the right, which corresponds to less right-sided cortical activation and, by contrast, relatively greater left-sided activation. Confusing the two is how a single asymmetry finding can appear to predict opposite clinical outcomes in different passages; this book keeps them separate by always specifying whether a statement is about alpha power or about inferred activation.

Bruder and colleagues translated this framework into a pharmaco-EEG prediction context. A 2001 study showed that FAA patterns at baseline differed between patients who went on to respond to SSRIs and those who did not (Bruder et al., 2001). Responders showed the expected pattern of relatively greater right-sided frontal alpha (consistent with greater left frontal activity), while nonresponders did not. The 2008 follow-up, however, introduced a complication: the responder/nonresponder asymmetry difference showed up at occipital rather than frontal sites, and the authors noted that the hemispheric difference had been stronger among women in their earlier, more female samples (Bruder et al., 2008).

The theoretical grounding is the strength of this lineage. FAA connects to a broader literature on affective neuroscience, giving it face validity that purely empirical markers lack. The weaknesses are equally clear. The Thibodeau 2006 meta-analysis found small-to-moderate effect sizes across FAA studies in depression, and those effects were sensitive to recording reference scheme (linked ears vs. average reference can flip the direction of findings). The sex dependency adds another source of heterogeneity. Across studies, FAA has not produced classification accuracies high enough for individual treatment decisions.

The evidence has continued to weaken. A 2025 meta-analysis of resting frontal alpha asymmetry in depression found a small pooled effect for the standard F4-F3 measure (mean difference −0.03, 95% CI −0.05 to −0.01) with high heterogeneity, and subgroup analyses by reference montage and severity did not account for that heterogeneity (Luo et al., 2025). The authors read this as a modest association between FAA and depression rather than a clinical test. That is enough to demote FAA from a promising-but-modest predictor to a group-level effect far too small to guide an individual medication choice. The sex-dependency findings have not been independently confirmed in adequately powered samples. FAA retains historical importance as the marker that connected the Davidson approach-withdrawal model to pharmacotherapy prediction, but clinicians should not treat resting FAA as an actionable predictor for medication selection.

20.4 Theta/Beta Ratio and Stimulant Response: Enthusiasm Meets Replication (Arns)

The theta/beta ratio (TBR) story in ADHD is the canonical cautionary tale in pharmaco-EEG. Initial work by Arns and colleagues in 2008 found that EEG phenotypes, including elevated TBR, predicted stimulant treatment outcome in children with ADHD (Arns et al., 2008). A 2012 study linked individual alpha peak frequency (iAPF) to stimulant nonresponse, adding a second EEG feature to the prediction model (Arns, 2012).

The 2013 meta-analysis, however, painted a more sober picture (Arns et al., 2013). Pooled across studies, TBR sensitivity for ADHD diagnosis was lower than the initial reports suggested, and the authors concluded that elevated TBR cannot be treated as a reliable diagnostic measure. The same analysis kept a prognostic role for excess theta and TBR in a subgroup of patients, where it has been associated with stimulant and neurofeedback outcomes. Boxum and colleagues (2024) reached a compatible conclusion through a different approach, separating a slow-alpha subgroup from a genuinely high-theta subgroup and finding no association between EEG subtype and behavioral traits (Boxum et al., 2024).

The trajectory has continued downward. Strzelczyk and colleagues' (2026) multiverse analysis directly challenged TBR's diagnostic value, demonstrating that analytic flexibility (epoch selection, band boundaries, artifact handling) can create or erase apparent TBR effects across reasonable pipeline variants (Strzelczyk et al., 2026). Payer policies as of 2025 continue to classify the NEBA system as investigational, with limited evidence of improved clinical outcomes. TBR's trajectory from biomarker candidate to cautionary tale is now largely complete; the ratio retains some group-level signal, but its clinical utility for individual treatment decisions is not supported by the current evidence base.

20.5 ATR Index: Composite Biomarker for Medication Selection (Leuchter, Greenwald)

The Antidepressant Treatment Response (ATR) Index grew out of Leuchter's cordance work and represents the most ambitious attempt to turn cordance-derived EEG features into a clinical decision tool. The ATR is a composite measure combining frontal alpha and theta features into a 0–100 probability score. It was tested in the BRITE-MD trial (n = 375), a randomized study comparing escitalopram with bupropion in major depressive disorder (Leuchter et al., 2009). Patients with ATR scores above a threshold (~58) predicted escitalopram remission with reported specificities of 82–91%. Patients with low ATR scores showed better outcomes when switched to bupropion, framing the ATR as a medication-selection tool rather than a simple response predictor.

The BRITE-MD trial is methodologically stronger than most work in this space: it was prospective, multi-site, and randomized. The ATR's claim is also more clinically actionable than cordance alone, because it answers "which drug?" rather than "will any drug work?" Those strengths are real. The limitations are equally clear. The classification thresholds have not been independently replicated outside Leuchter's group. The ATR measure is proprietary, limiting independent validation. The sample, though larger than most pharmaco-EEG studies, is still modest for a tool intended for individual-level prediction. The specificity numbers come from post-hoc threshold optimization on the same dataset, which inflates apparent accuracy. No subsequent RCT has tested ATR-guided treatment selection against standard care to show improved clinical outcomes.

For BoD's purposes, the ATR Index is a phenotype inference: a well-designed single-trial finding with plausible mechanism, awaiting independent replication and pragmatic-trial validation. Clinicians may reference the ATR as supporting evidence in prescriber conversations, but should not treat it as a validated clinical decision tool.

20.6 iSPOT-D: Large-Scale Response Prediction (Williams)

The International Study to Predict Optimized Treatment for Depression (iSPOT-D) was a large, multi-site, randomized trial comparing three antidepressants (escitalopram, sertraline, and venlafaxine) in adults with MDD (Williams et al., 2011). The study collected baseline EEG, cognitive, and clinical measures with the explicit goal of identifying pre-treatment predictors of differential response.

iSPOT-D's EEG findings partially overlap with other lineages. Frontal alpha asymmetry showed sex-dependent prediction of SSRI response, consistent with the Bruder FAA lineage but with larger samples. The study also found that a combination of EEG and cognitive features outperformed either alone in predicting response, suggesting that multi-modal approaches may be necessary for clinically useful accuracy. The Voetterl 2023 Brainmarker-I framework (see below) drew on the iSPOT-D dataset, making this trial the empirical substrate for the field's most methodologically advanced prediction model.

The iSPOT-D contribution is in its scale and multi-modal design. The limitations are that, despite its size, individual-level classification accuracy remained modest when EEG was used alone. The study demonstrated that the prediction problem is harder than early single-site work suggested, and that combining modalities is likely necessary. No subsequent pragmatic trial has tested iSPOT-derived algorithms in clinical decision-making.

20.7 Brainmarker-I: Pre-Registered and Prospective (Voetterl 2023)

The most recent entry in this lineage is Brainmarker-I, published by Voetterl and colleagues in *Nature Mental Health* (Voetterl, Sack, et al., 2023). The approach uses individual alpha peak frequency to stratify patients with major depressive disorder into those more likely to respond to sertraline (Zoloft) versus those more likely to respond to brain stimulation (rTMS, ECT). The study specified its analyses in advance, drew on a large pooled sample, and explicitly addressed methodological weaknesses that plagued earlier pharmaco-EEG work: reference-scheme sensitivity, lack of prospective validation, and small samples.

Brainmarker-I represents a genuine methodological step forward. The pre-registration alone distinguishes it from most prior work in this space, where analytic flexibility and post-hoc subgroup analyses were common. The sample size provides power that earlier studies lacked. And the focus on a binary stratification question (SSRI vs. stimulation) rather than continuous outcome prediction may be better matched to the actual information content of baseline EEG.

The limitations are scope and maturity. The framework is specific to MDD and does not yet extend to ADHD or anxiety prediction. Independent replication is ongoing but not yet published. And even within depression, the stratification is between two broad treatment categories, not among specific medications. Whether the approach generalizes beyond its initial validation cohort remains an open question.

As of early 2026, independent replication has arrived, but not for pharmacotherapy. A 2025 study validated iAPF as a predictor of rTMS response in depression in an independent sample (Baradits et al., 2026), and a 2024 analysis extended the Brainmarker-I logic to show that patients with 9 Hz alpha respond differently to 18 Hz deep TMS versus 10 Hz rTMS. These replications strengthen the case that iAPF captures something real about treatment-response heterogeneity. But the specific claim that iAPF predicts sertraline (Zoloft) response better than placebo has not been independently tested in a pharmacological trial. The distinction matters for this book: the drug-response prediction remains a single-study finding, and clinicians should frame it as the best-designed single trial in the field rather than as a replicated clinical tool.

20.8 Poor Stimulant-Response Subtypes: COMT Variants and Spindling Beta (Clarke, Arns)

Not all ADHD-presenting clients carry the frontal-theta phenotype that predicts stimulant response. Two well-characterized subtypes predict poor stimulant outcomes through distinct mechanisms, and distinguishing them from the stimulant-responsive phenotype changes what should be monitored and communicated to the prescriber.

Slowed alpha peak frequency (COMT variant). Some clients presenting with inattention and cognitive slowness show a dominant posterior alpha peak at 8–9 Hz rather than the age-expected 10–11 Hz. A common clinical reading attributes this pattern to the COMT Met/Met genotype, which produces slow dopamine metabolism in prefrontal cortex. That genotype link is a workflow heuristic: it is a mechanistic hypothesis, not a finding from the iAPF literature cited below. The "slowness" is not frontal theta excess but a constitutionally slowed alpha generator, and the distinction is clinically critical: stimulants increase beta activity and catecholaminergic drive but do not address the thalamocortical timing deficit that slowed alpha reflects. Clients with this pattern frequently report that stimulants increase anxiety without improving focus. The slowed-alpha phenotype overlaps with the Brainmarker-I slow-iAPF finding (see above), which showed that slow iAPF predicted superior sertraline response against placebo-controlled comparison data and poorer stimulant response in blinded out-of-sample validation (Voetterl, Sack, et al., 2023; Voetterl, Wingen, et al., 2023). The ADHD arm carries its own population limits: the stratification rule was specified for boys, and the blinded methylphenidate validation ran in 41 clients. When QEEG showed slowed posterior alpha rather than frontal theta excess in the study sample, the Brainmarker-I stratification placed these clients in the non-stimulant arm, where the studied treatment was sertraline. This is a group-level research association and is not validated to select or avoid medication for an individual.

Spindling excessive beta (Clarke ADHD subtype). Clarke and colleagues compared good and poor methylphenidate responders in ADHD and found that the poor responders were less cortically hypoaroused than the good responders (Clarke, Barry, McCarthy, et al., 2002). The clinical extension of that work, which is a workflow heuristic, describes an excess-beta subtype of roughly 10% of ADHD cases, marked by high-amplitude beta (20–30 Hz) with spindle morphology and frontal dominance, in which methylphenidate reduces beta slightly while the child stays over-aroused, with insomnia, anxiety, and agitation. The mechanism is straightforward: stimulants augment fast-frequency cortical activity, which amplifies the existing hyperarousal rather than correcting it. Neurofeedback (beta suppression, SMR training) is an in-scope non-pharmacological referral. No prospective trial has randomized excess-beta ADHD clients to stimulant versus non-stimulant treatment. The Clarke data and the mechanistic logic identify activation-related adverse effects (insomnia, anxiety, agitation) as the monitoring priority when a prescriber independently trials a stimulant in this subgroup.

20.9 GABAergic Response Prediction: LVF, Beta Spindles, and Addiction Vulnerability

The prediction literature identifies two QEEG phenotypes that converge on GABAergic medication-response prediction, each with distinct clinical implications.

Low-voltage fast (LVF) EEG. The LVF phenotype (low-amplitude, globally fast) has been linked to alcoholism and to GABAA receptor genes, and is otherwise described as a normal variant (Johnstone et al., 2005). Reading it as chronic cortical hyperarousal is a clinical interpretation laid on top of that link, not part of it. When LVF co-occurs with a family history of alcohol use disorder, the inference that the client will respond strongly to GABAergic agents and carries elevated addiction vulnerability is an extrapolation from that genetic link rather than a tested finding. The proposed mechanism follows from constitutionally underactive GABAergic inhibition: exogenous GABA enhancement (alcohol, benzodiazepines, neurosteroids) produces the subjective relief that drives both therapeutic response and dependence risk. Where LVF co-occurs with that family history, the dependence-vulnerability context is what the clinician can usefully pass to the prescriber. The expected-response half is an extrapolation the book does not make, and agent selection does not need it.

Beta spindles and thalamocortical GABAergic dysregulation. Spindling excessive beta (15–20 Hz bursts) reflects GABAergic dysregulation in thalamocortical circuits and correlates with the "can't turn brain off" phenomenology that predicts benzodiazepine sensitivity. The clinical prediction is response to GABAergic interventions broadly (alcohol, benzodiazepines, possibly cannabis), with the same addiction-risk caveat that applies to LVF. Gabapentinoids are sometimes named in this context and do not belong. They are alpha-2-delta calcium-channel ligands, and the gabapentin label states that the drug has no effect on GABA binding, uptake, or degradation, so grouping them with GABA enhancers misstates the mechanism. No QEEG marker predicts response to them, and they carry a labeled warning for serious respiratory depression when combined with opioids or other CNS depressants. Beta spindles are trainable: neurofeedback can reduce spindling without pharmacological tolerance, making this an actionable pattern for non-pharmacological intervention referral.

Neither LVF nor beta spindling has been tested as a medication-prediction marker in a controlled trial; the evidence is clinical-observation-grade with strong mechanistic backing. The composite prediction across these patterns is a phenotype inference for the LVF-alcoholism link (replicated in clinical populations) and a workflow heuristic for the broader GABAergic-response claim.

20.10 Limited-Response Lineage: Patterns Associated with Poor Pharmacotherapy Outcomes

The prediction literature also identifies patterns associated with poor medication response across drug classes at the group level. The clinical value is in recognizing when the population-level evidence suggests that first-line pharmacotherapy alone may be insufficient, so that monitoring and differential diagnosis can be planned accordingly.

Focal left anterior temporal slowing. Focal alpha-theta slowing at left temporal sites (T3/F7) appears in a subset of treatment-refractory depressed patients. In clinical case series, this group has shown poor antidepressant response alongside reports of benefit from neuromodulation (TMS, tDCS targeting the left temporal region, neurofeedback). The mechanism is unclear, and the pattern rests on clinical observation rather than trial data: localized temporal slowing is read as marking a dissociation between medication response and stimulation response at the group level. Suffin and Emory's original neurometric subgrouping defined its medication-response classes from frontal features rather than temporal ones, so it does not speak to this pattern directly (Suffin & Emory, 1995).

Diffuse low-voltage EEG. Low amplitudes across all bands, producing a flat or "encephalopathic" appearance, have been associated in clinical accounts with limited SSRI benefit and higher side-effect sensitivity. This pattern is consistent with a cortex operating at low energy that responds poorly to pharmacological perturbation. No prospective trial has tested alternative approaches in clients selected for this phenotype, so the association identifies a possible limit of SSRI monotherapy at the group level without indicating a specific next step.

Atypical multi-band dysregulation. Epileptiform discharges, extreme fast activity, or complex dysregulation across multiple bands have been associated at the group level with low rates of remission under conventional antidepressant monotherapy. These patterns suggest a complicated neurological substrate where multimodal treatment approaches or neurofeedback are commonly considered alongside pharmacotherapy, though no prospective trial has validated this sequencing.

The evidence for medication-resistance patterns is observational and retrospective. No prospective trial has enrolled clients selected by these QEEG features and randomized them to alternative treatments. The hypothesis is that identifying these patterns early may spare clients extended trials of monotherapy unlikely to succeed, but that hypothesis has not been tested prospectively.

20.11 The Honest Replication Picture

Every lineage surveyed here has produced group-level associations between EEG features and treatment outcomes that appear to be real. Cordance changes at week two predict antidepressant response better than chance. Frontal alpha asymmetry differs, on average, between SSRI responders and nonresponders. EEG phenotypes carry some information about stimulant outcomes in ADHD. These are genuine signals, not artifacts.

What makes TBR instructive is the trajectory. Early single-site studies with enthusiastic conclusions gave way to pooled analyses and independent replications that shrank the effects. The FDA's 2013 clearance of TBR as an aid to ADHD diagnosis (the NEBA system) added regulatory momentum at a point when the scientific literature was already moving toward caution. The lesson generalizes beyond ADHD: group-level associations in pharmaco-EEG often survive replication, but the effect sizes that matter for individual prediction frequently do not hold up to multicenter scrutiny.

The recent literature has sharpened this picture rather than resolved it. FAA has largely lost its signal under meta-analytic scrutiny. Cordance has failed to replicate as a prospective predictor in at least one independent sample. TBR's methodological fragility has been documented in detail. Brainmarker-I has been validated in neuromodulation but not yet in pharmacotherapy specifically. Machine-learning approaches report impressive in-sample accuracies, and where a validation cohort exists it can be five patients from the same hospital, a same-site holdout rather than out-of-sample generalization (Li et al., 2026). The field's methodology is improving; Brainmarker-I's preregistered, prospective design represents real progress. But the destination, reliable individual prediction for medication selection, has not been reached. The literature supports cautious engagement with these tools in clinical conversations, paired with honest acknowledgment that no QEEG biomarker is ready for standalone use in treatment decisions. QEEG findings should not be used to recommend medication discontinuation, dose changes, or pharmacologic substitution; those decisions rest with the prescriber.

For phenotype-by-phenotype pattern recognition guides and exemplar EEG plates organized by the same taxonomy used in this chapter and in Ch 21, see the companion Field Guide *Ch 6 phenotype atlas.*

Ch 21: Phenotype-by-Phenotype Treatment-Response Hypotheses

This chapter presents 45 entries: 41 phenotypes shared with the *QEEG Field Guide* taxonomy (31 individual phenotypes + 10 composite signatures) plus 4 medication-prediction constructs specific to this book (see Appendix G for the full crosswalk). Each entry describes a recognizable QEEG pattern, summarizes the published evidence linking that pattern to medication response or non-response, and identifies the claim type of the entry's central statement. The entries are organized by domain: Approach, Avoid, Cognitive, Social, Arousal, Sensorimotor, Learning, Symbols, and Stability.

Entry structure. Every entry opens with a prediction question: given a client presenting with this phenotype, what does the literature suggest about treatment response? The body summarizes treatment-response hypotheses, names the relevant prediction frameworks (Suffin & Emory, Arns TBR, Bruder FAA, Bares cordance, Brainmarker-I, and others as applicable), and frames the mechanism behind the predicted response. Caveats about group-to-individual translation follow. Each entry closes with a forward-direction cross-reference pointing the reader to the Part II chapter where the relevant drug class's EEG effects are cataloged.

Claim types. Entries carry one of three claim-type labels, following the taxonomy defined in Chapter 4. A spectral-effect label marks a claim about a directly measured spectral change under a drug; no inverse-direction entry in this chapter carries that label. A phenotype-inference label marks a claim about an empirical association between a measured phenotype and a treatment outcome, regardless of the association's strength. A workflow-heuristic label marks a claim about a clinical reasoning convention or interpretive procedure applied when the phenotype is encountered. The label names the kind of claim the entry makes. Evidence quality for the underlying association is discussed in words within each entry, not encoded in the label.

The group-to-individual caveat applies to every entry. Even spectral-effect associations describe statistical tendencies across samples, not deterministic predictions for individual clients. Chapter 19 discusses this gap and its limits in detail.

Cross-references. Each entry's closing line points to the relevant Part II chapter where the drug class's forward-direction EEG effects are described. The inverse direction raises a hypothesis; the forward direction provides monitoring parameters.

Scope boundary. QEEG findings should not be used to recommend medication discontinuation, dose changes, or pharmacologic substitution; those decisions rest with the prescriber. Every entry below is hypothesis-generating; none constitutes a treatment directive.

A note on precedent. This chapter presents an openly published, claim-type-rated, citation-anchored phenotype-to-treatment-response catalog in the pharmaco-EEG field. Commercial platforms (PEER Online, the proprietary rEEG/database-referenced pharmacotherapy prediction system developed from the Suffin and Emory neurometric subgroup work, and Brainmarker) carry proprietary versions of this logic. The academic prediction frameworks (Suffin and Emory 1995 (Suffin & Emory, 1995), Arns TBR, Bruder FAA, Bares cordance, Brainmarker-I) and the neurofeedback phenotype-classification tradition (Gunkelman and Johnstone 2003, 2005 (Gunkelman & Johnstone, 2005; Johnstone & Gunkelman, 2003)) are the direct intellectual predecessors of the entries here. This catalog synthesizes, extends, and rates those lineages by claim type in a single open clinical reference.

If you are reading this chapter as a reference lookup: You are likely here during a clinical case. Before using a Part III entry, confirm that forward-direction confidence for the phenotype is at least moderate (Step 9 of Chapter 26). If an active medication, state, or condition factor explains the phenotype, the inverse-direction inference is premature. Each entry assumes you have already done that check. Chapter 19 states the replication limits for the underlying prediction frameworks; those limits apply to every entry below.

21.1 Approach Domain

21.1.1 Frontal Alpha Asymmetry (Left > Right) [workflow heuristic]

Prediction question. For clients presenting with relatively greater left frontal alpha (consistent with reduced left frontal activation and possible approach deficit), what does the literature suggest about treatment response?

The Davidson approach-withdrawal model (Davidson, 2004; Davidson & Fox, 1982) provides the theoretical basis for interpreting this pattern. Greater left frontal alpha implies reduced left-hemisphere frontal activity, which in the approach-withdrawal framework indexes diminished approach motivation. The opposite direction of this asymmetry (right greater than left) has received more attention in the medication-prediction literature, including Bruder's work on SSRI response prediction (Bruder et al., 2001; Bruder et al., 2008). The left-greater-than-right direction, by contrast, has not been tested as a predictor of treatment outcome in any published pharmacotherapy trial.

Without direct medication-prediction data, clinical reasoning proceeds from the underlying model rather than from empirical outcome studies. If the mechanism involves reduced left frontal engagement, interventions that increase frontal activation (stimulants, activating antidepressants, behavioral activation) might theoretically address the pattern. However, this reasoning is mechanistic inference, not evidence-based prediction. No prospective study has examined whether clients carrying this specific asymmetry direction respond differentially to any drug class.

The practical implication is that this phenotype should not drive medication recommendations. Treatment decisions should be guided by symptom presentation and by other phenotype features that carry stronger evidence, not by the asymmetry score in isolation.

Forward-direction cross-reference. Stimulant and SSRI effects on frontal alpha distributions are cataloged in Part II Ch 5 (Stimulants) and Ch 6 (SSRIs and SNRIs); read those before forming a monitoring plan around this asymmetry direction.

Pattern recognition and differential diagnosis: see Field Guide Ch 6, Frontal Alpha Asymmetry (Left > Right) entry.

21.1.2 Frontal Alpha Excess [workflow heuristic]

Prediction question. For clients presenting with elevated alpha power over frontal regions relative to posterior sites, what does the literature suggest about treatment response?

Frontal alpha excess appears in the QEEG subtyping literature on ADHD as a pattern characterized by alpha intrusion over frontal leads rather than by the theta-excess profile more commonly associated with stimulant response (Chabot & Serfontein, 1996; Clarke et al., 2001). It is not one of the three clusters Clarke and colleagues enumerated, which were defined by slow-wave excess, high-amplitude theta with beta deficiency, and excess beta; treat frontal alpha excess as a phenotype of the broader subtyping tradition rather than as a replicated cluster. The pathophysiology of this pattern appears distinct from the classic frontal-theta ADHD phenotype: where theta excess suggests cortical underactivation, frontal alpha excess suggests inappropriate idling or disengagement of frontal networks.

This distinction matters for pharmacotherapy expectations. The theta-excess ADHD subtype has at least moderate evidence linking it to stimulant responsiveness (see entry for `frontal_theta_high`). The alpha-excess subtype lacks comparable medication-prediction data. No prospective study has tested whether stimulants, non-stimulant ADHD medications, or antidepressants produce differential outcomes in clients selected specifically for frontal alpha excess. The Brainmarker-I framework (Voetterl, Sack, et al., 2023; Voetterl, Wingen, et al., 2023) does not directly address this phenotype, though slow individual alpha peak frequency, which can co-occur with frontal alpha excess, is part of that model's stratification logic.

Clinically, the absence of prediction data does not mean the phenotype is irrelevant to the prescriber conversation. It means the conversation should be framed around the distinct pathophysiology rather than around predicted drug response. A client with frontal alpha excess who is being treated as a standard theta-excess ADHD case may be receiving an intervention matched to the wrong mechanism. That observation is hypothesis-generating, not prescriptive.

Forward-direction cross-reference. Because the alpha-excess subtype lacks a clean prediction signal, the prescriber conversation depends on knowing what stimulants and SSRIs do to alpha-band activity in the first place; that forward evidence sits in Part II Ch 5 (Stimulants) and Ch 6 (SSRIs and SNRIs).

Exemplar plates and normative reference: Field Guide Ch 6, Frontal Alpha Excess entry.

21.2 Avoid Domain

21.2.1 Frontal Alpha Asymmetry (Right > Left, Withdrawal) [phenotype inference]

Prediction question. For clients presenting with relatively greater right frontal alpha (consistent with right frontal hypoactivation and a withdrawal-motivation pattern), what does the literature suggest about treatment response?

This is the asymmetry direction most studied in the medication-prediction context. Bruder and colleagues demonstrated that baseline frontal alpha asymmetry patterns differed between patients who went on to respond to SSRIs and those who did not (Bruder et al., 2001). Responders showed relatively greater right-sided frontal alpha (indicating greater left frontal activation), which in the Davidson framework reflects preserved approach motivation. A 2008 follow-up, however, introduced a significant qualifier: frontal alpha asymmetry did not separate fluoxetine responders from nonresponders in that sample, and the responder/nonresponder difference appeared at occipital rather than frontal sites (Bruder et al., 2008). The authors noted that the hemispheric difference had been stronger among women in their earlier, more heavily female samples, so sex may account for part of the inconsistency.

Effect sizes across the FAA prediction literature are modest. The Thibodeau 2006 meta-analysis reported small-to-moderate effects for the FAA-depression relationship broadly, and the subset of studies examining medication response prediction produced even smaller effects. Reference-scheme sensitivity compounds the problem: linked ears, average reference, and Laplacian derivations can produce different asymmetry values from the same recording, and some studies have reported directional reversals depending on the reference chosen.

A 2025 meta-analysis of resting frontal alpha asymmetry in depression found a small grand mean effect size for the F4–F3 contrast (ES = −0.03, 95% CI −0.05 to −0.01), statistically significant but with high heterogeneity ($I^2 = 75.1\%$), and subgroup analyses by reference montage did not resolve the inconsistency (Luo et al., 2025). The authors read that as a modest diagnostic association. An effect of that size, measured against diagnosis rather than against treatment response, does not carry FAA as a standalone predictor. The Bruder findings remain historically instructive, but they should be read against a field that has not been able to replicate them consistently.

The literature suggests that FAA carries some information about SSRI response in depressed populations, but the signal is not strong enough to serve as a standalone predictor. Sex-dependent effects further limit generalizability. In practice, FAA should function as one data point among several in the clinician-prescriber conversation, with explicit acknowledgment that individual-level prediction accuracy has not been established. The sex-dependency finding is worth communicating to the prescriber, as it qualifies which clients the literature most directly applies to.

Forward-direction cross-reference. Before interpreting this asymmetry as an SSRI-response signal, read Part II Ch 6 (SSRIs and SNRIs) for what the drug does to frontal alpha distributions.

Visual reference and detection criteria: Field Guide Ch 6, Frontal Alpha Asymmetry (Right > Left, Withdrawal) entry.

21.2.2 Elevated Frontal High Beta [phenotype inference]

Prediction question. For clients presenting with elevated high-beta power localized to frontal sites, what does the literature suggest about treatment response?

Elevated frontal high beta is associated with cognitive hyperarousal, worry-dominant anxiety presentations, OCD, and the ADHD excess-beta subtype described by Clarke and colleagues (Clarke et al., 2001). The medication-prediction implications differ depending on the clinical context.

In the ADHD context, the excess-beta subtype presents a specific pharmacological concern. Stimulant medications increase catecholaminergic drive and tend to augment fast-frequency cortical activity. For a client whose ADHD presentation already features elevated frontal beta, stimulant exposure risks amplifying the hyperarousal component. Clarke's subtype literature identified this profile among poor stimulant responders, but no trial has tested dose adjustment or agent-class selection in clients prospectively identified by the excess-beta phenotype. Non-stimulant ADHD medications (atomoxetine (Strattera), guanfacine, clonidine) operate through mechanisms less likely to augment cortical fast-frequency activity; whether that mechanistic difference translates into better outcomes for this subtype has not been tested.

In the anxiety or OCD context, the elevated frontal beta pattern overlaps with the global hyperarousal phenotype addressed elsewhere in this chapter. SSRIs are commonly prescribed for these presentations and may reduce the hyperarousal component indirectly through anxiety reduction, but no study has examined whether baseline frontal beta levels predict SSRI response specifically.

What to say to the prescriber. "This client presents wound up and worry-driven, and the recording lines up with that: high beta is up at frontal sites, and conditions were stable enough that I don't think it's a benzodiazepine effect or a bad day. Clarke described this as a beta-heavy subtype of ADHD, and on average those clients have a rougher time on stimulants, though nobody has run the trial that would tell you whether this client is one of them. If a stimulant trial goes forward, activation-related side effects like anxiety or insomnia are the things I'd plan to monitor."

Forward-direction cross-reference. For how stimulants affect beta activity and how benzodiazepines produce beta signatures, see Part II Ch 5 (Stimulants) and Ch 8 (Benzodiazepines).

For clinical phenotype recognition, consult Field Guide Ch 6, Elevated Frontal High Beta entry.

21.2.3 Posterior Cingulate Hyperactivation [workflow heuristic]

Prediction question. For clients presenting with elevated theta and alpha power at Pz, consistent with posterior cingulate or posterior default-mode network overactivation, what does the literature suggest about treatment response?

No published study has directly examined whether this specific QEEG phenotype predicts differential medication response. The clinical reasoning here is entirely mechanistic, drawn from the broader default-mode network (DMN) literature rather than from EEG-based prediction studies.

The posterior cingulate cortex (PCC) is one of the regions whose task-related deactivation defined the default mode in the first place (Raichle et al., 2001). The onward associations between excessive DMN activation and rumination, self-referential processing, and treatment-resistant depression come from later fMRI work rather than from that founding paper. If PCC hyperactivation measured at Pz reflects DMN overengagement, then interventions that reduce DMN activity might be expected to benefit these clients. SSRIs and psychotherapy have both been shown to reduce DMN hyperconnectivity in some MDD samples, providing a mechanistic rationale for their use. Mindfulness-based interventions, which specifically target the disengagement of ruminative self-referential loops, have shown PCC deactivation in meditation studies and may serve as a useful adjunct.

However, linking scalp-level EEG findings at a single electrode to a specific cortical generator is inherently uncertain. Pz theta/alpha excess can reflect volume-conducted posterior alpha, drowsiness, or other sources unrelated to PCC function. The mechanistic chain from scalp measurement to DMN interpretation to medication prediction contains multiple uncertain steps, each of which reduces confidence. This entry is hypothesis-generating in the strongest sense of that qualifier: the hypothesis is plausible, but no element of it has been tested directly in a pharmacotherapy prediction design.

Forward-direction cross-reference. SSRI and SNRI spectral effects on alpha and theta are described in Part II Ch 6, which is the monitoring chapter to consult once a serotonergic agent has been started.

For pattern recognition and exemplar plates, see Field Guide *Ch 6, Posterior Cingulate Hyperactivation entry.*

21.3 Cognitive Domain

21.3.1 Elevated Frontal Theta [phenotype inference]

Prediction question. For clients presenting with elevated theta power at frontal sites, what does the literature suggest about treatment response?

Elevated frontal theta is the most studied phenotype in the ADHD medication-prediction literature. Suffin and Emory's 1995 work placed theta-excess patients into a neurometric subgroup that predicted favorable stimulant response (Suffin & Emory, 1995). Arns and colleagues' 2008 study found that children with ADHD carrying a frontal slow phenotype improved on a continuous-performance measure under stimulant treatment; that study classified by visually identified phenotype rather than by the theta/beta ratio, and argued against reading frontal theta through traditional band boundaries at all (Arns et al., 2008). The mechanism is straightforward: frontal theta excess reflects cortical underactivation in frontal networks, and stimulants increase catecholaminergic drive to those networks. When stimulants normalize the theta elevation, the client tends to experience clinical improvement.

The Suffin and Emory framework also used a medication challenge design: a single dose of stimulant was administered while EEG was recorded, and reduction in frontal theta under the drug was taken as evidence that the medication was engaging the relevant physiology. The mechanistic reasoning is that theta normalization reflects a catecholaminergic deficit that the stimulant corrects, while persistent theta may indicate a different mechanism of inattention. That design has not been validated in a controlled trial, and its individual-level accuracy is unknown.

The caveats are extensive. Arns's 2013 meta-analysis showed that TBR sensitivity for ADHD diagnosis was lower than initial reports suggested (Arns et al., 2013), and the Boxum 2024 EEG-subtyping meta-analysis, which separated a true high-TBR subgroup from a slow-alpha-peak-frequency subgroup, found only small and non-significant differences between those subgroups on behavioral measures (Boxum et al., 2024). Sleep deprivation elevates frontal theta independently of attention pathology and can push a non-ADHD client across the detection threshold for this phenotype, and the theta-beta profile itself shifts with age. Adult ADHD may present with theta excess but without the beta deficit seen in pediatric samples (Bresnahan et al., 1999). State confounds must be ruled out before interpreting frontal theta as a stable trait marker.

The literature supports a moderate association between frontal theta elevation and stimulant response at the group level, especially in studies that used a medication challenge to demonstrate theta normalization. Individual-level prediction remains limited. This finding should be presented to the prescriber as supporting evidence, not as a clinical directive.

What to say to the prescriber. "I screened sleep and state before I read this one, so I have decent confidence that the elevated frontal theta here is a stable feature rather than sleep debt. In ADHD samples this pattern has gone along with a better stimulant response, but that's an average across groups, and later work narrowed it, so on its own it won't tell you much about this client. Does that add anything to what you're already weighing? If a trial goes forward, I can record again and track theta against this one."

Forward-direction cross-reference. Stimulant pharmacology and its effect on frontal theta and the theta/beta ratio are covered in Part II Ch 5; pair this hypothesis with that chapter when discussing dosing or formulation choices with the prescriber.

Amplitude, distribution, and exemplar plates: Field Guide Ch 6, Elevated Frontal Theta entry.

21.3.2 Suppressed Frontal Theta [workflow heuristic]

Prediction question. For clients presenting with suppressed theta power at frontal sites, what does the literature suggest about treatment response?

No published medication-prediction study has examined this phenotype directly. Suppressed frontal theta is associated with hypervigilance and overactivation in the clinical QEEG literature, and it occupies the opposite end of the frontal-theta dimension from the well-studied theta-excess phenotype. If elevated frontal theta predicts stimulant response through a cortical underactivation mechanism, suppressed frontal theta might theoretically predict poor stimulant tolerance or paradoxical activation from stimulant exposure. The frontal cortex in these clients appears tonically engaged rather than underactivated, which conflicts with the catecholaminergic deficit that stimulants are designed to correct. That inference, however, has not been tested in any prospective design.

The absence of prediction data means this phenotype should not inform medication selection. It may be clinically relevant as a marker of hypervigilance, and the clinician might reasonably flag it for the prescriber as a pattern inconsistent with classical stimulant-responsive ADHD, but that observation is qualitative clinical reasoning, not evidence-based prediction. In the anxiety context, the pattern often co-occurs with reduced posterior alpha, reinforcing a broader hyperarousal interpretation that may point toward anxiolytic consideration rather than stimulant initiation.

Arousal-domain interventions exist for this pattern but are outside the scope of this book; the medication-prediction literature is empty.

Forward-direction cross-reference. Theta-band effects of stimulants are catalogued in Part II Ch 5; benzodiazepine effects in Ch 8. These are the two forward chapters most relevant to monitoring this hypothesis.

Pattern recognition and differential diagnosis: Field Guide Ch 6, Suppressed Frontal Theta entry.

21.3.3 Frontal Slowing (Delta + Theta) [workflow heuristic]

Prediction question. For clients presenting with elevated delta and theta power at frontal sites, consistent with frontal slowing, what does the literature suggest about treatment response?

Frontal slowing involving both delta and theta bands is a broader pattern than isolated frontal theta elevation. When it appears in the context of traumatic brain injury, the neurofeedback literature has addressed this pattern, but the medication-prediction question is less well studied.

In the TBI context, no published pharmaco-EEG study has specifically tested whether baseline frontal delta-theta power predicts differential response to any medication class. The relevant clinical question is often not which medication to choose, but whether the slowing reflects a structural or functional injury that requires neurological workup before any medication strategy is pursued. When frontal slowing appears without known TBI history, the first clinical step is to rule out undiagnosed head injury, sleep apnea, substance effects, or other neurological conditions.

For clients with documented TBI and frontal slowing, the prescriber conversation should address the pattern's likely mechanism (frontal lobe dysfunction from diffuse axonal injury, contusion, or metabolic disruption) rather than a specific medication prediction. Stimulants are sometimes used off-label for post-TBI attentional deficits, and the logic of matching stimulant treatment to frontal underactivation applies here as it does in the theta-excess ADHD phenotype. The evidence base is much thinner in TBI than in ADHD, and the presence of structural injury introduces variables that the ADHD prediction models did not account for.

Forward-direction cross-reference. When this hypothesis is taken to the prescriber, expected forward-direction effects on frontal slow-wave activity are documented for stimulants in Part II Ch 5 and for atypical antipsychotics in Part II Ch 10.

Exemplar plates and normative reference: Field Guide Ch 6, Frontal Slowing (Delta + Theta) entry.

21.3.4 Low SMR (12–15 Hz) [workflow heuristic]

Prediction question. For clients presenting with reduced sensorimotor rhythm power at central sites, what does the literature suggest about treatment response?

SMR (12–15 Hz at C3/C4) has received more research attention in the neurofeedback literature than in pharmaco-EEG prediction, and the medication-prediction question for low SMR specifically is unanswered. The SMR rhythm reflects thalamic inhibition of the sensorimotor strip during rest; reduced SMR suggests that the thalamocortical loop governing motor inhibition is not engaging efficiently, which may underlie motor restlessness and poor sustained stillness.

Low SMR co-occurs with elevated frontal theta in many ADHD presentations (the classic attention constellation described in the composite-signature literature), and the combination may predict stimulant response more reliably than either feature alone. However, no published study has tested SMR power specifically as a predictor of medication outcome independent of the other features in the constellation.

For the prescriber conversation, the value of identifying low SMR is contextual. When low SMR co-occurs with frontal theta elevation in a client being considered for stimulants, the combination strengthens the case that the client's attentional issues involve cortical underactivation. When low SMR appears as an isolated finding with prominent sleep-onset difficulty or motor restlessness, the clinical picture may point toward sensorimotor regulation deficits that the medication-prediction literature does not directly address.

Forward-direction cross-reference. For how benzodiazepines and stimulants affect SMR-range activity, see Part II Ch 5 (Stimulants) and Ch 8 (Benzodiazepines).

For pattern recognition and exemplar plates, see Field Guide *Ch 6, Low SMR (12–15 Hz) entry.*

21.3.5 Elevated SMR (12–15 Hz) [workflow heuristic]

Prediction question. For clients presenting with elevated sensorimotor rhythm power at central sites, what does the literature suggest about treatment response?

No medication-prediction framework targets elevated SMR for reduction. This pattern is generally considered favorable; higher baseline SMR power is associated with better seizure control in the epilepsy literature (Sterman, 1996) and with good self-regulation capacity in the neurofeedback outcome literature. In healthy individuals, strong resting SMR reflects efficient thalamocortical gating of the sensorimotor strip and is not typically associated with clinical complaints.

When elevated SMR appears in a clinical recording, the interpretation should consider whether the finding reflects a constitutional trait, a medication effect (benzodiazepines can increase spindle-like activity in the SMR range), or an artifact of the recording conditions. If the finding is constitutional, it is unlikely to require intervention and does not carry medication-prediction implications. If the elevation is benzodiazepine-driven, the clinical question shifts to whether the medication is producing an iatrogenic signature rather than to whether a new drug should be added.

The practical guidance is negative: this phenotype should not drive medication recommendations in either direction. If a client with elevated SMR presents with clinical complaints, those complaints are likely explained by other phenotype features in the recording rather than by the SMR finding.

Forward-direction cross-reference. Part II Ch 8 (Benzodiazepines) catalogs the forward-direction story for SMR-range beta and spindle-like activity.

For pattern recognition and exemplar plates, see Field Guide *Ch 6, Elevated SMR (12–15 Hz) entry.*

21.3.6 Elevated Theta/Beta Ratio [phenotype inference]

Prediction question. For clients presenting with an elevated theta/beta ratio at midline and frontal sites, what does the literature suggest about treatment response?

TBR has the most cautionary trajectory in the ADHD medication-prediction literature. Early work placed it at the center of ADHD identification and stimulant-response prediction (Monastra et al., 1999; Snyder & Hall, 2006), and the FDA's 2013 clearance (NEBA system) gave the metric regulatory status. The caution arrived early. Arns and colleagues' 2008 phenotype study argued that ADHD research should move away from traditional frequency bands and should separate slowed alpha peak frequency from frontal theta rather than treat TBR as a unitary marker (Arns et al., 2008). Subsequent replication data have steadily eroded confidence further. Ogrim and colleagues found that the theta/beta ratio at Cz, and theta and beta separately, did not discriminate significantly between patients and matched controls (Ogrim et al., 2012), and a later randomized pilot from the same group comparing neurofeedback against stimulant medication found theta and beta power unchanged in both arms (Ogrim & Hestad, 2013). Neither study tested TBR as an individual-level predictor of stimulant response, which is itself part of the point: the metric's diagnostic base is thinner than its prediction reputation. Arns's 2013 meta-analysis showed weaker sensitivity than originally claimed (Arns et al., 2013). The Boxum 2024 EEG-subtyping study separated a genuinely high-theta subgroup from a slow-alpha-peak subgroup and found no association between EEG subtype and behavioral traits (Boxum et al., 2024), and a 2026 multiverse analysis by Strzelczyk and colleagues demonstrated that analytic choices about epoch selection, band boundaries, and artifact handling can create or erase TBR significance across reasonable pipeline variants (Strzelczyk et al., 2026).

TBR retains some group-level signal: clients with elevated TBR are, on average, somewhat more likely to respond to stimulants. But "somewhat more likely on average" does not translate to reliable individual prediction. The clinical guidance is to treat TBR as one data point, decompose the ratio into its constituent parts (high theta, low beta, or both?) before drawing inference, and present the finding to the prescriber with explicit qualification about limited individual-level accuracy.

What to say to the prescriber. "I'm going to hand you something and then tell you not to lean on it. The theta/beta ratio is up at midline and frontal sites. It used to be tied to stimulant response and it hasn't held up, and how you clean and slice the data can make it show up or disappear, so I don't think it should weigh on your decision. I've broken the ratio apart so you can see whether it's high theta, low beta, or both, which tells you more than the ratio does."

Forward-direction cross-reference. Part II Ch 5 (Stimulants) covers the forward-direction story: how stimulants act on theta and beta independently, and why TBR change does not always mean both bands moved.

Amplitude, distribution, and exemplar plates: Field Guide Ch 6, Elevated Theta/Beta Ratio entry.

21.3.7 Low-Voltage Fast EEG [workflow heuristic]

Prediction question. For clients presenting with globally low-amplitude EEG dominated by fast frequencies, what does the literature suggest about treatment response?

The low-voltage fast (LVF) phenotype is one of the Gunkelman EEG phenotypes. It was among the phenotypes cataloged in Arns and colleagues' 2008 study of children with ADHD, but the low-voltage group there was too small to enter the treatment analysis, so that study carries no stimulant-response result for this pattern (Arns et al., 2008). It does support one thing: the phenotype is not disorder-specific, appearing in both the ADHD and the control samples. The clinical profile attached to LVF in the phenotype tradition, chronic high arousal, a "wired-but-tired" presentation, anxiety, and substance vulnerability, comes from clinical description rather than from that study.

The medication-prediction implication is primarily cautionary, and it is mechanistic rather than tested. Stimulants increase cortical activation and shift spectral content toward lower amplitude and faster frequencies, which reinforces the characteristics that define the LVF phenotype. For a client already in a chronically over-aroused state with suppressed slow-wave activity, adding a catecholaminergic agonist works against the presenting physiology. Prescribers will weigh this against clinical indication; no published study has tested stimulant outcome in a prospectively identified LVF group, so the concern rests on mechanism, not on outcome data.

This is a high-caution phenotype for monitoring. If a prescriber independently trials a stimulant, anxiety, insomnia, and subjective distress are the adverse effects to track. The finding should be communicated explicitly to the prescriber as a monitoring context, not as a prediction about the individual client's response.

What to say to the prescriber. "Whole head is running low and fast, which is the low-voltage fast pattern, and the data are clean enough that I'm confident in the pattern itself. Nobody has actually tested how this group does on stimulants, so I wouldn't let the pattern weigh much on its own. The mechanism at least lines up: stimulants push arousal further in the direction this client already sits, so if a stimulant trial goes forward, anxiety or trouble sleeping are what I'd plan to track on re-recording."

Forward-direction cross-reference. Read Part II Ch 5 (Stimulants) before taking this phenotype to the prescriber. The fast-frequency activation picture establishes the rationale for the caution.

Pattern recognition and differential diagnosis: Field Guide Ch 6, Low-Voltage Fast EEG entry.

21.3.8 GABAergic Response Patterns [phenotype inference]

Prediction question. For clients presenting with low-voltage fast EEG, beta spindling, or related patterns of GABAergic dysregulation, what does the literature suggest about response to GABAergic agents?

Several QEEG phenotypes converge on observations about GABAergic medication response. The strongest link is the LVF phenotype described above. The phenotype literature ties the low-voltage fast pattern to alcoholism and to GABAA receptor genes (Johnstone et al., 2005); it does not go on to test GABAergic medication response. When LVF co-occurs with a family history of alcoholism, the further inference that the client will respond strongly to GABAergic agents and carries elevated addiction vulnerability is an extrapolation from that genetic link rather than a finding, and it is among the more clinically consequential extrapolations in this chapter. The proposed mechanism is straightforward: a constitutionally underactive GABAergic system responds vigorously to exogenous GABA enhancement (alcohol, benzodiazepines, neurosteroids), producing the subjective relief that drives both therapeutic response and dependence risk.

Beta spindling (18–25 Hz bursts with characteristic morphology) suggests a complementary GABAergic pathway. Thalamocortical GABAergic circuits regulate spindle generation; dysregulation produces the "can't turn brain off" phenomenology that correlates with benzodiazepine sensitivity. Gabapentinoids (gabapentin (Neurontin), pregabalin (Lyrica)) are sometimes named in this context and do not belong here. They are alpha-2-delta calcium-channel ligands, and the gabapentin label states that the drug has no effect on GABA binding, uptake, or degradation, so grouping them with GABA enhancers misstates the mechanism. No QEEG marker predicts response to them. They also carry a labeled warning for serious respiratory depression when combined with opioids or other CNS depressants, along with documented misuse, and a client showing this pattern is frequently already carrying one of those co-prescriptions.

The evidence base is mixed across the subtypes. LVF as a marker of GABAergic sensitivity is well-replicated in clinical observation but has not been tested in a controlled medication-prediction trial. Beta spindling and GABAergic sensitivity are linked by mechanism rather than by prospective outcome data. The neurosteroid angle (allopregnanolone, brexanolone (Zulresso)) is too new for any QEEG-prediction work. The entry carries a phenotype-inference label because the LVF-alcoholism genetic link has been replicated in clinical populations; the broader GABAergic-response claim that extends beyond that link rests on clinical reasoning rather than on outcome data, and that limitation is stated in the text.

The clinical message is risk-aware rather than prescriptive. What the pattern supports passing to the prescriber is the dependence-vulnerability context, which is the half with a genetic and clinical literature behind it. The book does not forecast a therapeutic response from this pattern, and the prescriber does not need one from a QEEG to select an agent.

Forward-direction cross-reference. When this hypothesis goes to the prescriber, the forward-direction pharmacology for each contributing agent sits in separate chapters: benzodiazepines in Part II Ch 8, gabapentinoids and anticonvulsant-class sedatives in Part II Ch 11, alcohol in Part VI Ch 31, and GABAergic withdrawal patterns in Part V Ch 28.

Exemplar plates and normative reference: Field Guide Ch 6, GABAergic Response Patterns entry.

21.3.9 Elevated Midline Theta (ACC/DMN) [phenotype inference]

Prediction question. For clients presenting with elevated theta power across midline sites (Fz, Cz, Pz), consistent with anterior cingulate cortex or default-mode network involvement, what does the literature suggest about treatment response?

Midline theta differs from frontal-only theta in its topographic distribution and its putative generators. The anterior cingulate cortex generates task-related theta activity involved in error monitoring, conflict detection, and cognitive control (Cavanagh & Frank, 2014; Cohen, 2011). Elevated resting midline theta may reflect dysregulated ACC function and correlates with OCD, perseveration, and altered midline connectivity in MDD.

Arns's 2012 work is sometimes read as support here, but its predictive claims rest on individual alpha peak frequency rather than on midline theta: a slow iAPF, not a theta elevation, is what that paper links to nonresponse across stimulant medication, rTMS, and antidepressants (Arns, 2012). The paper does note that excess theta has been associated with stimulant response, which is a pharmacotherapy observation about frontal theta rather than a midline-theta result. For medication prediction specifically, the evidence is limited. Stimulants and SSRIs both modulate ACC activity and can normalize task-evoked theta patterns, but whether baseline midline theta elevation predicts differential response to either class has not been tested prospectively.

In the OCD context, a clinician should be aware of a paradoxical effect: theta suppression protocols targeting midline sites can sometimes increase anxiety rather than reduce obsessive symptoms. If midline theta reflects hyperactive error monitoring, suppressing it may disrupt a compensatory mechanism. This observation comes from clinical reports rather than from controlled studies, and it warrants caution in extrapolating the finding to medication expectations. SSRIs remain the first-line pharmacotherapy for OCD regardless of EEG phenotype; the midline theta finding does not change that.

Forward-direction cross-reference. Part II Ch 5 (Stimulants) and Ch 6 (SSRIs and SNRIs) catalog the forward-direction effects on midline and frontal theta.

Visual reference and detection criteria: Field Guide Ch 6, Elevated Midline Theta (ACC/DMN) entry.

21.3.10 Theta Cordance (Early SSRI Response Predictor) [phenotype inference]

Prediction question. For clients whose prefrontal theta cordance decreases within the first one to two weeks of SSRI or SNRI treatment, does this early biomarker predict eventual clinical response?

Theta cordance is a derived EEG measure that combines absolute and relative power at prefrontal sites in a way that correlates with regional cerebral perfusion (Leuchter et al., 1994). The measure is not raw theta power. Cordance applies a normalization algorithm that blends absolute power (amplitude) with relative power (proportion of total spectral energy), producing a composite that tracks cerebral blood flow more closely than either component alone. Conflating cordance with raw theta power is a common misreading and produces incorrect clinical inferences.

Bares and colleagues provided the core replication data. A 2007 study showed that prefrontal cordance at week one separated eventual responders from nonresponders to antidepressants (Bares et al., 2007). The 2008 follow-up reported the same week-one relationship in 25 inpatients with treatment-resistant depression, all of them on venlafaxine (Bares et al., 2008). The BRITE-MD trial, a randomized study led by Leuchter's group, tested cordance prospectively and supported the association at the group level (Leuchter et al., 2009). A 2024 Indian prospective trial, however, found no significant predictive value for early theta cordance changes in an MDD sample ($p = 0.37$) (Singh et al., 2024), raising questions about generalizability across populations and clinical settings.

The clinical value of cordance, if it holds, is timing: the biomarker operates at a clinically useful window (one to two weeks), potentially allowing clinicians to identify nonresponse and switch medications weeks before conventional symptom-based assessment would reveal the same information. The practical barriers are real. Computing cordance requires specific recording parameters and analysis pipelines. The measure is sensitive to reference scheme, recording conditions, and analysis choices. No commercial QEEG platform currently provides validated cordance output, and individual-level classification accuracy in the BRITE-MD trial was modest.

Theta cordance is best understood as a treatment-tracking marker rather than a pre-treatment predictor. A marker that changes when treatment works is clinically informative but does not answer the pre-treatment question of who will respond before treatment starts. For pre-treatment prediction, the ATR Index and Brainmarker-I frameworks address the question more directly (see Ch 20). The cordance signal should be communicated to the prescriber as a potential monitoring tool, not as a prescriptive indicator.

What to say to the prescriber. Because this measure is about timing, the offer comes before the finding. "If you start a serotonergic agent, I can record again at one to two weeks and compute prefrontal theta cordance. An early drop in it has tracked with eventual response in several studies, but a 2024 trial found nothing, and even in the studies that worked it wasn't accurate enough to call any one person. No platform computes it for me either, so I'd be doing it by hand. It's a tracking signal at best, not a way to know in advance who will respond. Would something at two weeks be worth anything to you, against waiting on symptom report?"

Forward-direction cross-reference. For how SSRIs and SNRIs affect frontal theta and alpha power distributions, see Part II Ch 6 (SSRIs and SNRIs). For the broader cordance prediction lineage, see Ch 20.

For clinical phenotype recognition, consult Field Guide Ch 6, Theta Cordance (Early SSRI Response Predictor) entry.

21.3.11 Elevated Temporal Beta [phenotype inference]

Prediction question. For clients presenting with elevated beta and high-beta power at temporal sites, what does the literature suggest about treatment response?

Elevated temporal beta is read clinically as a marker of temporal irritability, emotional reactivity, and episodic dysphoria, and, when sufficiently marked or accompanied by sharp transients, of seizure risk. The published support for that reading is indirect and comes from an adjacent phenotype: focal spindling beta, which the phenotype literature describes in terms of cortical irritability and notes in areas associated with pre-epileptic auras (Johnstone et al., 2005). The pattern is taken to overlap with the ADHD excess-beta subtype when frontal high beta is also present, and with temporal lobe dysrhythmia phenotypes when lower-frequency temporal abnormalities co-occur; both overlaps are conventions of the phenotype tradition rather than tested relationships.

The medication-prediction implications depend heavily on severity and lateralization. Mild bilateral temporal beta elevation in an anxiety or irritability context does not carry specific pharmacotherapy prediction data. Markedly elevated temporal beta, especially when accompanied by clinical features suggestive of temporal lobe instability (sudden mood shifts, deja vu, depersonalization, memory disturbances), warrants neurological referral and possible anticonvulsant evaluation before pharmacological decisions are made. The clinical question shifts from "which medication will work best?" to "does this pattern require neurological workup?"

For the clinician-prescriber conversation, temporal beta elevation should be flagged when it is marked (z-scores above 2.0) or lateralized. If the prescriber is considering stimulants for co-occurring ADHD, the same caution that applies to the frontal excess-beta subtype applies here: stimulants can augment fast-frequency activity and may worsen temporal irritability. Anticonvulsants (carbamazepine (Tegretol), oxcarbazepine (Trileptal), lamotrigine (Lamictal), levetiracetam (Keppra)) reduce temporal spikes and may dampen temporal beta, though this use falls outside their labeled indications for most clients.

Forward-direction cross-reference. Read Part II Ch 11 (Anticonvulsants and Mood Stabilizers) and Ch 5 (Stimulants) before framing the prescriber conversation around this pattern.

Amplitude, distribution, and exemplar plates: Field Guide Ch 6, Elevated Temporal Beta entry.

21.4 Social Domain

21.4.1 Elevated Mu Rhythm (Central Alpha) [workflow heuristic]

Prediction question. For clients presenting with elevated mu rhythm (8–13 Hz alpha-range activity at C3/C4 that persists during action observation), what does the literature suggest about treatment response?

Mu rhythm is the sensorimotor cortex's idling oscillation, typically suppressed (desynchronized) during both motor execution and motor observation (Pfurtscheller & Lopes da Silva, 1999). Persistent mu activity during action observation has been studied in the mirror neuron system literature and has drawn attention in autism spectrum disorder (ASD) research, where some studies report reduced mu suppression during social-cognitive tasks (Oberman et al., 2005; Pineda, 2005). Whether this scalp-level finding reliably indexes mirror neuron dysfunction remains debated, but the association between elevated resting mu and reduced social-perceptual processing has generated a body of intervention-oriented work.

No published pharmaco-EEG study has tested whether baseline mu amplitude predicts medication response. No medication class has demonstrated selective mu-suppression effects, and the pattern does not map onto established pharmacological prediction frameworks. The clinical implication is that elevated mu carries no pharmacological signal to follow. It belongs in the broader phenotype picture, not in the medication decision.

Forward-direction cross-reference. When this question goes to the prescriber, the relevant monitoring chapters are Part II Ch 5 (Stimulants) and Ch 11 (Anticonvulsants and Mood Stabilizers).

For pattern recognition and exemplar plates, see Field Guide *Ch 6, Elevated Mu Rhythm (Central Alpha) entry.*

21.5 Arousal Domain

21.5.1 Elevated Left Temporal Alpha [workflow heuristic]

Prediction question. For clients presenting with elevated alpha power localized to left temporal sites (T3/T5), what does the literature suggest about treatment response?

No established prediction framework addresses this phenotype. Left temporal alpha elevation suggests relative deactivation or idling of left temporal cortex, a region heavily involved in language processing, verbal memory, and auditory comprehension. Clinicians have observed this finding in clients with word-finding difficulty, reduced verbal fluency, and language-processing complaints, though no prospective study has validated these associations with sufficient rigor to treat them as diagnostic markers.

The medication-prediction picture is empty. No published study has tested whether left temporal alpha levels predict response to any drug class. The theoretical reasoning would be that activating language circuits might reduce temporal alpha, but this has not been translated into a testable pharmacotherapy hypothesis. Stimulants increase cortical activation broadly and might reduce temporal alpha as part of a global arousal effect, but that general mechanism does not constitute a specific prediction for this phenotype.

Speech-language therapy is more directly indicated than pharmacological interventions when the clinical picture centers on language dysfunction. If medication is being considered for co-occurring conditions (ADHD, depression), the left temporal alpha finding may inform the conversation but cannot tell the prescriber which drug to choose. The evidence base is too thin for that.

Forward-direction cross-reference. Part II Ch 5 (Stimulants) and Ch 6 (SSRIs and SNRIs) catalog broad-activation effects on temporal and regional alpha; neither chapter addresses left-lateralized prediction specifically.

For pattern recognition and exemplar plates, see Field Guide *Ch 6, Elevated Left Temporal Alpha entry.*

21.5.2 Elevated Right Temporal Alpha [workflow heuristic]

Prediction question. For clients presenting with elevated alpha power localized to right temporal sites (T4/T6), what does the literature suggest about treatment response?

No established prediction framework addresses this phenotype. Right temporal alpha elevation suggests relative deactivation of right temporal cortex, a region involved in prosody perception, nonverbal auditory processing, emotional tone recognition, and some aspects of social cognition. Clinically, this pattern has been observed in clients with reduced pragmatic language skills and difficulty interpreting emotional context from voice, though these associations lack prospective validation.

The pharmacotherapy literature has nothing to say here. Drug-class response has not been tested against right temporal alpha levels in any published trial. Theoretical reasoning would parallel the left temporal case: activating the deactivated cortex might reduce alpha locally, but no hypothesis specific to this lateralization has been tested. Stimulants increase cortical activation broadly and might reduce temporal alpha as part of a general arousal effect, but a global mechanism is not a specific prediction.

If medication is being considered for co-occurring conditions (ADHD, depression, social anxiety), the right temporal alpha finding adds to the clinical picture but carries no pharmacological prescription of its own. The evidence base is too thin to point in any direction for this lateralization.

Forward-direction cross-reference. Read Part II Ch 5 (Stimulants) and Ch 6 (SSRIs and SNRIs) before the prescriber conversation; neither chapter carries a right-lateralized prediction, but both catalog the broad-activation effects that apply.

For pattern recognition and exemplar plates, see Field Guide *Ch 6, Elevated Right Temporal Alpha entry.*

21.5.3 Elevated High Beta (Global Hyperarousal) [phenotype inference]

Prediction question. For clients presenting with globally elevated high-beta power (>20 Hz) across multiple scalp regions, what does the literature suggest about treatment response?

Global high-beta elevation is the QEEG pattern most often read as cortical hyperarousal. Clinically it is reported across anxiety disorders, chronic insomnia, PTSD, obsessive-compulsive spectrum presentations, and stimulant overmedication, though the published phenotype work behind that list is narrower than the list itself: an excess-beta cluster within ADHD samples (Clarke et al., 2001), and a spindling excessive beta phenotype most often traced to a sedative medication effect and otherwise treated as a nonspecific sign of dysfunction (Johnstone et al., 2005). The proposed mechanism is diffuse: widespread cortical overactivation produces excessive fast-frequency activity that can be measured at virtually every scalp location.

The medication-prediction reasoning varies by etiology. If global high beta reflects an anxiety-driven hyperarousal state, SSRIs and buspirone may reduce the pattern indirectly as the anxious state remits. The closest evidence is not an anxiety result and does not run in the expected direction: in 70 patients with major affective disorder treated openly with paroxetine, greater pretreatment fast activity at frontal sites went with greater symptom improvement (V. J. Knott et al., 2000). Baseline high-beta amplitude has not been tested prospectively as a predictor of SSRI response in an anxiety sample. If the high beta reflects stimulant overmedication, the pattern is often iatrogenic, which is the first thing to tell the prescriber rather than reaching for a second medication; whether the stimulant dose changes is their call. Clinicians should always rule out iatrogenic causes before attributing global high beta to a primary neurophysiological trait. Benzodiazepines can suppress high-beta power during acute exposure, but this reflects pharmacological override of the arousal state rather than normalization of the underlying circuit, and gains are state-dependent rather than durable.

For the prescriber conversation, the key message is that global high beta is a treatable signature, but treatment should be matched to the cause. If the cause is iatrogenic (stimulant dose too high, excessive caffeine), that is the first thing to tell the prescriber, and it points away from adding pharmacotherapy; whether the dose changes is their decision. If the cause is a primary anxiety or hyperarousal state, anxiolytic pharmacotherapy is something the prescriber may weigh.

Forward-direction cross-reference. When the prescriber asks about monitoring parameters, Part II Ch 5 (Stimulants) and Ch 8 (Benzodiazepines) document what to expect from each pharmacological approach on high-beta power.

For pattern recognition and exemplar plates, see Field Guide *Ch 6, Elevated High Beta (Global Hyperarousal) entry.*

21.5.4 Elevated Posterior Alpha (Hypoarousal) [phenotype inference]

Prediction question. For clients presenting with elevated posterior alpha power (8–12 Hz at P3 / P4 / Pz / O1 / O2), consistent with cortical hypoarousal, what does the literature suggest about treatment response?

Elevated posterior alpha reflects an abundance of the brain's default resting oscillation, suggesting that posterior cortical networks remain in an idling state more than expected. The clinical picture that reading points toward has support in the arousal-regulation literature: among 102 MDD patients with fatigue, 23.5% were classified as hypoaroused on a 15-minute resting EEG scored with VIGALL, and that subgroup scored higher on the Beck Depression Inventory items for loss of energy and concentration difficulty, and reported higher trait and state sleepiness, than the non-hypoaroused patients (Surova et al., 2021).

Read that finding carefully before carrying it into a report, because "hypoarousal" does not mean the same thing in the two traditions this entry stands between. In the neurofeedback alpha-idling reading, hypoarousal means more posterior alpha. In the VIGALL arousal-regulation framework that Surova and colleagues used, alpha-dominant EEG is stage A and counts as adequate vigilance, and hypoarousal means the alpha drops out and the record slides toward theta, drowsiness, and sleep (Olbrich et al., 2009). The two words point at opposite EEG appearances, so when a paper reports a hypoarousal result, check which one it measured before mapping it onto a posterior alpha finding.

No published study has isolated posterior alpha elevation as an independent predictor of stimulant outcome. The activation rationale parallels the frontal theta phenotype: if the cortex is underactivated, catecholaminergic agents should increase activation. But the posterior alpha phenotype is less well studied than frontal theta, and the mechanistic parallel does not constitute prediction evidence. The nearest prediction evidence is adjacent rather than direct: in 28 adult ADHD patients, a baseline arousal-stability score from a 15-minute record scored with VIGALL 2.1 predicted methylphenidate response (OR 1.28, 95% CI 1.0-1.65, $p = 0.027$), with less stable arousal regulation, meaning a faster decline toward drowsiness, raising the odds of response (Strauß et al., 2020). The predictor there is arousal stability across the record, not posterior alpha power, and the authors call the study a pilot at $n = 28$. The association is reasonable but hypothesis-generating.

In the MDD context, the mechanistic picture suggests that the hypoarousal component is relevant to the prescriber's choice among antidepressant classes, because activating and sedating agents push arousal in opposite directions. No prospective study has tested whether baseline posterior alpha levels predict differential response to any specific antidepressant. The pattern is worth communicating to the prescriber as context for their independent decision, not as a basis for the clinician to recommend one agent over another.

Forward-direction cross-reference. Part II Ch 5 (Stimulants) and Ch 7 (TCAs, MAOIs, and Atypical Antidepressants) catalog the forward-direction arousal effects for activating agents on posterior alpha.

For pattern recognition and exemplar plates, see Field Guide *Ch 6, Elevated Posterior Alpha (Hypoarousal) entry.*

21.5.5 Deficient Posterior Alpha (Hypervigilance) [phenotype inference]

Prediction question. For clients presenting with reduced posterior alpha power, consistent with cortical hypervigilance and failure to generate the resting alpha rhythm, what does the literature suggest about treatment response?

Reduced posterior alpha is the inverse of the hypoarousal phenotype and reflects a cortex that does not idle efficiently. The empirical anchor for that reading is narrow: mean alpha level tracks resting-state arousal in healthy adults under both eyes-closed and eyes-open conditions (Barry et al., 2007). The clinical extension to anxiety, PTSD, chronic pain, and hypervigilance states, where the brain remains in a tonically activated posture rather than cycling between task-engaged and resting modes, is clinical observation carried onto that arousal finding rather than a result from it. Clients with this profile often report difficulty relaxing, poor sleep quality, and a subjective sense of being "always on."

The medication-prediction reasoning centers on the alpha-generation deficit, and the direct evidence cuts against the most appealing version of it. Alpha does not appear to behave as a treatment-tracking measure: neither alpha power nor alpha asymmetry changed across 12 weeks of fluoxetine treatment in depressed patients, and alpha power was close to unchanged on retest. What that work found instead was a baseline effect, with responders showing greater pretreatment alpha, and the paroxetine work likewise reports pretreatment spectral correlates of outcome rather than post-treatment normalization (Bruder et al., 2008; V. J. Knott et al., 2000). Alpha in this literature behaves like a stable trait-level predictor, not like a signal that recovers as the client improves. Whether a baseline alpha deficit predicts which anxious clients respond to SSRIs has not been tested prospectively at all.

Benzodiazepines increase alpha power acutely but through a pharmacological override rather than through restoration of endogenous alpha-generation capacity. The alpha increase under benzodiazepines is state-dependent and reverses on discontinuation. This distinction matters for the prescriber conversation: benzodiazepines mask the deficit rather than building durable alpha-generation capacity.

Forward-direction cross-reference. Read Part II Ch 6 (SSRIs and SNRIs) and Ch 8 (Benzodiazepines) before the prescriber conversation. The distinction between durable alpha recovery and pharmacological override is documented in both chapters.

For pattern recognition and exemplar plates, see Field Guide *Ch 6, Deficient Posterior Alpha (Hypervigilance) entry.*

21.5.6 Slow Individual Alpha Peak Frequency [phenotype inference]

Prediction question. For clients presenting with a slowed individual alpha peak frequency (iAPF below age-expected norms), what does the literature suggest about treatment response?

This is the Brainmarker-I phenotype, and it carries the strongest treatment-stratification evidence of any single QEEG metric in the Brainmarker program's published work. Voetterl and colleagues' 2023 work was an observational, prospective accuracy study rather than a trial of its own, and it found that slow iAPF predicted superior response to sertraline (Zoloft) relative to placebo when the model was tested blinded and out-of-sample against the placebo-controlled EMBARC dataset (Voetterl, Sack, et al., 2023). Testing a QEEG stratification model out-of-sample against randomized data is unusual in this literature, but it is not the same thing as a prospective trial designed around the biomarker. The same study also reported better electroconvulsive therapy remission in its slow-iAPF subgroup, in separate datasets with their own blinded check. Neuromodulation is outside this volume's scope, and the finding is recorded here as evidence about the marker rather than as a route to a referral.

The complementary finding is equally informative: slow iAPF predicted poorer stimulant response (Voetterl, Wingen, et al., 2023). If iAPF is interpreted as an index of thalamocortical processing speed (with slower frequencies reflecting reduced thalamocortical loop velocity), the medication-prediction logic becomes mechanistic. Sertraline, through serotonergic modulation, may stabilize thalamocortical timing in a way that benefits clients whose alpha generators are running slowly. Stimulants, which drive the cortex toward faster activation through catecholaminergic mechanisms, may not address the thalamocortical timing deficit and may produce activation without the processing-speed improvement the client needs.

The strength of this evidence relative to other entries in this chapter is worth emphasizing. The Brainmarker-I design included a placebo control, prospective phenotype identification, and replication across independent samples. These design features are absent from most other QEEG prediction studies. The group-to-individual caveat still applies: slow iAPF predicts a higher probability of sertraline response at the population level, not a guarantee for any individual client. But the evidence places iAPF in a different confidence category than phenotypes supported only by retrospective or uncontrolled data.

As of 2026, however, the sertraline stratification remains a single-trial finding. No independent laboratory has published a pharmacological replication of the iAPF-sertraline association. Independent work has validated iAPF as a predictor of rTMS response (Baradits et al., 2026), extending the Brainmarker-I logic to neuromodulation, but the drug-response claim specifically rests on one study. The study's design (prospective, placebo-controlled, out-of-sample validation) is stronger than most work in this space, but design quality does not substitute for independent replication.

The Brainmarker-I framework treats iAPF as a stratification variable (which treatment class showed better group-level outcomes in the studied population). That group-level stratification should be communicated to the prescriber as research context, not as an instruction to choose one treatment over another for an individual client.

Forward-direction cross-reference. For how SSRIs and stimulants affect alpha peak frequency and thalamocortical dynamics, see Part II Ch 5 (Stimulants) and Ch 6 (SSRIs and SNRIs).

For pattern recognition and exemplar plates, see Field Guide *Ch 6, Slow Individual Alpha Peak Frequency entry.*

21.5.7 Fast Individual Alpha Peak Frequency [phenotype inference]

Prediction question. For clients presenting with a fast individual alpha peak frequency (iAPF above age-expected norms), what does the literature suggest about treatment response?

Fast iAPF is the Brainmarker-I complement. Where slow iAPF predicts better sertraline and ECT response, a higher iAPF predicted better methylphenidate remission in the Brainmarker-I stratification (Voetterl, Sack, et al., 2023; Voetterl, Wingen, et al., 2023). The iAPF literature reaches this from the other direction, reporting that a slow iAPF goes with nonresponse to stimulants, to rTMS, and to antidepressants (Arns, 2012), so a normal-to-fast peak is at least as much the absence of a risk marker as it is a positive predictor. The mechanistic interpretation follows from the thalamocortical processing-speed model. If alpha frequency indexes thalamocortical loop velocity, clients with fast iAPF have intact or accelerated thalamocortical timing, and the stimulant mechanism of increasing catecholaminergic drive aligns with their neurophysiological profile rather than overriding it.

The prognostic picture for clients with fast iAPF is generally favorable. The rTMS association runs through the same iAPF logic rather than through a trial designed around fast peaks, and it is consistent with the broader observation that clients with faster cortical dynamics may tolerate and benefit from inhibitory stimulation protocols, where the intervention calms overactive circuits without compromising baseline processing capacity.

As with the slow-iAPF entry, the fast-iAPF prediction rests on the Brainmarker-I trial and has not been independently replicated in a separate pharmacological study. The neuromodulation extension (iAPF predicting rTMS outcome) has been validated independently (Baradits et al., 2026), but the drug-response claim for methylphenidate specifically awaits replication. The entry carries a phenotype-inference label because the association comes from a prospective study with out-of-sample validation; the absence of independent replication is a limitation of the evidence, stated here, not encoded in the label.

The clinical message for the prescriber is straightforward: fast iAPF is not a red flag. When a client with fast iAPF presents with ADHD symptoms, the Brainmarker-I data do not conflict with the conventional prescribing pathway. The finding's value is primarily in the contrast with the slow-iAPF case, where the Brainmarker-I data showed a lower group-level probability of stimulant response.

Forward-direction cross-reference. For how stimulants affect alpha peak frequency, see Part II Ch 5 (Stimulants). Neuromodulation approaches (rTMS) and their interaction with iAPF are outside this volume's scope; see *QEEG Field Guide* Ch 6 for the iAPF-rTMS evidence base.

For pattern recognition and exemplar plates, see Field Guide *Ch 6, Fast Individual Alpha Peak Frequency entry.*

21.6 Sensorimotor Domain

21.6.1 Beta Spindling (Cortical Irritability) [workflow heuristic]

Prediction question. For clients presenting with beta spindling (rhythmic bursts of high-amplitude beta activity, often at 18–25 Hz), what does the literature suggest about treatment response?

Beta spindling is a high-caution phenotype. The waveform consists of brief, rhythmic beta bursts that stand out from background activity and are morphologically distinct from the continuous low-amplitude beta seen in normal recordings. The phenotype literature treats it most commonly as a sedative medication effect, benzodiazepines being the class most often behind it in outpatient practice, and otherwise as a nonspecific sign of dysfunction, including the cortical irritability that may overlap with seizure susceptibility (Johnstone et al., 2005). Confirm on the raw trace that the pattern is cortical and not temporalis or frontalis EMG before treating it as a finding at all. Identifying the cause is the essential first step and must precede any medication-prediction discussion.

No medication-prediction framework addresses beta spindling directly, and the clinical reasoning here is entirely cause-dependent. If the spindling reflects current benzodiazepine use, the "prediction" is straightforward: the waveform is iatrogenic and usually resolves if the medication is tapered under medical supervision. If the spindling persists after benzodiazepine discontinuation or appears without benzodiazepine history, a neurological evaluation is indicated to assess for cortical irritability or subclinical seizure activity. Whether anticonvulsant treatment is warranted is a question for the neurologist, not a conclusion the QEEG finding can reach on its own.

The core message for the prescriber is that beta spindling raises a medical question, not a prediction question.

Forward-direction cross-reference. When the prescriber needs to understand what these drug classes do to beta-range activity, Part II Ch 8 (Benzodiazepines) and Ch 11 (Anticonvulsants and Mood Stabilizers) have the forward-direction picture.

For pattern recognition and exemplar plates, see Field Guide *Ch 6, Beta Spindling (Cortical Irritability) entry.*

21.6.2 Deficient Mu Rhythm [workflow heuristic]

Prediction question. For clients presenting with reduced mu rhythm at central sites (C3/C4), what does the literature suggest about treatment response?

No validated prediction framework addresses deficient mu rhythm specifically. Reduced mu has received less attention than elevated mu, in part because reduced mu is harder to distinguish from a general absence of central alpha activity or from the effects of tonic motor activation, fidgeting, or arousal-driven alpha suppression. The interpretive challenge is signal attribution: low mu at C3/C4 could reflect deficient sensorimotor inhibition, or it could reflect hyperarousal suppressing all alpha-range activity across the scalp, with central sites merely participating in a global phenomenon.

The clinical approach depends on context. If deficient mu co-occurs with global alpha suppression and the broader hypervigilance phenotype, the mu finding is likely secondary to the arousal disturbance, and the arousal domain is the more useful target: relaxation training sits within the clinician's scope, and anxiolytic pharmacotherapy is an option a prescriber may weigh.

No medication class has demonstrated selective effects on mu generation, and this phenotype should not drive prescribing decisions. The value of identifying deficient mu lies in understanding the broader phenotype profile: is this a primary sensorimotor finding, or is it a downstream consequence of a hyperarousal state that has more direct treatment implications?

Forward-direction cross-reference. Part II Ch 5 (Stimulants) and Ch 8 (Benzodiazepines) catalog central-site oscillatory effects for the drug classes most relevant to monitoring this phenotype.

For pattern recognition and exemplar plates, see Field Guide *Ch 6, Deficient Mu Rhythm entry.*

21.7 Learning Domain

21.7.1 Low Central Beta [workflow heuristic]

Prediction question. For clients presenting with reduced beta power at central sites (C3/C4/Cz), what does the literature suggest about treatment response?

No medication-prediction study has specifically addressed low central beta as an independent predictor of treatment outcome. The pattern overlaps with the low-SMR phenotype (SMR spans the 12–15 Hz portion of the beta range) and shares mechanistic territory with sensorimotor underactivation presentations. Low central beta can co-occur with attentional deficits, but the association is less specific than the frontal-theta-to-attention link, and the clinical literature has not carved out a distinct pharmacotherapy prediction role for central beta deficiency.

The prescriber conversation should distinguish this phenotype from attention-domain deficits that carry more specific medication implications. A client with low central beta and co-occurring frontal theta excess falls into the well-studied ADHD attention phenotype, and the frontal theta finding drives the medication-prediction reasoning. A client with isolated low central beta and no frontal theta excess presents a less informative picture for medication selection. In that case, the phenotype does not point toward a specific medication class.

Forward-direction cross-reference. Read Part II Ch 5 (Stimulants) before this phenotype enters the prescriber conversation; the central-beta effects establish the monitoring baseline.

For pattern recognition and exemplar plates, see Field Guide *Ch 6, Low Central Beta entry.*

21.8 Symbols Domain

21.8.1 Posterior Slowing (Delta + Theta) [workflow heuristic]

Prediction question. For clients presenting with elevated delta and theta power at posterior sites (P3/P4/Pz/O1/O2), consistent with posterior cortical slowing, what does the literature suggest about treatment response?

Posterior slowing in the delta and theta ranges differs from the posterior alpha-excess hypoarousal phenotype in an important respect: where alpha excess suggests cortical idling, delta-theta excess at posterior sites suggests a deeper processing deficit, potentially involving reduced posterior cortical efficiency, impaired visual processing speed, or compromised posterior network integrity. The pattern can appear in traumatic brain injury, neurodegenerative processes, toxic exposures, and chronic sleep deprivation.

No published medication-prediction study has examined posterior delta-theta elevation as a predictor of pharmacotherapy outcome.

The absence of medication-prediction evidence means the prescriber conversation should center on the pattern's clinical significance rather than on a specific drug recommendation. Medical workup to rule out treatable causes (sleep apnea, medication effects, metabolic abnormalities, early neurodegenerative process) should precede any intervention commitment. If posterior slowing resolves with correction of an underlying cause, the finding was secondary and the treatment implication was medical, not neurotherapeutic. If the pattern persists after correctable factors are addressed, pharmacotherapy plays a supportive role for co-occurring symptom domains rather than targeting the slowing directly.

Forward-direction cross-reference. For how stimulants affect slow-wave activity, see Part II Ch 5 (Stimulants). Cholinesterase inhibitors and memantine are disease-specific prescribing considerations outside this volume's QEEG-prediction scope.

For pattern recognition and exemplar plates, see Field Guide *Ch 6, Posterior Slowing (Delta + Theta) entry.*

21.9 Stability Domain

21.9.1 Globally Low Beta (Underactivation) [workflow heuristic]

Prediction question. For clients presenting with globally reduced beta power across the scalp, consistent with diffuse cortical underactivation, what does the literature suggest about treatment response?

Globally reduced beta power reflects a widespread decrease in fast-frequency cortical activation. The pattern differs from localized beta deficits (central or frontal) in its diffuseness, which suggests a systemic rather than circuit-specific cause. Sleep deprivation, sedating medications, metabolic disorders (hypothyroidism, hypoglycemia), chronic fatigue conditions, and post-concussive states can all produce globally low beta. Identifying and addressing these correctable factors is a clinical prerequisite before attributing the pattern to a primary neurophysiological trait.

No prediction framework links global beta deficiency to differential medication response, and the practical reason is that this finding is usually downstream of something else. The client whose low global beta tracks an undertreated thyroid problem needs thyroid hormone replacement, and the QEEG is irrelevant to the prescription. The client whose low global beta tracks a sedating medication needs a medication review, and again the QEEG is reporting on the existing prescription rather than predicting a new one. Low global beta is a flag for differential diagnosis upstream of pharmacology.

For the prescriber, the key message is evaluative rather than predictive. Low global beta raises a question about what is suppressing cortical activation. The answer may involve medication side effects, medical comorbidity, sleep pathology, or constitutional factors. The QEEG finding is a prompt for medical differential diagnosis, not a pointer toward a specific drug class.

Forward-direction cross-reference. When the differential includes medication-suppressed cortical activation, the forward-direction effects of the contributing agents are documented in Part II Ch 5 (Stimulants), Ch 8 (Benzodiazepines), and Ch 10 (Atypical Antipsychotics).

For pattern recognition and exemplar plates, see Field Guide *Ch 6, Globally Low Beta (Underactivation) entry.*

21.9.2 Global Hypercoherence [workflow heuristic]

Prediction question. For clients presenting with globally elevated coherence values across multiple electrode pairs, what does the literature suggest about treatment response?

Global hypercoherence indicates excessive phase-coupling between cortical regions, suggesting that distributed networks are synchronizing more tightly than expected. This finding correlates with diffuse connectivity disruptions and has been observed in seizure-prone populations, post-TBI presentations, and some neurodevelopmental conditions. In the Thatcher normative database, global hypercoherence is defined relative to age-matched norms and can involve multiple frequency bands (Thatcher, 2010).

The medication-prediction literature does not address hypercoherence directly. Anticonvulsants reduce cortical synchrony and may reduce hypercoherence as a secondary effect of their mechanism of action. Carbamazepine, valproate, and lamotrigine measurably alter the resting QEEG, shifting alpha frequency and broadband power (Clemens et al., 2006), and their ion-channel and synaptic-coupling mechanisms could plausibly reduce excessive inter-regional phase-locking. That last step is inference: the spectral work does not report coherence outcomes. Prediction data is absent for this phenotype; the clinical reasoning is mechanistic inference rather than evidence from prediction studies.

In seizure-prone populations, the treating neurologist's assessment of seizure management takes priority over any intervention targeting cortical synchrony.

Forward-direction cross-reference. Part II Ch 11 (Anticonvulsants and Mood Stabilizers) catalogs the coherence and synchrony effects that form the monitoring rationale for anticonvulsant consideration.

For pattern recognition and exemplar plates, see Field Guide *Ch 6, Global Hypercoherence entry.*

21.9.3 Frontal Hypocoherence [workflow heuristic]

Prediction question. For clients presenting with reduced inter-hemispheric or intra-hemispheric coherence at frontal sites (commonly F3-F4 or F7-F8 below age-matched norms), what does the literature suggest about medication response?

Frontal hypocoherence reflects diminished functional coupling between frontal cortical regions. The pattern is reported in traumatic brain injury, especially diffuse axonal injury affecting frontal white matter, and in some attention and executive-function presentations, though the coherence methodology literature cautions that a measured coherence value depends on the reference scheme used to derive it (Thatcher, 2010). Drug-class response has not been tested against baseline frontal coherence levels in any published trial, so the medication-prediction literature is empty for this phenotype as a stand-alone signature.

The drug-relevant clinical work centers on iatrogenic worsening rather than positive prediction. Sedating medications (benzodiazepines, sedating anticholinergics, muscle relaxants, certain anticonvulsants, sedating tricyclics) reduce cortical activation broadly and can further degrade frontal coupling. Anticholinergic burden is associated with worsened frontal-network integrity in older adults and post-TBI populations. Before any pharmacotherapy decision is made for a client with marked frontal hypocoherence, a careful medication review for sedative and anticholinergic exposure is the appropriate first step. In TBI populations the clinical question is rarely "which drug should we add?" and more often "which drug should we taper or remove?"

When frontal hypocoherence appears without TBI history, the absence of a specific medication-prediction framework means the prescriber conversation should focus on the symptom-level presentation and on other phenotype features that carry stronger prediction evidence. Stimulants are sometimes used off-label for post-TBI attentional deficits, with the same activation rationale as in classical ADHD; whether baseline coherence predicts differential stimulant outcome has not been tested.

Forward-direction cross-reference. For how benzodiazepines, anticholinergics, and stimulants affect frontal coherence and connectivity, see Part II Ch 5 (Stimulants), Ch 8 (Benzodiazepines), and Ch 11 (Anticonvulsants and Mood Stabilizers).

For pattern recognition and exemplar plates, see Field Guide *Ch 6, Frontal Hypocoherence entry.*

21.9.4 Diffuse Slowing (Elevated Delta) [workflow heuristic]

Prediction question. For clients presenting with globally elevated delta power across the scalp during a relaxed-wakeful eyes-closed recording, what does the literature suggest about medication response?

Diffuse delta elevation in the awake EEG functions as a differential-diagnostic signal rather than a drug-selection biomarker. The pattern appears in toxic-metabolic encephalopathies, post-concussive states, neurodegenerative processes, hepatic and renal dysfunction, hypothyroidism, and as an effect of several drug classes. Sedating anticonvulsants (phenobarbital, valproate (Depakote) at higher doses, topiramate (Topamax) at higher doses), opioids, sedating antipsychotics, benzodiazepines, and sedating antidepressants can all produce or contribute to globally elevated delta in waking recordings. Identifying iatrogenic contributors is the essential first step.

Where medication is contributing, that is a question for the prescriber and not an instruction the QEEG can issue. The recording cannot say which of the causes above is operating, or that any of them is causal at all, and decisions about dose, substitution, or taper rest on clinical grounds. Several of the agents named here, opioids and sedating anticonvulsants among them, carry withdrawal and seizure risk that no spectral finding can weigh. What the pattern does support is caution in the other direction. Where waking delta is elevated and a sedating tricyclic, a high-dose anticonvulsant, or an opioid burden is on board, the sedating load is itself a candidate explanation for the delta. Adding an activating agent does not address that load, and whether to do so is the prescriber's judgement, not a reading the trace supplies. Adding activating medications on top of a pharmacologically suppressed cortex risks producing activation without clinical benefit and can mask the contribution of the suppressing agents.

When iatrogenic causes are excluded, no published prediction framework links global delta elevation to differential response to any specific drug class. In neurodegenerative or post-TBI contexts, cognitive enhancers (cholinesterase inhibitors, memantine) may be considered for diagnoses that carry a pharmacological indication, but this reflects standard disease-specific prescribing rather than QEEG-driven selection. The prescriber conversation for this phenotype should center on differential diagnosis (sleep evaluation, metabolic workup, medication audit) rather than on phenotype-to-drug matching.

Forward-direction cross-reference. For how sedating medications and opioids affect delta power, see Part II Ch 8 (Benzodiazepines), Ch 7 (TCAs, MAOIs, and Atypical Antidepressants), Ch 10 (Atypical Antipsychotics), Ch 11 (Anticonvulsants and Mood Stabilizers), and Ch 14 (Opioids).

For pattern recognition and exemplar plates, see Field Guide *Ch 6, Diffuse Slowing (Elevated Delta) entry.*

21.9.5 Mixed Fast-Slow (Encephalopathic) [workflow heuristic]

Prediction question. For clients presenting with simultaneously elevated slow-wave (delta, theta) and elevated fast-wave (beta, high beta) activity across multiple regions, what does the literature suggest about medication response?

The mixed fast-slow pattern is most often a polypharmacy signature. The classic configuration is benzodiazepine-induced beta activity layered on top of background slowing produced by sedating co-prescribed agents (older antipsychotics, sedating tricyclics, opioids, sedating anticonvulsants). The pattern can also reflect toxic or metabolic encephalopathy, in which case it functions as a medical-workup prompt rather than a medication-selection signal.

The pattern is not a candidate for medication addition, and it is not a basis for medication subtraction either. It is nonspecific: sedative polypharmacy, toxic or metabolic illness, drowsiness, and muscle or movement artifact all produce it, and neither the raw EEG nor the quantitative record separates them or establishes that a regimen is causal. Whether simplifying a regimen changes the pattern, and on what timescale, has not been studied. Where sedative load is in fact contributing, adding drugs works against the mechanism: the existing regimen is already producing both ends of the spectral distortion, and additional pharmacological pressure compounds the problem rather than relieving it. This pattern warrants caution about any prescriber move that increases pharmacological load. The pharmacotherapy literature has nothing to say about positive medication selection for this phenotype because the clinical literature treats it as an iatrogenic or medical signature rather than as a candidate for prescription matching.

The clinical message for the prescriber is direct. When this pattern is identified, the appropriate sequence is raw-EEG review, medical workup to exclude toxic-metabolic etiology, and an accurate medication inventory handed to the treating team. Any change to the regimen is a clinical decision made on clinical grounds, not on the basis of a QEEG feature. If the regimen does change and the pattern is reassessed, any residual phenotype features can be considered against the standard prediction frameworks. Approaching a mixed fast-slow recording as a candidate for positive medication selection inverts the appropriate clinical priority.

Forward-direction cross-reference. For how benzodiazepines produce beta activity and how sedating antipsychotics and tricyclics produce background slowing, see Part II Ch 8 (Benzodiazepines), Ch 7 (TCAs, MAOIs, and Atypical Antidepressants), Ch 9 (Typical Antipsychotics), and Ch 10 (Atypical Antipsychotics).

For pattern recognition and exemplar plates, see Field Guide *Ch 6, Mixed Fast-Slow (Encephalopathic) entry.*

21.9.6 Temporal Theta Dysrhythmia [workflow heuristic]

Prediction question. For clients presenting with elevated theta power at temporal sites (T3/T4/T5/T6), especially when intermittent or rhythmic in morphology, what does the literature suggest about medication response?

Temporal theta dysrhythmia overlaps clinically and electrophysiologically with the temporal-lobe instability spectrum: episodic mood shifts, depersonalization, deja vu phenomena, intrusive imagery, and, at the more abnormal end, subclinical or clinical seizure activity (Johnstone et al., 2005). Severity drives clinical priority. Mild bilateral elevation without paroxysmal features in an anxiety or PTSD context does not direct medication choice. Marked elevation (z-scores above 2.5 to 3.0), lateralized findings, or any sharp or paroxysmal features warrant neurological referral before pharmacological decisions are made.

The drug-prediction literature for this phenotype is anchored to anticonvulsant pharmacology rather than to a controlled-trial prediction study. Carbamazepine, oxcarbazepine, lamotrigine, and levetiracetam are established anticonvulsants, and the first-line effectiveness data in newly diagnosed epilepsy covers carbamazepine, valproate, and lamotrigine (Kwan & Brodie, 2001). The further expectation that they dampen temporal slow-wave activity and abnormal temporal discharges is pharmacological reasoning rather than an EEG-outcome result from that literature. This pharmacological logic is mechanistic; no controlled study has tested whether baseline temporal theta predicts differential anticonvulsant outcome at the individual level. If a clinical EEG confirms epileptiform activity, antiseizure medication becomes the treating neurologist's question. The QEEG finding does not itself indicate one, and a quantitative power elevation is not epileptiform morphology.

In the PTSD or dissociation context, where temporal theta dysrhythmia can accompany the broader trauma-spectrum presentation, SSRIs remain the first-line pharmacotherapy for PTSD itself, and the temporal theta finding does not alter that calculus. The same caution that applies to the temporal beta phenotype applies here: stimulants increase cortical activation broadly and can amplify temporal irritability in clients with underlying instability. When ADHD is being considered alongside a marked temporal dysrhythmia, the clinical sequence is to evaluate the temporal pattern first and to address that question before initiating a stimulant trial.

Forward-direction cross-reference. For how anticonvulsants reduce temporal slow activity, how SSRIs are used in PTSD, and how stimulants can augment temporal irritability, see Part II Ch 5 (Stimulants), Ch 6 (SSRIs and SNRIs), and Ch 11 (Anticonvulsants and Mood Stabilizers).

For pattern recognition and exemplar plates, see Field Guide *Ch 6, Temporal Theta Dysrhythmia entry.*

21.9.7 Limited-Response Signatures [workflow heuristic]

Prediction question. For clients presenting with QEEG patterns historically associated with treatment-refractory depression or poor medication response, what does the literature suggest about pharmacotherapy outcomes?

Several QEEG patterns have been linked to medication resistance in the depression and attentional-disorder literatures, though none has been validated as a prospective predictor of treatment refractoriness in a controlled trial. The Suffin and Emory lineage identified neurometric subgroups whose membership correlated with responsivity to particular pharmacologic agent classes, which carries the implication that a client matched to the wrong class responds poorly (Suffin & Emory, 1995). That work compared medication classes against each other; it did not test non-pharmacological alternatives. The specific patterns linked to limited pharmacotherapy response in that work included focal left anterior temporal slowing, diffuse low-voltage EEG, and atypical multi-band dysregulation.

Focal left anterior temporal slowing (alpha-theta range at T3/F7) has appeared in subsets of treatment-refractory depressed patients who respond poorly to antidepressant monotherapy but may respond to neuromodulation (TMS, tDCS targeting that region). The mechanism is unclear, but the consistent finding across clinical case series is that localized temporal slowing predicts a dissociation between medication response and stimulation response.

Diffuse low-voltage EEG with low amplitudes across all bands produces a different limited-response profile. These clients have been described in clinical accounts as reporting minimal benefit from SSRIs combined with higher side-effect sensitivity, a pattern read as consistent with a cortex already operating at low energy. The description carries no denominator and no prospective test, and nothing in this phenotype indicates what to try instead.

Complex multi-band dysregulation, where the EEG shows abnormalities across delta, theta, alpha, and beta simultaneously without a clear pattern, suggests either a complicated neurological substrate or heavy polypharmacy. The likelihood of remission with conventional antidepressant monotherapy is low in this profile, and multimodal approaches are typically required.

The evidence for these patterns is observational and retrospective. No prospective trial has enrolled clients selected by these QEEG features and randomized them to alternative treatments. The hypothesis is that identifying these patterns early may spare clients extended trials of monotherapy unlikely to succeed, but that hypothesis has not been tested prospectively, and the patterns do not indicate which alternative to pursue.

Forward-direction cross-reference. For how various medication classes produce the patterns described here, see Part II Ch 6 (SSRIs and SNRIs) and Ch 7 (TCAs, MAOIs, and Atypical Antidepressants). Neuromodulation approaches (rTMS, ECT) are outside this volume's scope.

21.10 Composite Signatures

The remaining entries describe constellations: phenotypes defined by the joint presence of two or more of the single-feature patterns cataloged above. Composites carry their own medication-prediction implications when the literature has examined the joint pattern, and they often guide the prescriber conversation more reliably than any single component because they constrain the differential diagnosis more tightly. The same group-to-individual caveat applies; the same claim-type conventions apply.

21.10.1 Hyperarousal Constellation [phenotype inference]

Prediction question. For clients presenting with the joint pattern of globally elevated high beta and reduced posterior alpha (component phenotypes `high_beta_global_high` and `alpha_posterior_low`), what does the literature suggest about medication response?

This constellation is the QEEG correlate of the chronic hyperarousal state seen across generalized anxiety, panic disorder, PTSD, OCD-spectrum presentations, and chronic insomnia. Both component patterns have been replicated in anxiety-spectrum samples; the joint occurrence is more specific to a sustained activation state than either feature alone (Johnstone et al., 2005; V. J. Knott et al., 2000). The medication-prediction reasoning combines the SSRI literature for the underlying anxiety phenotype with mechanistic reasoning about which pharmacological approaches address the activation state durably versus those that only override it.

SSRIs and SNRIs are the conventional pharmacotherapy for the underlying anxiety state, but the EEG evidence does not show the constellation resolving as the client improves. Alpha power did not change across 12 weeks of fluoxetine treatment in depressed patients (Bruder et al., 2008), and the paroxetine work reports pretreatment spectral correlates of outcome rather than post-treatment normalization (V. J. Knott et al., 2000). Buspirone, a partial 5-HT1A agonist, may produce a similar profile through serotonergic modulation without direct GABAergic effect. Whether baseline hyperarousal-constellation severity predicts differential SSRI response has not been tested prospectively, and mechanism-to-target alignment is not a substitute for that test. The composite does not indicate a drug or a drug class, and whether pharmacotherapy is indicated at all is a clinical decision it does not contribute to. Benzodiazepines reduce high beta and increase alpha acutely through GABAergic suppression, but the effect is state-dependent rather than reflective of restored endogenous regulation, and tolerance, dependence, and rebound complicate long-term use. The acute-versus-durable distinction matters and should be communicated explicitly to the prescriber when benzodiazepines are being considered.

Two clinical preconditions warrant attention before any drug is added. Stimulant overmedication, including over-the-counter and prescription stimulants and excessive caffeine, can produce the constellation iatrogenically, which is the first thing to tell the prescriber; whether the dose comes down, rather than pharmacotherapy being added, is their call. Sleep architecture should also be assessed, because chronic sleep restriction sustains the hyperarousal pattern and undermines treatment response across drug classes.

Forward-direction cross-reference. Read Part II Ch 6 (SSRIs and SNRIs) and Ch 8 (Benzodiazepines) before the prescriber discussion. The durable-versus-override distinction documented in those chapters is essential context for this recommendation.

For pattern recognition and exemplar plates, see Field Guide *Ch 6, Hyperarousal Constellation entry.*

21.10.2 Classic Attention Constellation [phenotype inference]

Prediction question. For clients presenting with the joint pattern of elevated frontal theta and reduced central SMR (component phenotypes `frontal_theta_high` and `smr_low`), what does the literature suggest about medication response?

This constellation is the canonical attention-deficit QEEG signature in the Suffin and Emory and Arns frameworks, though neither framework tested the two components jointly. Suffin and Emory reported that their frontal theta excess subgroup was responsive to stimulants across that retrospective series, while their frontal theta excess with hypercoherence subgroup responded mostly to anticonvulsants instead, so the subgrouping turns on what accompanies the theta (Suffin & Emory, 1995). Arns and colleagues' 2008 study found that children with a frontal slow phenotype improved on a continuous-performance measure under stimulant treatment, classifying by visually identified phenotype rather than by the theta/beta ratio (Arns et al., 2008). The mechanistic reading is consistent across frameworks: elevated frontal theta with reduced SMR points to combined cortical underactivation and sensorimotor underregulation, both of which catecholaminergic stimulation addresses directly.

When the constellation is identified in a client carrying the symptom-level ADHD diagnosis, it is consistent with a presentation that, at the group level, often responds to stimulants; that is context for the prescriber, not a drug selection. The prediction studies used methylphenidate; amphetamine-class stimulants share the catecholaminergic mechanism but were not tested in this literature. The association is qualified by the iAPF finding: if iAPF is also slowed, the Brainmarker-I data showed lower group-level stimulant response in that subgroup (see the slowed-modality entry below). When iAPF is in the normal-to-fast range, the EEG and the clinical picture are consistent rather than in tension. The Suffin and Emory tradition also used a single-dose stimulant challenge design with intra-test EEG monitoring, where frontal theta normalization on a single dose was taken as evidence of mechanism engagement. That design has not been tested in a controlled trial.

The replication and reliability caveats from the frontal theta and TBR entries apply here. The Boxum 2024 EEG-subtyping study found no association between EEG subtype and behavioral traits, and the Arns 2013 meta-analysis reduced confidence in TBR as a stand-alone diagnostic while keeping a prognostic role for excess theta in a subgroup (Arns et al., 2013; Boxum et al., 2024). The constellation has been associated with a higher group-level probability of stimulant response, not with a guaranteed outcome for any individual client. The finding can be communicated to the prescriber as supporting evidence, with explicit acknowledgment that individual-level prediction confidence is limited.

Forward-direction cross-reference. When the prescriber is considering stimulant titration, the forward-direction theta and SMR effects sit in Part II Ch 5 (Stimulants).

For pattern recognition and exemplar plates, see Field Guide *Ch 6, Classic Attention Constellation entry.*

21.10.3 Sensory Sensitivity Composite [workflow heuristic]

Prediction question. For clients presenting with the joint pattern of globally elevated high beta, reduced posterior alpha, and elevated temporal beta (component phenotypes `high_beta_global_high`, `alpha_posterior_low`, and `temporal_beta_high`), what does the literature suggest about medication response?

This three-component constellation extends the hyperarousal pattern with a temporal-beta component that raises the clinical question of cortical irritability. The composite presentation overlaps with sensory-sensitivity complaints, hyperreactivity to ambient stimuli, autonomic reactivity, and, in some clients, atypical sensory processing of the kind described in the autism spectrum and developmental-trauma literatures. Drug-class response has not been tested against this composite as a medication-prediction signature; the entry is structured around mechanism-driven reasoning rather than prediction evidence.

The clinical sequence is differential-diagnostic before pharmacological. The temporal-beta component should prompt evaluation for epileptiform activity, paroxysmal features, or temporal-lobe instability, because the presence of any of those findings shifts the conversation toward anticonvulsant consideration and away from the hyperarousal-anxiety pharmacology that the rest of the constellation suggests (Johnstone et al., 2005). Once epileptiform activity is excluded, the SSRI-and-buspirone reasoning from the hyperarousal entry applies for the anxiety component, with the same caveat that no controlled trial has tested baseline composite severity as a response predictor. Stimulants augment fast-frequency activity at the sites that are already overactive in this profile, so activation-related adverse effects are the monitoring priority if a prescriber independently trials a stimulant; the same caution that applies to the LVF and excess-beta phenotypes applies here.

The honest summary is that this composite is hypothesis-generating rather than prescriptive. The component patterns each carry some literature signal; the joint occurrence sharpens the clinical picture but does not produce a controlled-trial prediction beyond what the components individually provide.

Forward-direction cross-reference. For how SSRIs reduce hyperarousal-related fast activity, how anticonvulsants address temporal irritability, and how stimulants can augment beta, see Part II Ch 5 (Stimulants), Ch 6 (SSRIs and SNRIs), and Ch 11 (Anticonvulsants and Mood Stabilizers).

For pattern recognition and exemplar plates, see Field Guide *Ch 6, Sensory Sensitivity Composite entry.*

21.10.4 ADHD Excess-Beta Subtype [phenotype inference]

Prediction question. For clients presenting with the joint pattern of elevated frontal high beta and fast individual alpha peak frequency (component phenotypes `high_beta_frontal_high` and `alpha_peak_freq_high`) in the context of an ADHD presentation, what does the literature suggest about medication response?

This composite captures one of the more clinically consequential medication-prediction tensions in the ADHD subtype literature. The fast-iAPF component carries the Brainmarker-I prediction of better methylphenidate remission, on the reading that a faster alpha peak reflects faster information processing in thalamocortical pathways (Voetterl, Wingen, et al., 2023). The frontal high-beta component maps onto the excess-beta cluster Clarke and colleagues identified within ADHD samples (Clarke et al., 2001); the expectation that the same stimulant exposure may augment an already-elevated fast-frequency activation state, increasing anxiety, irritability, sleep disruption, and somatic activation, is mechanistic and was not tested in that work.

The clinical decision often becomes a balance between focus improvement and worsened anxiety. Methylphenidate and amphetamine-class stimulants may produce the cognitive benefit that fast iAPF predicts while also amplifying the hyperarousal that the frontal beta component flags. What this composite raises is one question worth handing to the prescriber: whether activation risk is a live concern for this client. It does not indicate a dose, a titration rate, or a drug class. Non-stimulant agents operate through mechanisms less likely to augment cortical fast-frequency activity, but no randomized trial has compared stimulant and non-stimulant outcomes in clients prospectively identified by this composite, and mechanism is not a substitute for that comparison.

The prescriber conversation should present the research picture. The fast-iAPF component is associated at the group level with better stimulant response in the Brainmarker-I data, while the frontal high-beta component is the pattern Clarke described among poor stimulant responders. Communicating both associations, rather than relying on either alone, gives the prescriber context for the clinical decision. This is a group-level research association and is not validated to select or avoid medication for an individual.

Forward-direction cross-reference. For how stimulants and non-stimulant ADHD medications affect frontal beta and alpha peak frequency, see Part II Ch 5 (Stimulants).

For pattern recognition and exemplar plates, see Field Guide *Ch 6, ADHD Excess-Beta Subtype entry.*

21.10.5 ADHD Excess-Alpha Subtype [phenotype inference]

Prediction question. For clients presenting with the joint pattern of frontal alpha excess and slow individual alpha peak frequency (component phenotypes `frontal_alpha_excess` and `alpha_peak_freq_low`) in the context of an ADHD presentation, what does the literature suggest about medication response?

This composite is one of the more commonly reported QEEG profiles in clients whose history includes poorly tolerated stimulant trials. The slow-iAPF component is the Brainmarker-I phenotype, and the Voetterl 2023 ADHD work found that a slower iAPF predicted poorer methylphenidate remission (Voetterl, Wingen, et al., 2023), and the companion depression work found superior sertraline response for slow iAPF when the model was checked blinded and out-of-sample against the placebo-controlled EMBARC data (Voetterl, Sack, et al., 2023). The frontal alpha excess component, which sits in the ADHD subtyping tradition rather than in a named Clarke cluster (Clarke et al., 2001), picks out a subgroup whose ADHD-like presentation involves frontal disengagement rather than the cortical underactivation that classical stimulant-responsive ADHD reflects. In the available data, both components were independently associated with poorer stimulant response at the group level.

Clients with this composite have been reported to show poor cognitive response, paradoxical activation, or both under stimulant trials. The mechanistic reading is that catecholaminergic drive does not address the slowed thalamocortical timing that the slow iAPF reflects; stimulating an already alpha-saturated frontal cortex risks producing activation without targeted improvement in attention and processing speed. Sertraline was the better-responding arm in the Brainmarker-I stratification, which is relevant when depression or anxiety is also present and a serotonergic agent is clinically appropriate. The same stratification reported better electroconvulsive therapy remission in slow-iAPF clients, but neuromodulation sits outside this volume's scope and a QEEG finding is not a reason to raise it. Bupropion and other activating non-stimulant antidepressants have not been tested prospectively in this composite, and the activation logic that supports their use in posterior-alpha-excess presentations may apply less cleanly here because frontal disengagement is mechanistically distinct from posterior idling.

The prescriber message is direct. When this composite is identified in a client whose history includes failed or poorly tolerated stimulant trials, that history is consistent with the group-level QEEG association rather than with poor effort or noncompliance. Communicating that consistency to the prescriber provides context for their clinical reasoning without directing what they prescribe next.

Forward-direction cross-reference. For how stimulants and SSRIs affect frontal alpha and alpha peak frequency, see Part II Ch 5 (Stimulants) and Ch 6 (SSRIs and SNRIs).

For pattern recognition and exemplar plates, see Field Guide *Ch 6, ADHD Excess-Alpha Subtype entry.*

21.10.6 Frontal Disconnect (TBI Pattern) [phenotype inference]

Prediction question. For clients presenting with the joint pattern of reduced frontal coherence and elevated frontal slow activity (component phenotypes `coherence_frontal_low` and `frontal_delta_theta_high`), what does the literature suggest about medication response?

The combined pattern is a recognizable post-TBI signature in the clinical QEEG tradition, where reduced frontal coupling alongside elevated frontal delta-theta activity is read as white-matter or functional disconnection accompanied by underactivation of frontal cortex after diffuse axonal injury. Read that against the source literature, which is less tidy. Thatcher's discriminant work found frontal and frontotemporal coherence and phase changes after mechanical head injury, but in the direction of increased coherence and decreased phase rather than reduced coupling, alongside reduced posterior alpha and flattened anterior-posterior power differences (Thatcher et al., 1989); the later methodological work makes the further point that measured coherence depends heavily on the reference scheme used to compute it (Thatcher, 2010). The composite should be held loosely on that account. Prediction data is absent for this composite as a medication-prediction signature; the literature treats it as a structural-functional finding rather than as a candidate for pharmacological matching.

The drug-relevant clinical priority is iatrogenic harm reduction rather than positive prediction. Sedating medications and anticholinergic-burden agents worsen the pattern through the same mechanisms described in the frontal hypocoherence and global delta entries. Common offenders in post-TBI populations include sedating antidepressants, sedating muscle relaxants for chronic pain, anticholinergic bladder medications, sedating sleep agents, and certain anticonvulsants prescribed for headache or mood. A medication review focused on these categories is the appropriate first step before any new prescription is initiated.

When the medication review is complete and the client remains symptomatic, the pharmacological choices are guided by the symptom-level presentation rather than by the QEEG composite. Stimulants are sometimes used off-label for post-TBI attentional deficits, with the same activation rationale that applies to classical ADHD; cognitive enhancers (cholinesterase inhibitors, memantine) may be considered in clients whose presentation overlaps with cognitive-decline indications. Neither pathway has prospective prediction evidence specific to this composite, and the prescriber conversation should frame the QEEG finding as a structural-functional context for symptom-driven prescribing rather than as a drug-class selection signal.

Forward-direction cross-reference. For how sedating medications and anticholinergics affect frontal slow activity and coherence, see Part II Ch 5 (Stimulants), Ch 8 (Benzodiazepines), and Ch 7 (TCAs, MAOIs, and Atypical Antidepressants). Cognitive enhancers (cholinesterase inhibitors, memantine) used post-TBI are disease-specific prescribing considerations outside this volume's QEEG-prediction scope.

For pattern recognition and exemplar plates, see Field Guide *Ch 6, Frontal Disconnect (TBI Pattern) entry.*

21.10.7 Rumination Constellation [workflow heuristic]

Prediction question. For clients presenting with the joint pattern of elevated posterior cingulate theta and alpha and right-greater-than-left frontal alpha asymmetry (component phenotypes `pcc_theta_alpha_high` and `frontal_alpha_asymmetry_right_high`), what does the literature suggest about medication response?

This composite is mechanism-driven rather than prediction-tested. The posterior cingulate component implicates default-mode network overengagement; the posterior cingulate is one of the regions whose task-related deactivation defined the default mode (Raichle et al.,

2001), and the link from sustained DMN activity to rumination in MDD comes from later fMRI work rather than from that paper. The right-greater-than-left frontal alpha asymmetry component is the Bruder phenotype linked, with sex-dependent effects, to differential SSRI response in depression (Bruder et al., 2001; Bruder et al., 2008). The pharmacotherapy literature has nothing to say about the joint pattern as a stand-alone medication-prediction signature, and the entry accordingly carries workflow-heuristic confidence.

The drug-prediction signal that does exist comes from the FAA component alone. In Bruder's 2001 sample, the right-greater-than-left alpha power direction (indicating relatively greater left frontal activation) was associated with better SSRI response, not poorer. The 2008 follow-up did not replicate that finding at frontal sites; the responder/nonresponder difference appeared at occipital sites instead, and the effect was stronger in women. Reference-scheme sensitivity and modest effect sizes further constrain the inference; this is hypothesis-generating evidence rather than a clinical directive. The composite as a whole has not been tested as a medication-prediction signature. SSRIs remain a reasonable first-line consideration for the depressive symptomatology this composite often accompanies; the FAA component does not argue against that choice.

The rumination-process component of this composite may respond more reliably to non-pharmacological interventions than to medication adjustment alone. Mindfulness-based cognitive therapy and rumination-focused CBT have demonstrated efficacy in reducing rumination and lowering relapse risk in MDD, and they are reasonable adjuncts when this composite is identified. The clinical message for the prescriber is that pharmacotherapy alone may underperform expectations in the rumination-dominant presentation, and that combined-modality care often produces better outcomes than medication monotherapy.

Forward-direction cross-reference. For how SSRIs affect frontal alpha asymmetry and posterior alpha-theta distributions, see Part II Ch 6 (SSRIs and SNRIs).

For pattern recognition and exemplar plates, see Field Guide *Ch 6, Rumination Constellation entry.*

21.10.8 Encephalopathic Composite [workflow heuristic]

Prediction question. For clients presenting with the joint pattern of mixed fast-slow activity and globally elevated delta (component phenotypes `mixed_fast_slow` and `delta_global_high`), what does the literature suggest about medication response?

The encephalopathic pattern reproduces and intensifies the message of its components. The joint occurrence of mixed fast-slow activity with diffuse delta elevation is nonspecific. Sedative polypharmacy, toxic or metabolic illness, drowsiness, and artifact all produce it, and neither the raw EEG nor the quantitative record distinguishes them or establishes that a regimen is causal. The pattern raises polypharmacy and toxic-metabolic encephalopathy as questions, and it functions as a medical-workup and medication-inventory prompt rather than as a candidate for additional pharmacological matching.

The appropriate response is raw-EEG review, medical referral for differential diagnosis, and an accurate medication inventory handed to the treating team. Whether tapering or consolidating the contributing agents changes the QEEG, and over what interval, has not been studied, so no timeline should be offered to a client or a prescriber. Adding any drug to the regimen on the basis of the QEEG composite is not supported either. Taper and consolidation decisions belong entirely to the prescriber and rest on clinical grounds; several of the agents that contribute to this picture, benzodiazepines and sedating anticonvulsants among them, carry withdrawal risk that no QEEG feature can weigh.

No published prediction framework supports positive medication selection for this composite, and the entry should not inform prescribing decisions in that direction. The clinical priority is identifying and addressing the cause. If the regimen changes and the systemic workup is complete, any residual phenotype features can be reassessed against the standard prediction frameworks. Until that point, the QEEG finding is a prompt for clinical and medical reassessment rather than a guide to pharmacotherapy.

Forward-direction cross-reference. For how the contributing drug classes produce the component patterns, see Part II Ch 8 (Benzodiazepines), Ch 7 (TCAs, MAOIs, and Atypical Antidepressants), Ch 9 (Typical Antipsychotics), Ch 10 (Atypical Antipsychotics), and Ch 11 (Anticonvulsants and Mood Stabilizers).

For pattern recognition and exemplar plates, see Field Guide *Ch 6, Encephalopathic Composite entry.*

21.10.9 OCD Signature Composite [workflow heuristic]

Prediction question. For clients presenting with the joint pattern of elevated midline theta and elevated frontal high beta (component phenotypes `midline_theta_high` and `high_beta_frontal_high`), what does the literature suggest about medication response?

Two recognizable OCD-spectrum electrophysiological features converge here: midline theta elevation associated with anterior cingulate hyperactivity (Cavanagh & Frank, 2014; Cohen, 2011), and frontal high-beta elevation, which is read clinically as cognitive hyperarousal and worry-dominant cognition. The excess-beta cluster behind that second reading was described in ADHD samples rather than in OCD ones (Clarke et al., 2001), so the transfer across populations is an assumption of this entry. The composite appears in OCD, generalized anxiety with prominent worry, and some perfectionism-driven clinical presentations. No prospective prediction trial has tested this composite as a stand-alone signature for differential medication response.

The drug-prediction conversation is anchored to established OCD pharmacotherapy rather than to QEEG-based stratification. SSRIs are the established first-line treatment for OCD across diagnostic guidelines. The composite neither supports nor argues against that choice, because nothing has tested it against treatment outcome; the guideline stands on its own evidence. OCD treatment guidelines specify SSRI dosing and trial-duration requirements that differ from depression treatment; those specifics sit in the prescriber's guideline reference, not in a QEEG phenotype entry. Clomipramine (Anafranil), a serotonergic tricyclic, retains a role for SSRI non-responders, with its broader pharmacological profile producing greater side-effect burden but, in some clients, superior response.

The treatment-resistance literature describes augmentation with atypical antipsychotics (risperidone (Risperdal), aripiprazole (Abilify)) and, with a smaller evidence base, glutamatergic agents (memantine, riluzole, N-acetylcysteine) for refractory cases. None of these augmentation strategies has been linked prospectively to the QEEG composite, and this entry provides no basis for choosing among them. Exposure and response prevention (ERP) therapy is the established psychotherapy for OCD and produces effect sizes comparable to or exceeding SSRI monotherapy in head-to-head comparisons; combined ERP-and-SSRI care is the standard for moderate-to-severe presentations. These treatment decisions belong with the prescribing team, and none of them follows from the QEEG. The composite is not a route to an alternative pathway, and it is not evidence for the standard one either.

Forward-direction cross-reference. For how SSRIs, tricyclics, and atypical antipsychotics affect midline theta and frontal beta, see Part II Ch 6 (SSRIs and SNRIs), Ch 7 (TCAs, MAOIs, and Atypical Antidepressants), and Ch 10 (Atypical Antipsychotics).

For pattern recognition and exemplar plates, see Field Guide *Ch 6, OCD Signature Composite entry.*

21.10.10 Slowed-Modality Composite (Brainmarker-I Underarousal) [phenotype inference]

Prediction question. For clients presenting with the joint pattern of slow individual alpha peak frequency and elevated frontal theta (component phenotypes `alpha_peak_freq_low` and `frontal_theta_high`), what does the literature suggest about medication response?

This composite is the central treatment-stratification signature in the Brainmarker-I framework. The slow-iAPF component carries the strongest QEEG-based medication-prediction evidence in the current literature: Voetterl and colleagues' 2023 accuracy study found that slow iAPF predicted superior sertraline response in depression, a result that held up blinded and out-of-sample against randomized placebo-controlled data, and the same lineage links slow iAPF to better ECT response (Voetterl, Sack, et al., 2023). The companion ADHD paper reports the other side of the stratification, with slower peaks going to poorer methylphenidate remission and better outcomes from combined non-pharmacological care (Voetterl, Wingen, et al., 2023). The frontal theta component, in isolation, has a long history as a putative stimulant-response predictor in ADHD (Arns et al., 2008; Suffin & Emory, 1995). In combination, the two components produce a clinically consequential research finding: in the Brainmarker-I sample, the composite was associated with lower group-level stimulant response and higher serotonergic response.

The composite signature is the major reason the "stimulants made me worse" complaint should be taken seriously rather than reframed as poor effort or motivation. In the Brainmarker-I sample, slow iAPF was associated with poorer methylphenidate remission, and the addition of a frontal theta excess does not rescue the prediction. The mechanistic reading is that catecholaminergic drive does not address the thalamocortical timing deficit the slow iAPF reflects. In the studied populations, the slow-iAPF group showed lower methylphenidate remission rates; anxiety and sleep disruption are the adverse effects to monitor if a prescriber independently trials a stimulant in a client carrying this composite. In the Brainmarker-I stratification, the slow-iAPF component placed this profile in the sertraline-responding arm when depression was the presenting condition. The same stratification reported better ECT remission in slow-iAPF clients. Whether ECT is considered at all is a psychiatric decision about illness severity and treatment history, not one this composite contributes to.

In a client presenting with mixed depression and inattention, the conventional pathway might trial a stimulant first for the inattention or an SSRI first for the depression on the basis of symptom prominence. The Brainmarker-I data associate this composite with lower group-level stimulant response and higher serotonergic response in the populations studied. That association is anchored in a placebo-controlled trial, which distinguishes it from most other entries in this chapter, but the drug-response claim rests on a single study and has not been independently replicated in a pharmacotherapy trial. This is a group-level research association and is not validated to select or avoid medication for an individual.

Forward-direction cross-reference. For how SSRIs and stimulants affect alpha peak frequency, frontal theta, and thalamocortical dynamics, see Part II Ch 5 (Stimulants) and Ch 6 (SSRIs and SNRIs). ECT and other neuromodulation approaches are outside this volume's scope; see *QEEG Field Guide* Ch 6 for the Brainmarker-I iAPF evidence base.

For pattern recognition and exemplar plates, see Field Guide *Ch 6, Slowed-Modality Composite (Brainmarker-I Underarousal) entry.*

21.11 Methodological Note: Aperiodic Decomposition

The treatment-response literature underlying the entries in this chapter was produced largely before aperiodic spectral decomposition became a standard analytical step. Most studies report band-power metrics (theta, alpha, TBR) that combine periodic oscillatory activity with the aperiodic 1/f background of the EEG. The consequence is that group-level prediction signals attributed to "elevated theta" or "slow alpha peak" may partially reflect aperiodic exponent or offset shifts rather than purely oscillatory features. This does not invalidate the directional claims (the prediction signals exist in the data as processed), but it means that specific mechanistic interpretations and magnitude thresholds should be held with additional caution. The Brainmarker-I iAPF metric is less susceptible to this issue because individual alpha peak frequency is a peak-frequency estimate rather than a band-power sum, but even iAPF estimation can be influenced by aperiodic slope in lower-frequency ranges. When this chapter is revised for a second edition, translating the empirical base into specparam-consistent terms will be a priority.

Part IV

Complex Cases

Ch 22: Polypharmacy in NFB Practice

22.1 Why this class matters in NFB practice

Polypharmacy is the rule, not the exception, in real neurofeedback practice. Mojtabai and Olfson documented that office-based psychiatric visits increasingly involved multiple psychotropics, with the median number of psychotropics per visit rising from one to two and visits involving two or more medications increasing over the study window (Mojtabai & Olfson, 2010). That trend matches what clinicians see: SSRI plus stimulant, stimulant plus sleep aid, antipsychotic plus mood stabilizer, benzodiazepine plus antidepressant, pain medication plus psychotropic, and medical medications layered on top.

Strongest evidence	Psychotropic polypharmacy is common in psychiatric practice, but direct QEEG evidence for realistic medication stacks is sparse.
Biggest interpretation trap	Applying single-drug rules to stacks: A methylphenidate chapter cannot explain a stimulant plus SSRI plus benzodiazepine plus cannabis stack.
Default clinical action	Use single-drug evidence only as a starting point, lower confidence for 4-6 drug stacks, and document the full exposure state before making attributions.

The problem is that pharmaco-EEG evidence rarely follows the client into that reality. Most studies examine one drug, one diagnosis, one dose window, and a cleaned-up sample. The client in front of the clinician may have ADHD, anxiety, pain, sleep apnea, cannabis use, caffeine, an SSRI, a stimulant, a benzodiazepine PRN, and an antihistamine at night.

This chapter is therefore not a claim that every stack has a known signature. It is the opposite. Realistic 4-6 drug stacks have almost no direct pharmaco-EEG literature. The task is to interpret conservatively, document thoroughly, and use the book's four interaction modes: masking, mimicry, exaggeration, and transformation.

22.2 Mechanism (clinician-level pharmacology)

Polypharmacy alters EEG through pharmacodynamic and pharmacokinetic pathways. Pharmacodynamic interactions occur when drugs push the brain in similar or opposing directions. A stimulant and a benzodiazepine can create simultaneous activation and sedation signals. An antipsychotic and an anticonvulsant can both contribute to slowing. An SSRI and caffeine can both affect arousal, sleep, and beta interpretation.

Pharmacokinetic interactions occur when one drug changes the exposure of another. CYP inhibition can raise concentration; induction can lower it; renal or hepatic impairment can prolong exposure. A medication with a mild EEG effect alone may become more visible when another drug increases its level. A medication expected to be active may look weak if metabolism is accelerated or adherence is inconsistent.

PRN medications matter because they can dominate the recording day. A daily SSRI may be steady, but a benzodiazepine taken that morning, diphenhydramine taken the night before, cannabis used the evening before, or caffeine skipped that day can shift vigilance more than the chronic medication.

Comorbidity drives much of this. Polypharmacy is not usually random. A client with ADHD plus anxiety often ends up on stimulant plus SSRI or SNRI. Bipolar disorder plus insomnia may lead to mood stabilizer, antipsychotic, and sleep medication. Chronic pain plus depression may lead to SNRI, gabapentinoid, opioid, cannabis, or antihistamine. The EEG reflects the stack and the conditions that produced the stack.

Medication	Phenotype	Confounder/State	Mode	Confidence
SSRIs	Polypharmacy composite context	Psychotropic polypharmacy	transformation	reduced
Benzodiazepines	Medication-stack masking context	PRN medication overlay	masking	substantially reduced
Antipsychotics	Polypharmacy composite context	Psychotropic polypharmacy	exaggeration	reduced
Methylphenidate	Medication-stack masking context	PRN medication overlay	transformation	reduced
Opioids	Comorbidity-driven polypharmacy evidence gap	Multi-diagnosis medication stack	exaggeration	substantially reduced

Figure 22.1: Polypharmacy interaction matrix: common medication stacks with interaction modes and confidence adjustments.

22.3 Known spectral effects

There are few true polypharmacy QEEG studies. Hyun and colleagues provide useful evidence that psychotropic medication status can affect QEEG interpretation in psychiatric populations, but the literature does not resolve realistic medication stacks into clean additive components (Hyun et al., 2011). Zandstra and colleagues reinforce the broader problem that psychotropic exposure and clinical complexity complicate EEG interpretation (Zandstra et al., 2023).

The strongest empirical statement is epidemiologic and methodological: multiple psychotropics are common (Mojtabai & Olfson, 2010), while direct medication-stack pharmaco-EEG evidence is sparse. The clinician then infers from single-drug signatures and downgrades confidence.

Common stack expectations should remain qualitative. SSRI plus stimulant may combine antidepressant-related alpha/beta changes with stimulant-related attention-state effects. SSRI plus benzodiazepine may combine chronic antidepressant exposure with acute or intermittent sedative effects. Antipsychotic plus mood stabilizer may increase slowing or reduce alpha clarity. Stimulant plus sleep aid may create a day-night alternation: daytime activation with residual morning sedation. Pain medication plus psychotropic may mix pain arousal, sedative load, and sleep disruption.

22.4 Phenotype interaction effects

The four interaction modes from Chapter 1 (masking, mimicry, exaggeration, and transformation) apply to polypharmacy stacks, but with a complication: multiple drugs can activate different modes simultaneously. A stimulant may mask theta while a benzodiazepine mimics beta excess and untreated OSA exaggerates slowing, all in the same recording. A normal-looking map in a heavily medicated client may reflect masking rather than absence of clinical concern.

22.5 Common Medication Stacks

Each drug in a stack can produce its own spectral effects during a recording. This book does not predict a net composite direction for any combination, because stacks do not add as vectors; some mask, some exaggerate, some transform the individual signatures in ways that cannot be decomposed from a single recording (see "Assuming additive effects" in the interpretation traps below). The twelve stacks listed here are the ones clinicians encounter most often. For each, the example regimen is illustrative, the interaction mode names how the drugs relate, the primary trap names the attribution error most likely to follow, and the confidence ceiling reflects how far phenotype interpretation can go.

SSRI + benzodiazepine. Sertraline 100 mg QD + clonazepam 0.5 mg QHS or PRN. Mimicry and masking: benzo-beta mimics anxiety beta while masking the SSRI-responder phenotype. Trap: calling benzo-beta endogenous hyperarousal without documenting benzo timing. Confidence reduced.

Stimulant + SSRI. Lisdexamfetamine 50 mg QAM + sertraline 100 mg QD. Masking plus mimicry: stimulant suppresses theta phenotype; SSRI activation can mimic hyperarousal beta. Trap: reading a "normalized" TBR as a clean phenotype when it reflects near-peak stimulant coverage. Confidence moderate if timing is documented; reduced otherwise.

SSRI + benzodiazepine + cannabis. Escitalopram 10 mg QD + lorazepam 0.5 mg PRN + cannabis edible 5-10 mg THC nightly. Exaggeration and masking: three sedative-adjacent exposures reduce alpha reactivity through different mechanisms. Trap: missing cannabis because the intake asked about "marijuana" but not edibles; edibles carry a longer pharmacokinetic window. Confidence reduced to substantially reduced depending on cannabis recency.

Antipsychotic + mood stabilizer. Quetiapine 200 mg QHS + valproate 1000 mg BID. Exaggeration: both are clinically sedating. Trap: reading diffuse slowing as a mood-disorder phenotype without accounting for medication load; the reverse is as costly when next-morning quetiapine sedation becomes the default explanation for slowing that has a medical cause. Confidence reduced to substantially reduced.

Dual stimulant + caffeine. Methylphenidate XR 36 mg QAM + armodafinil 150 mg QAM + caffeine 400 mg. Exaggeration: three arousal-pathway activators suppress any hypoarousal phenotype. Trap: using this recording to "confirm" no attention phenotype when TBR is normalized by triple coverage. Confidence low for unmedicated phenotype claims.

Gabapentinoid + opioid. Gabapentin 600 mg TID + oxycodone ER 20 mg BID + PRN oxycodone IR 5 mg. Exaggeration: both reduce arousal through different mechanisms. Trap: assigning the slow-wave profile to the pain condition rather than the medication stack. Confidence substantially reduced; useful as a current-state baseline, not for phenotype labeling.

Three-drug attention stack. Amphetamine XR 20 mg QAM + buspirone 10 mg BID + zolpidem 5 mg QHS. Masking with possible zolpidem mimicry if the 8-hour window was not met. Trap: missing zolpidem timing; document the drug, dose, and clock time rather than inferring clearance. Confidence moderate if timings documented; reduced if zolpidem timing is unknown.

SSRI + stimulant + benzodiazepine. Fluoxetine 20 mg QD + methylphenidate ER 27 mg QAM + alprazolam 0.25 mg PRN. Multiple modes simultaneous: stimulant masking theta, benzo mimicking anxiety beta, SSRI transforming FAA. Trap: phenotype labeling without documenting alprazolam timing; PRN benzos are frequently taken before appointments because the appointment triggers anxiety. Confidence reduced; substantially reduced for FAA.

Antipsychotic + mood stabilizer + antidepressant. Lurasidone 40 mg QD + lamotrigine 150 mg BID + venlafaxine 150 mg QD. Complex composite with offsetting vectors; two of three agents are resting-QEEG gaps. Trap: treating the recording as a stable phenotype baseline when any dose change will shift the composite picture. Confidence reduced.

Gabapentinoid + antidepressant + sleep aid. Pregabalin 150 mg BID + duloxetine 60 mg QD + trazodone 50 mg QHS. Exaggeration partially offset by duloxetine activation. Trap: attributing reduced alpha and possible slow iAPF to fibromyalgia rather than the medication stack; pain severity and sleep quality on recording day are first-order variables. Confidence reduced.

Maintenance opioid + SSRI + benzodiazepine. Buprenorphine/naloxone 16 mg SL QD + sertraline 50 mg QD + clonazepam 0.5 mg QHS. Exaggeration combined with mimicry (benzo-beta mimicking anxiety). Trap: using QEEG findings to question the clinical appropriateness of buprenorphine maintenance. Buprenorphine and naloxone are stabilizing treatments for opioid use disorder; a report implying these produce a "problematic" brain state without naming the clinical indication introduces harmful framing. Confidence reduced; critically reduced for any interpretation implying medication questioning.

Steroid burst + psychiatric baseline. Prednisone 40 mg QD x 7 days overlaid on sertraline 100 mg QD + bupropion 150 mg QD. Exaggeration and mimicry: prednisone-related activation mimics anxiety or stimulant-class phenotypes. Trap: missing the steroid course because the intake asks only about psychiatric medications; clients frequently do not mention short-course steroids. Confidence reduced to substantially reduced during any active course and for at least one week after.

22.6 Claim-Type Discipline

Most comorbidity-specific pharmaco-EEG is a workflow heuristic unless directly supported. The exceptions are limited and should not be inflated into general rules. A clozapine (Clozaril) monotherapy finding in schizophrenia is not evidence for a clozapine plus valproate (Depakote) plus benzodiazepine plus cannabis stack. An ADHD stimulant response study is not evidence for stimulant plus SSRI plus insomnia medication in an anxious adult.

This does not make the interpretation useless. It makes it conditional. The clinician can say: "The stack plausibly exaggerates sedative load" or "the stimulant may mask theta during active dosing." The clinician should not say: "This exact QEEG pattern is caused by the stack."

22.7 Decision Workflow

Start by identifying the dominant exposure on the recording day. This is not always the medication with the highest clinical importance. A daily antidepressant may be less visible than a benzodiazepine taken that morning, a cannabis edible taken the night before, or a first-generation antihistamine taken for sleep.

Next, identify directionally aligned agents. If several exposures increase sedation, slow activity, or sleep fragmentation, the interpretation should emphasize exaggeration. If several exposures increase arousal, beta, insomnia, or task engagement, the interpretation should emphasize arousal-state complexity rather than a single anxious phenotype.

Then identify opposing agents. Stimulant plus sedative, caffeine plus sleep deprivation, SSRI activation plus benzodiazepine PRN, and cannabis plus stimulant can all produce mixed maps. Mixed maps are not necessarily mysterious; they may reflect competing exposures at different time scales.

Then identify high-risk attribution errors. If a finding would lead to a major clinical conclusion, ask whether any medication or substance in the stack could plausibly mimic it. Diffuse slowing should trigger a sedative-load check. Beta excess should trigger stimulant, caffeine, nicotine, withdrawal, and benzodiazepine checks. Low alpha or poor alpha block should trigger drowsiness, visual engagement, medication timing, and migraine checks.

Finally, assign confidence. A clean single-drug context may allow moderate confidence. A stable two-drug context may allow cautious interpretation. A changing 4-6 drug stack should usually be low-confidence for medication attribution unless the finding is gross, time-locked, or medically obvious.

22.8 Pharmacokinetic Interactions

CYP interactions are rarely visible as a neat QEEG signature, but they matter because they change exposure. A CYP inhibitor may make a medication act like a higher dose. An inducer may make it act like a lower dose. Poor metabolism can turn an ordinary dose into a high-exposure state, while rapid metabolism can make a medication look ineffective.

The clinician does not need to become a pharmacologist. The minimum standard is to flag when the medication list includes known inhibitors, inducers, narrow-therapeutic-index drugs, or pharmacogenetic results. Atomoxetine (Strattera) and CYP2D6 are the clean teaching example elsewhere in this book, but the principle applies more broadly.

The report language should remain modest: "The stack includes agents with possible pharmacokinetic interactions; medication-attribution confidence is reduced." That sentence is often more defensible than naming a specific enzyme interaction from memory.

22.9 When to Defer Interpretation

Sometimes the right answer is not a clever synthesis. If the medication list is incomplete, if PRN timing is unknown, if the client is in active withdrawal, if recent dose changes occurred, or if the recording day included unusual sleep or substance use, the report should defer strong medication interpretation.

Deferral does not mean the QEEG has no value. It means the QEEG documents the client in a particular unstable state. The clinician can still use raw EEG safety observations, artifact review, vigilance notes, and cautious symptom-linked planning. What should be deferred is high-confidence phenotype labeling and medication attribution.

22.10 Case vignette

Six active substances, four diagnoses, one 32-year-old: methylphenidate XR, sertraline (Zoloft), clonazepam (Klonopin) PRN, nightly gabapentin (Neurontin), several-times-per-week cannabis, daily morning caffeine, against a backdrop of ADHD, panic symptoms, insomnia, and chronic pain. The QEEG shows variable beta, intermittent frontal theta, and drowsiness during eyes closed.

There is no single-drug answer. The stimulant may improve task engagement. Sertraline may affect arousal and sleep. Clonazepam timing may suppress task response. Gabapentin and cannabis may increase drowsiness. Caffeine may increase fast activity while masking sleep debt. The correct report describes a polypharmacy context with reduced medication-attribution confidence. The bottle is not the only thing moving the trace. In this case, six different things are moving it simultaneously, and any report that names one of them as the explanation has chosen narrative coherence over clinical honesty.

A second client with bipolar disorder takes lithium, quetiapine (Seroquel), lamotrigine (Lamictal), and a sleep aid. Diffuse slowing is present. The report should not label the slowing as a tidy "bipolar phenotype" without naming sedative and anticonvulsant load; medication questions stay with the prescriber (see Clinical recommendations).

22.11 Interpretation traps

- **Applying single-drug rules to stacks.** A methylphenidate chapter cannot explain a stimulant plus SSRI plus benzodiazepine plus cannabis stack by itself.
- **Ignoring PRN timing.** The as-needed medication may dominate the recording day.
- **Counting only psychiatric drugs.** OTC antihistamines, cannabis, caffeine, nicotine, pain medications, and sleep agents matter.
- **Assuming additive effects.** Some stacks mask or transform effects rather than adding them.
- **Overclaiming causality.** Most stack interpretations are workflow-heuristic clinical synthesis.
- **Forgetting comorbidity.** The conditions that led to polypharmacy are also EEG confounders.

22.12 Intake questions

When this chapter's topic appears on the intake form, ask:

- **List every prescription medication.** Include dose, formulation, last dose, duration, and indication.
- **List every PRN medication.** Include the last time it was taken.
- **List OTC and supplements.** Include antihistamines, sleep aids, melatonin, magnesium, kava, valerian, and nootropics.
- **List substances.** Caffeine, nicotine, cannabis, alcohol, psychedelics, stimulants, and kratom need timing.
- **What changed recently?** New starts, dose changes, discontinuations, generic switches, missed doses, and holidays.

- **Which symptoms drove each medication?** ADHD, anxiety, insomnia, psychosis, mood instability, pain, migraine, fatigue, or sleep disorder.
- **Any known CYP or pharmacogenetic results?** Note CYP2D6, CYP2C19, and major inhibitors or inducers if known.
- **Any prescriber concerns?** Sedation, activation, seizure risk, QT concerns, falls, or cognitive adverse effects.

22.13 Clinical recommendations

Treat polypharmacy as a confidence reducer. The more CNS-active agents and relevant conditions present, the less confidently a QEEG finding can be assigned to one drug or phenotype.

Name the stack in the report. "Current CNS-relevant exposures include sertraline, methylphenidate XR, clonazepam PRN, gabapentin, cannabis, and caffeine" is better than "on medication."

Use the four interaction modes. State whether the stack may mask, mimic, exaggerate, or transform the phenotype. If the mode is uncertain, say that.

Separate chronic from acute exposure. A daily SSRI and a PRN benzodiazepine taken two hours before recording are not equivalent metadata.

Recommend matched-state follow-up when feasible. If a baseline was collected after PRN sedative use, a follow-up without PRN use may not be comparable.

> **Scope of practice.** QEEG interpretation does not direct prescribing. Medication decisions, including discontinuation, dose changes, and substitution, rest with the prescriber.

22.14 Evidence summary

- **Spectral effect:** Psychotropic polypharmacy is common in psychiatric practice, but direct QEEG evidence for realistic medication stacks is sparse.
- **Phenotype inference:** Medication stacks can mask, mimic, exaggerate, or transform phenotype interpretation, especially when PRN timing, sleep, pain, substances, and comorbidity are undocumented.

- **Workflow heuristic:** Use single-drug evidence only as a starting point, lower confidence for 4-6 drug stacks, and document the full exposure state before making phenotype claims.

Ch 23: Paradoxical Responses

23.1 Why this class matters in NFB practice

Population-level medication signatures are useful until a client reports that the medication does the opposite. A sedative causes agitation. A stimulant causes sleepiness. An antidepressant causes activation. An antipsychotic causes akathisia that looks like anxiety. Diphenhydramine makes a child wired. Caffeine makes an adult calm.

Strongest evidence	Paradoxical-response clinical phenomena are documented for several drug classes, but direct QEEG signatures are largely absent.
Biggest interpretation trap	Dismissing the client's report: Paradoxical response history is clinically relevant even when QEEG evidence is thin.
Default clinical action	Ask directly about opposite reactions, document them, screen timing / genetic / developmental context, and treat paradoxical responders as lower-confidence interpretations.

Paradoxical responses are uncommon, but they are clinically important because they invalidate simple class-level interpretation. If a benzodiazepine usually increases beta and sedation, but the client becomes disinhibited and agitated, the QEEG cannot be interpreted only through the ordinary benzodiazepine chapter. If methylphenidate usually improves alertness, but the client becomes sedated, the ordinary stimulant model is incomplete.

The evidence base is mostly clinical, not QEEG. Mancuso and colleagues review paradoxical benzodiazepine reactions (Mancuso et al., 2004). De Leon and colleagues describe CYP2D6 ultra-rapid metabolism as a mechanism for paradoxical diphenhydramine excitation (Leon & Nikoloff, 2008). Recent case literature describes methylphenidate-induced sedation (Naguy et al., 2024; Yadav & Garg, 2025). Developmental-variant contexts, including Down syndrome populations, must be framed respectfully and biologically, not pathologized.

23.2 Mechanism (clinician-level pharmacology)

Paradoxical response is a clinical observation, not a single mechanism. Several pathways can produce an opposite-looking effect.

First, receptor biology can differ. GABA-A receptor subunit variation, altered inhibitory control, or network-level disinhibition are among the proposed mechanisms by which a sedative might produce behavioral activation in a vulnerable person. Mancuso and colleagues document that paradoxical benzodiazepine agitation and disinhibition occur but conclude that the mechanism remains unclear, naming a genetic link, a history of alcohol abuse, and psychological disturbance as contributing factors (Mancuso et al., 2004).

Second, pharmacokinetics can produce unexpected exposure. Ultra-rapid or poor metabolism can change concentration, timing, active metabolites, and side-effect profile. Diphenhydramine excitation in CYP2D6 ultra-rapid metabolizers is the clean example in this chapter (Leon & Nikoloff, 2008).

Third, baseline arousal matters. A stimulant may calm a low-arousal ADHD presentation but sedate a rare responder through mechanisms that remain poorly mapped. A caffeine response may feel calming when it improves attention or reduces mental restlessness. These are subjective and behavioral effects, not established QEEG signatures.

Fourth, comorbidity and developmental neurobiology matter. Autistic individuals, people with Down syndrome, clients with TBI, older adults, children, and people with substance-use histories may have different vulnerability profiles. The correct language is developmental variant, condition, population, or neurobiology, not pathologizing framing.

23.3 Known spectral effects

The key QEEG finding is the gap: paradoxical responders are rarely characterized with pharmaco-EEG. Most literature documents behavior, adverse events, or pharmacogenomics without paired EEG.

Benzodiazepine paradoxical reactions include agitation, disinhibition, aggression, emotional lability, and hyperactivity in a small subset of users (Mancuso et al., 2004). There is no validated QEEG signature separating typical benzodiazepine responders from paradoxical responders.

Diphenhydramine paradoxical excitation can occur in children and in some adults with CYP2D6 ultra-rapid metabolism (Leon & Nikoloff, 2008). Whether the EEG looks stimulant-like, anticholinergic, or nonspecific is unknown.

Methylphenidate-induced sedation has been described in recent case literature (Naguy et al., 2024; Yadav & Garg, 2025). These reports are important because they warn clinicians not to assume that every stimulant exposure increases arousal. They do not establish a QEEG phenotype.

SSRI activation, antidepressant-induced switching, antipsychotic akathisia, and cannabis paradoxical anxiety are clinically recognized, but QEEG evidence is sparse. These phenomena should be treated as workflow-heuristic interpretation modifiers unless a specific study directly supports the claim.

Paradoxical response workflow. When a client reports the opposite of the expected drug effect: (1) document the reported response and timing, (2) check dose, formulation, and last-dose timing, (3) screen for pharmacogenomic context (CYP2D6 poor/ultra-rapid metabolizer, CYP2C19 status), (4) check for drug-drug interactions or recent switches, (5) consider developmental or diagnostic context (age, diagnosis, prior paradoxical history), (6) lower confidence in class-level EEG predictions for this client, and (7) coordinate medication questions with the prescriber. Paradoxical responses are workflow heuristics and should not be modeled algorithmically.

23.4 Phenotype interaction effects

Paradoxical responses transform medication interpretation. A beta excess under benzodiazepine exposure may not mean ordinary anxiolytic sedation. It may reflect agitation, disinhibition, withdrawal overlap, or paradoxical activation.

Paradoxical responses can mimic non-medication phenotypes. SSRI activation can look like anxiety, bipolar activation, insomnia, or stimulant excess. Antipsychotic akathisia can look like panic, agitation, or restlessness. Cannabis paradoxical anxiety can look like primary anxiety or withdrawal.

Paradoxical responses can mask expected effects. A stimulant that causes sedation may fail to reduce theta or improve task engagement. An antihistamine that causes activation may fail to produce the expected sedative slowing. A caffeine response that feels calming may improve task performance while still altering arousal markers.

Paradoxical responses can exaggerate existing vulnerability. A client with TBI, sleep deprivation, developmental-variant neurobiology, substance-use history, or pharmacogenomic exposure differences may show outsized or directionally unexpected effects.

23.5 Risk Contexts

Children and older adults already differ from middle-aged norms in both EEG and pharmacokinetics, so paradoxical reports in these groups deserve careful documentation. TBI and concussion histories add another layer, since behavioral disinhibition or fatigue from injury can be amplified by medications that are predictable in uncomplicated adults. In Down syndrome populations, cholinergic-system differences may alter anticholinergic response (Russell et al., 2025). In autistic individuals, stimulant and SSRI tolerability can vary. When response is surprising, extreme, or inconsistent with dose, consider pharmacogenomics. A QEEG cannot identify CYP status, but it can flag that prescriber review of pharmacogenetic context may be relevant.

23.6 Interpretive Workflow

Start by believing the report enough to document it. "Benadryl wires me" and "stimulants make me sleepy" are clinically relevant data, not contradictions to dismiss. Separate subjective effect from EEG effect; a client may feel calm on caffeine while EEG shows activation. Check timing, dose, formulation, co-exposures, and sleep context. Then lower confidence in class-level prediction. A paradoxical report does not prove the EEG will be opposite, but it prevents confident use of the ordinary signature.

23.7 Class-Specific Notes

Benzodiazepines are the canonical paradoxical-reaction class. The ordinary expectation is anxiolysis, sedation, and increased fast activity, but paradoxical reactions can include agitation, impulsivity, aggression, emotional lability, or disinhibition (Mancuso et al., 2004). A QEEG recorded during such a reaction should not be interpreted as a simple sedative-on-board state. The report should mention that behavioral response is atypical and that ordinary benzodiazepine class expectations may not apply.

First-generation antihistamines are common enough that every intake form should ask about them. Diphenhydramine is often assumed to be a benign sleep aid, but paradoxical excitation can occur, especially in children and in some pharmacogenomic contexts (Leon & Nikoloff, 2008). If a client used diphenhydramine the night before QEEG and reports activation rather than sedation, the recording may reflect poor sleep, anticholinergic effects, rebound fatigue, or activation.

Stimulants produce another interpretive trap. Calming with stimulants is not necessarily paradoxical in ADHD; it may reflect improved regulation. Sedation or sleepiness on stimulants is different and should be documented separately. Recent methylphenidate case literature is useful as a warning that sedation can occur (Naguy et al., 2024; Yadav & Garg, 2025), but it is not a basis for claiming a known QEEG pattern.

SSRIs and SNRIs can produce activation, insomnia, agitation, emotional lability, akathisia-like restlessness, or switching in vulnerable clients. The EEG may show nonspecific arousal or sleep disruption, but there is no validated "SSRI activation QEEG." When a client reports activation after initiation or dose increase, timing and symptom cluster are more important than band-power speculation.

Antipsychotic paradox is often not true paradox but expectation mismatch. A drug expected to calm may cause akathisia, inner restlessness, insomnia, or subjective activation. Aripiprazole (Abilify) and other partial agonist or activating profiles are especially important to document. QEEG should not equate akathisia with primary anxiety.

Cannabis can calm one client and provoke panic, derealization, tachycardia, or insomnia in another. Route, THC/CBD ratio, dose, tolerance, withdrawal, and anxiety vulnerability all matter. Cannabis paradoxical anxiety is clinically common enough to screen for, but QEEG signatures are heterogeneous and should not be overclaimed.

Caffeine can feel focusing or calming in some ADHD clients and anxiogenic in others. CYP1A2 and ADORA2A variation may affect subjective response, but clinical QEEG interpretation should stay practical: document dose, timing, habitual use, skipped use, and the client's reported response.

23.8 Report Language

Use conditional phrasing. "The client reports paradoxical agitation with benzodiazepines; therefore benzodiazepine-related findings should not be interpreted solely through the expected sedative profile." This is better than "benzodiazepines caused the beta excess."

Use gap language when needed. "No validated QEEG signature of methylphenidate-induced sedation is established; the present finding should be interpreted as a low-confidence medication-attribution context." That sentence protects the clinician from overreading a case report.

Use developmental language carefully. "In this client with Down syndrome" or "in Down syndrome populations" is appropriate. "Autistic individuals" or "on the autism spectrum," per the client's preference, is appropriate. Avoid language that pathologizes a developmental variant.

Use prescriber-coordination language when the response is risky. Akathisia, severe agitation, suicidal ideation, mania, dangerous sedation, delirium, or seizure-like symptoms should not be processed as ordinary QEEG interpretation.

23.9 Case vignette

A client reports that alprazolam (Xanax) makes him angry and restless rather than calm. The QEEG shows fast activity and poor task tolerance. The clinician should not write "benzodiazepine expected sedative effect present." A better report says the client reports paradoxical activation on benzodiazepines; medication attribution is therefore atypical and class-level expectations are low-confidence.

A parent reports that diphenhydramine makes a child with Down syndrome "wired." The QEEG was recorded the morning after a nighttime dose and shows poor sleep-state stability. The correct interpretation documents developmental-variant context, anticholinergic paradox report, and sleep disruption. It does not use outdated pathologizing language or infer a validated QEEG signature.

A young adult with ADHD reports sedation after methylphenidate. The map shows persistent theta and low task engagement. The report should not assume nonadherence or laziness. It should label a possible paradoxical stimulant response and recommend prescriber coordination.

23.10 Interpretation traps

- **Dismissing the client's report.** Paradoxical response history is clinically relevant even when QEEG evidence is thin.
- **Inventing an opposite EEG signature.** Opposite behavior does not prove opposite band-power change.
- **Using outdated developmental language.** Down syndrome and autism should be framed as developmental or neurodevelopmental variants, conditions, or populations.
- **Confusing akathisia with anxiety.** Antipsychotic activation can mimic anxiety but has different medication implications.
- **Missing pharmacogenomics.** Extreme metabolism can make ordinary dose-response assumptions fail.
- **Overgeneralizing case reports.** Case reports warn; they do not define population signatures.

23.11 Intake questions

When this chapter's topic appears on the intake form, ask:

- **Have any medications ever had the opposite effect?** Sedatives causing agitation, stimulants causing sedation, antihistamines causing activation, antidepressants causing activation.

- **Which medication, dose, and timing?** Record onset, duration, route, formulation, and co-exposures.
- **Was there a developmental, neurologic, or injury context?** Autism, Down syndrome, TBI, seizure history, sleep disorder, or aging context.
- **Any pharmacogenetic results or family history of unusual drug reactions?** Include CYP2D6, CYP2C19, CYP1A2 when known.
- **What did observers notice?** Agitation, aggression, sleepiness, disinhibition, akathisia, panic, insomnia, or emotional lability.
- **Did stopping or changing the medication resolve it?** Document only what happened; do not recommend changes.

23.12 Clinical recommendations

When a paradoxical response is reported, lower confidence in ordinary medication-class interpretation. Do not erase the class-level evidence; qualify it.

Document the paradoxical response in the QEEG report if it affects interpretation. Use language such as: "Client reports paradoxical activation with benzodiazepines; therefore typical sedative benzodiazepine EEG expectations may not apply."

Do not infer a validated QEEG paradox signature unless a direct study exists. Most paradoxical-response interpretation is a workflow heuristic.

When paradoxical activation, akathisia, suicidal ideation, mania, severe agitation, confusion, or dangerous sedation is reported, coordinate with the prescriber or advise appropriate medical follow-up.

Scope of practice. QEEG interpretation does not direct prescribing. Medication decisions, including discontinuation, dose changes, and substitution, rest with the prescriber.

23.13 Evidence summary

- **Spectral effect:** Paradoxical-response clinical phenomena are documented for several drug classes, but direct QEEG signatures are largely absent.
- **Phenotype inference:** Reported paradoxical responses can invalidate ordinary class-level expectations and reduce confidence in medication attribution.

- **Workflow heuristic:** Ask directly about opposite reactions, document them, screen timing/genetic/developmental context, and treat paradoxical responders as low-confidence cases for population-level QEEG prediction.

Ch 24: Comorbidity and Clinical Presentation Patterns

24.1 Why this class matters in NFB practice

Diagnosis is not EEG phenotype. A client does not arrive as "ADHD" or "depression" in isolation. They arrive as ADHD plus anxiety, depression plus chronic pain, bipolar disorder plus substance-use history, PTSD plus TBI, insomnia plus stimulant treatment, or schizophrenia-spectrum symptoms plus antipsychotic and mood-stabilizer exposure.

Strongest evidence	Direct comorbidity-specific pharmaco-EEG is limited; clozapine (Clozaril) in schizophrenia is the strongest medication-specific anchor.
Biggest interpretation trap	Treating diagnosis as phenotype: A billing diagnosis is not a QEEG mechanism.
Default clinical action	Interpret real clients by presentation pattern, not diagnosis label, and downgrade confidence when multiple diagnoses, substances, or sleep issues coexist.

Comorbidity changes both the baseline EEG and the medication context. It also explains why polypharmacy is so common. Mojtabai and Olfson show that multiple psychotropic prescribing is not rare in psychiatric practice (Mojtabai & Olfson, 2010). The reason is often clinical presentation: more than one symptom domain requires treatment.

Only a few comorbidity-adjacent pharmaco-EEG findings have direct support, including clozapine work in schizophrenia (V. Knott et al., 2001), EEG prediction of valproate (Depakote) versus lithium response in mania (Reeves et al., 2001), and baseline EEG findings in borderline personality disorder (De la Fuente et al., 1998). Most other comorbidity-specific pharmaco-EEG claims are workflow heuristics unless explicitly supported.

24.2 Mechanism (clinician-level pharmacology)

Comorbidity affects QEEG through three routes. First, each condition may carry its own EEG tendencies. Anxiety can add high arousal. Pain can add sleep disruption and muscle artifact. OSA can add daytime slowing. TBI can add focal or network disruption. Substance-use history can add trait-like recovery signatures.

Second, comorbidity drives medication selection. ADHD plus anxiety may lead to stimulant plus SSRI or SNRI. Depression plus pain may lead to SNRI, gabapentinoid, cannabis, opioid, or sleep medication. Bipolar disorder plus insomnia may lead to mood stabilizer, antipsychotic, and hypnotic. PTSD plus nightmares may lead to SSRI/SNRI, prazosin, sedative-hypnotic, or cannabis.

Third, comorbidity changes the meaning of response. A stimulant that improves task performance may worsen anxiety or sleep. An antidepressant that improves mood may worsen activation. An antipsychotic that reduces agitation may slow cognition. The QEEG is an intersection of presentation, medication, sleep, timing, and pipeline.

Papakostas and colleagues illustrate how anxious depression affects medication interpretation in clinical outcome data, even without QEEG endpoints (Papakostas et al., 2007). That pattern repeats across this chapter: clinical comorbidity is well known, but direct pharmaco-EEG is sparse.

24.3 Known spectral effects

The strongest schizophrenia-spectrum pharmaco-EEG example is clozapine. Knott and colleagues showed QEEG differences in chronic schizophrenia and changes with clozapine treatment (V. Knott et al., 2001). This is useful spectral-effect evidence for a medication in a serious psychiatric population. It is not evidence for every antipsychotic stack or schizoaffective polypharmacy presentation.

Reeves and colleagues studied EEG prediction of valproate versus lithium response in mania (Reeves et al., 2001). This is one of the

Medication	Phenotype	Confounder/State	Mode	Confidence
Antipsychotics	Frontal theta elevated	TBI / concussion history	exaggeration	substantially reduced
Benzodiazepines	Post-concussive slowing	TBI / concussion history	mimicry	substantially reduced
Methylphenidate	Frontal theta elevated	TBI / concussion history	masking	reduced
SSRIs	Long COVID alpha disruption	Long COVID / PASC	transformation	substantially reduced
Methylphenidate	ME/CFS cortical hypoactivation	ME/CFS	masking	reduced
Anticonvulsants and mood stabilizers	Fibromyalgia pain-network pattern	Fibromyalgia	exaggeration	substantially reduced
Z-drugs and non-benzodiazepine sleep medications	OSA-related daytime slowing	Untreated obstructive sleep apnea	mimicry	substantially reduced

Figure 24.1: Comorbidity presentation matrix: multi-diagnosis presentations with medication-stack overlaps and confidence adjustments.

few examples where EEG may help with mood-stabilizer selection. It should be presented as a phenotype inference and not generalized to all bipolar comorbidity patterns.

De la Fuente and colleagues found EEG abnormalities in borderline personality disorder, including nonspecific slowing, and carbamazepine (Tegretol) did not modify the EEG in that sample (De la Fuente et al., 1998). This helps distinguish baseline presentation findings from medication-effect claims.

For anxious depression, Papakostas and colleagues provide medication-outcome context but not EEG markers (Papakostas et al., 2007). For ADHD plus anxiety, PTSD plus TBI, depression plus chronic pain, bipolar plus SUD, and sleep disorder plus ADHD, direct pharmaco-EEG is mostly absent. Interpretations should be clinical synthesis with explicit workflow-heuristic framing.

24.4 Phenotype interaction effects

ADHD plus anxiety can mask the classic theta/beta story. Anxiety, caffeine, sleep loss, SSRI activation, or stimulant timing can add beta and reduce the appearance of a simple hypoarousal pattern. A normal TBR does not rule out ADHD in an anxious client.

Depression plus chronic pain can mimic medication slowing. Pain, poor sleep, gabapentinoids, opioids, cannabis, SNRIs, and antihistamines can all influence vigilance and slow activity. A "depression map" may be a pain-sleep-medication composite.

Bipolar disorder plus SUD changes relapse and medication-risk interpretation. Alcohol, cannabis, stimulant history, benzodiazepines, mood stabilizers, antipsychotics, and sleep aids can all affect EEG. A map cannot decide which diagnosis is primary.

PTSD plus TBI is a high-risk attribution context. Hypervigilance, dissociation, headache, sleep disruption, sedative exposure, cannabis use, and injury-related slowing can coexist. Protocol decisions should not be based on a single label.

Sleep disorder plus ADHD is especially common. Untreated OSA, delayed sleep phase, insomnia, stimulant treatment, caffeine, and sedating nighttime medications can create theta, beta, and vigilance findings that look like ADHD medication failure.

24.5 High-Frequency Clinical Patterns

ADHD plus anxiety is the most common trap. Anxiety, caffeine, sleep restriction, stimulant timing, and SSRI activation can all push the map toward faster activity and mask the classic theta/beta story. Beta excess does not prove anxiety when stimulant, nicotine, caffeine, or withdrawal is active.

Depression plus chronic pain is often a medication composite disguised as a mood presentation. Duloxetine (Cymbalta), gabapentin (Neurontin), pregabalin (Lyrica), opioids, cannabis, and diphenhydramine may all be present. Slowing or poor alpha organization should be read as a pain-mood-sleep-medication picture.

Bipolar spectrum plus substance-use history requires timeline context. Mood stabilizers and antipsychotics slow spectra; antidepressants and stimulants activate; withdrawal adds instability. Without temporal framing, the map cannot separate bipolar physiology from substance recovery or medication effect.

PTSD plus TBI stacks hypervigilance, dissociation, sleep disruption, cannabis, benzodiazepine exposure, prazosin, and antidepressants.

A beta/theta pattern here should not be read as generic anxiety or ADHD.

Sleep disorder plus ADHD confuses because both produce attention-relevant EEG changes. If sleep is unstable, stimulant response cannot be interpreted cleanly from resting QEEG.

Schizophrenia spectrum is often treated with antipsychotic plus mood stabilizer plus additional agents. Knott's clozapine data are useful (V. Knott et al., 2001), but real clients carry more complex exposure. QEEG slowing may reflect antipsychotic burden, illness course, sleep, substance use, or seizure-threshold context.

24.6 Medication Stack as Presentation Clue

Medication lists often reveal the clinical presentation better than diagnosis labels do. SSRI plus stimulant suggests attention plus mood/anxiety. SNRI plus gabapentinoid suggests mood plus pain. Antipsychotic plus mood stabilizer suggests bipolar, psychosis-spectrum, severe depression augmentation, or sleep/agitation management. Benzodiazepine PRN plus antidepressant suggests anxiety, panic, insomnia, or acute distress. Topiramate (Topamax) plus antidepressant plus triptan suggests migraine plus mood.

The medication list is not proof of diagnosis, but it tells the clinician what problem the prescriber was trying to solve. That matters because the QEEG is shaped by both the drug and the target symptom. A sedating medication prescribed for insomnia may indicate sleep instability before the drug ever enters the picture. A stimulant prescribed for fatigue may indicate sleep, depression, Long COVID, OSA, or ADHD.

When a medication appears mismatched to the diagnosis, ask why. Quetiapine (Seroquel) may be used for psychosis, bipolar disorder, anxiety, sleep, or off-label sedation. Gabapentin may be used for seizures, pain, anxiety, insomnia, or alcohol recovery. Propranolol may be used for blood pressure, tremor, performance anxiety, migraine, or akathisia. The indication changes the interpretation.

24.7 How to Write the Impression

A weak impression says: "Findings are consistent with ADHD." A stronger impression says: "Findings are interpreted in the context of

ADHD symptoms, anxiety, chronic sleep restriction, morning stimulant exposure, and current SSRI treatment; medication and sleep factors reduce confidence in assigning theta/beta findings to a single ADHD phenotype."

A weak impression says: "Diffuse slowing suggests depression." A stronger impression says: "Diffuse slowing and unstable vigilance occur in a client with depression, chronic pain, gabapentinoid use, cannabis exposure, and poor sleep; this pattern should be interpreted as a pain-sleep-medication context rather than a depression-specific marker."

A weak impression says: "Beta excess indicates anxiety." A stronger impression says: "Beta elevation is present during a recording obtained after caffeine and stimulant exposure in a client with anxiety symptoms and poor sleep; anxiety is one possible contributor, but medication/substance timing and sleep state are major confounders."

This style tells the reader why confidence is reduced and what information would improve the next recording.

24.8 Follow-Up Strategy

When comorbidity is high, the best comparison is within-person and matched-state. Match sleep, medication timing, caffeine, and recording conditions across sessions; otherwise the apparent change may reflect a different presentation state rather than treatment response. Collect brief symptom ratings (attention, anxiety, pain, sleepiness, fatigue) before acquisition to identify the state being sampled. If a comorbidity factor is unstable, say so directly in the report. For protocol selection, favor targets that remain plausible across the full presentation pattern and persist across eyes-open, task, and stable vigilance.

24.9 Case vignette

A 41-year-old client is referred for ADHD protocol planning. The medication list includes amphetamine XR, sertraline (Zoloft), trazodone (Desyrel), cannabis several nights per week, and caffeine. The history includes panic symptoms, delayed sleep phase, and possible OSA. The QEEG shows frontal theta and beta variability.

Calling this "ADHD theta/beta phenotype" is too narrow. The presentation is ADHD plus anxiety plus sleep disruption plus stimulant/SSRI/sedative/cannabis/caffeine exposure. The report should state that stimulant response, sleep debt, anxiety arousal, and sedating nighttime exposures all reduce confidence in single-phenotype interpretation.

A second client with chronic pain and depression takes duloxetine, pregabalin, hydrocodone PRN, and diphenhydramine for sleep. The QEEG shows diffuse slowing and unstable vigilance. The interpretation should not attribute slowing to depression alone. It is a pain-sleep-medication presentation.

24.10 Interpretation traps

- **Treating diagnosis as phenotype.** A billing diagnosis is not a QEEG mechanism.
- **Ignoring the medication stack that follows comorbidity.** Comorbid presentations often explain polypharmacy.
- **Overusing single-diagnosis literature.** Clean samples do not generalize automatically to real clients.
- **Missing sleep and pain.** These often dominate EEG more than the psychiatric label.
- **Inflating workflow-heuristic synthesis.** Most comorbidity-specific pharmaco-EEG is not directly studied.
- **Forgetting substance history.** Alcohol, cannabis, nicotine, caffeine, and stimulant-use history reshape interpretation.

24.11 Intake questions

When this chapter's topic appears on the intake form, ask:

- **What are the top three current symptom domains?** Attention, anxiety, mood, sleep, pain, trauma, psychosis, substance recovery, fatigue, cognition.
- **Which medication treats which symptom?** Map every drug to an indication.
- **What medical conditions affect brain state?** TBI, OSA, migraine, pain, Long COVID, ME/CFS, fibromyalgia, hormonal state, aging.
- **What substances are current or recent?** Alcohol, cannabis, caffeine, nicotine, stimulants, psychedelics, opioids, kratom.
- **What changed recently?** Diagnosis, dose, sleep, pain flare, substance pattern, trauma exposure, infection, concussion, or surgery.

- **Which symptom was present during recording?** Pain severity, anxiety level, fatigue, sleepiness, headache, dissociation, cravings, or medication side effects.

24.12 Clinical recommendations

Write presentation-based interpretations. Instead of "ADHD QEEG," write "ADHD/anxiety/sleep-restriction presentation under stimulant plus SSRI exposure."

Label comorbidity claims by type. If the claim is extrapolated from single-diagnosis or single-drug studies, call it a clinical heuristic.

Use comorbidity to reduce attribution confidence. The more active symptom domains and CNS exposures present, the less confidently a finding belongs to one condition.

When longitudinally tracking clients, keep presentation context stable or document changes. A pain flare, new sleep medication, or substance relapse can change the QEEG as much as neurofeedback.

Coordinate safety issues with prescribers and medical clinicians when comorbidity raises risk: bipolar activation, psychosis, withdrawal, seizure risk, delirium, severe sleep apnea, or medication toxicity.

Scope of practice. QEEG interpretation does not direct prescribing. Medication decisions, including discontinuation, dose changes, and substitution, rest with the prescriber.

24.13 Evidence summary

- **Spectral effect:** Direct comorbidity-specific pharmaco-EEG is limited; clozapine in schizophrenia is the strongest medication-specific anchor.
- **Phenotype inference:** EEG may help in selected contexts, such as valproate versus lithium response prediction in mania, but these findings do not generalize to broad comorbidity stacks.
- **Workflow heuristic:** Interpret real clients by presentation pattern, not diagnosis label, and downgrade confidence when multiple diagnoses, substances, sleep problems, pain, and medications overlap.

Ch 25: When It's Not the Drug

Most of this book is about what drugs do to the EEG. But real clients take drugs because something else is wrong. Head injury, post-viral illness, untreated sleep apnea, pain, and circadian collapse can land on the same spectral families as benzodiazepines, antipsychotics, antidepressants, stimulants, and gabapentinoids. Chapter 18 built the receptor-to-spectrum vocabulary for those families; this chapter applies it to the differential question. This chapter is a differential guide, not a condition primer. For underlying condition signatures, see the Field Guide or the future *Dynamic Brain* volume.

Four blocks follow, each built on the same structure: what drug class does the condition mimic, a short mechanism, how to separate condition from drug, and what happens if you get it wrong. Real clients stack these conditions. A post-concussive client with untreated apnea, post-viral fatigue, and a short sleep night before the recording can mimic half the drug classes in this book without touching a single prescription. If you know your client's bupropion (Wellbutrin) dose but have not screened for apnea, you are not doing medication-QEEG work. You are doing brand-name storytelling.

25.1 TBI and Concussion

Looks like a sedative or antipsychotic. Post-concussive physiology can produce excess slow activity, reduced posterior alpha, slowed or labile alpha peak, and connectivity changes. The pattern overlaps quetiapine (Seroquel), nocturnal cannabis, benzodiazepine hangover, and opioid sedation. A client prescribed methylphenidate for post-traumatic cognitive fatigue may still show a dominant post-concussive pattern; the map does not support a clean ADHD-off-stimulant read (Haneef et al., 2013; Modarres et al., 2017; Thatcher, 2010).

Here's why. TBI is not one state. Mild, repetitive, and moderate-to-severe injuries produce different network loads. Post-concussive sleep disruption, autonomic shift, and headache move the same frequency knobs that sedatives, antipsychotics, and CNS depressants move.

How to tell. Lead with history, not z-scores. Count injuries. Document loss of consciousness, hospitalization, imaging, seizures, and blast or repetitive subconcussive exposure. Weigh current post-concussive symptoms (headache, screen intolerance, dizziness, irritability, cognitive fatigue) ahead of any remote one-concussion label. Moderate-to-severe injury with hospitalization, abnormal imaging, or neurosurgery increases the likelihood that brain-injury physiology is a primary contributor to the map. A single remote uncomplicated concussion may be a minor caveat; persistent symptoms after multiple injuries are a central interpretive context.

TBI rarely arrives alone. Check for untreated OSA, chronic pain, migraine, cannabis or alcohol, and post-viral fatigue in the same file. If snoring, weight gain, or marked daytime sleepiness sit alongside a concussion history, do not assign slowing to the sedating medication list until sleep-disordered breathing is ruled out. Repetitive impact deserves its own question. A former athlete may deny "concussion" but endorse years of collisions. A service member may report blast exposure but no loss of consciousness.

Read indications. Stimulants for post-TBI fatigue are not the same interpretive frame as idiopathic ADHD. Anticonvulsants after structural injury or seizures carry a different safety envelope than routine mood or pain use. Log last dose, recent titration, and whether the visit was a stable-medication, rested day. A stimulant-day QEEG is valid data, but it answers a different question than a drug-holiday recording. If the map cannot separate lamotrigine (Lamictal) from injury from sleep loss, the report should say so rather than picking a winner.

Consequence if you get it wrong. The report blames citalopram (Celexa), gabapentin (Neurontin), or nightly cannabis for frontal theta when untreated apnea, mood disorder, and injury physiology are stacked underneath. A prescriber gets a defensible but false single-cause story. A stimulant is read as failing because the map did not normalize, and training locks onto a stimulant-responsive phenotype that was never the right question. Seizure risk or structural lesion context gets collapsed into "too many sedatives." When a client asks, "Is this from my concussion or my medication?" the honest answer is often "The QEEG cannot separate those cleanly." That answer is clinically useful. It prevents false causal claims and directs attention toward stable repeatable conditions for follow-up.

25.2 Post-Viral Fatigue, Long COVID, ME/CFS, and Fibromyalgia

Looks like an SSRI, a gabapentinoid, or stimulant undertreatment. Long COVID and PASC can read as sedative slowing and alpha disruption. ME/CFS can read as depression-like hypoarousal, or as stimulant undertreatment when fatigue dominates. Fibromyalgia can read as a gabapentinoid or SNRI profile layered on pain-network shifts that overlap medication signatures (Cecchetti et al., 2022; Fallon et al., 2018; Kopanska et al., 2022; Vanneste et al., 2017; Zinn et al., 2018). In practice, that often means sertraline (Zoloft), methylphenidate, or pregabalin (Lyrica) get causal credit the map cannot support.

Here's why. Post-viral and central-sensitivity states alter vigilance, alpha reactivity, low-frequency load, and connectivity in directions that overlap SSRIs, SNRIs, tricyclics, stimulants, and gabapentinoids. No adequate pharmaco-EEG literature deconvolves a combined state like "Long COVID plus sertraline plus intermittent modafinil (Provigil)" into labeled components. The QEEG arrives as a composite measurement; the medication list does not unmix it.

How to tell. Infection-related onset, relapse pattern, and exertional or autonomic symptoms pull toward Long COVID over a pure SSRI read. If brain fog tracks illness course rather than dose timing, condition weight increases. If cognitive symptoms began after COVID rather than after starting the antidepressant, say so. Long COVID versus sedative burden: both can load low frequencies and feel cognitively slow; infection-linked onset and dysautonomia argue for condition weight, whereas dose- or timing-locked change argues for the drug.

Post-exertional malaise differentiates ME/CFS from depression in clinical criteria. The EEG cannot do that job alone. Ask what happens after physical, cognitive, or emotional exertion. A recording after a crash may represent a post-exertional state, not baseline. ME/CFS versus stimulant undertreatment is a specific trap: improved alertness on methylphenidate or modafinil does not diagnose a primary ADHD phenotype. Stimulant response is not diagnostic.

For fibromyalgia, log pain and sleep on test day. A flare changes muscle tone, vigilance, and PRN analgesic use. Pregabalin and gabapentin are prescribed because pain and sleep are severe; slowing in that setting is entangled, not a clean drug demonstration. Beta excess in fibromyalgia may reflect arousal, pain, medication, muscle artifact, or all four. Do not reduce pain beta to "anxiety."

Map medications as clusters. Long COVID commonly carries SSRIs, modafinil, beta-blockers, antihistamines, and sleep aids. ME/CFS often includes low-dose naltrexone (Vivitrol), antidepressants, and wake-promoting agents. Fibromyalgia often stacks duloxetine (Cymbalta), low-dose tricyclics, pregabalin, gabapentin, and sometimes opioids. Polypharmacy is typical. One-drug blame is usually dishonest.

Consequence if you get it wrong. An SSRI gets accused of producing the post-COVID alpha loss. A modafinil response is mistaken for primary ADHD. A fibromyalgia map on pregabalin is read as pure gabapentinoid sedation while pain and sleep debt are written out of the report. The recording may look like a fatigue-state sample rather than a clean medication-effect sample, and if the report does not say so, the prescriber reads a single-cause conclusion that was never warranted. Training inherits those false culprits.

25.3 OSA, Migraine, and Chronic Pain

Looks like a benzodiazepine, an anticonvulsant, or an opioid-gabapentinoid composite. Untreated OSA mimics daytime benzodiazepine, Z-drug, antipsychotic, opioid, or alcohol burden: frontal slowing, fatigue, inattention, unstable vigilance. Wake-promoting agents can mask sleepiness while sleep-pressure signatures stay in the trace (D. Wang et al., 2015). Interictal or peri-ictal migraine states can mimic topiramate (Topamax)-like cognitive slowing or anxiety-linked beta, as if the drug and the headache day were interchangeable (Perucca & Gilliam, 2012; W. W. Wang et al., 2003). Chronic pain can couple high-frequency muscle contamination with slow load, so the z-score output resembles stimulant, antidepressant, and opioid layers at once.

Here's why. OSA fragments sleep and loads homeostatic pressure into the waking record. Migraine changes interictal versus post-attack state, and rescue medications add their own half-life problem. Pain seizes attention, tenses muscle, fragments sleep, and forces irregular PRN dosing of opioids, gabapentinoids, and muscle relaxants.

How to tell. Screen for sleep-disordered breathing first. Ask about snoring, witnessed apneas, morning headache, and unrefreshing sleep. "On CPAP" means nothing until you ask: how many nights per week, was it used last night, any mask leak, and did daytime sleepiness improve. If untreated or inconsistent OSA is plausible, slow frequencies must not be assigned to mirtazapine (Remeron) or clonazepam (Klonopin) alone.

OSA and sedatives are mutually worsening. Opioids, benzodiazepines, Z-drugs, alcohol, cannabis, and sedating antihistamines can deepen sleep-disordered breathing or next-day sleep pressure even when each prescription is defensible. Newly started or restarted CPAP is a treatment-transition state, not a binary "fixed" label.

For migraine, document time since last full attack, current headache level, prodrome or postdrome status, and timing of rescue medications. The morning after a severe attack is not interictal baseline. Name preventives (topiramate, valproate (Depakote), beta-blockers, tricyclics) as active agents in the report header, not as silent covariates. CGRP-targeted preventives are an open gap for resting QEEG but still belong in the medication list.

For chronic pain, record the pain score that day and the sedating stack: pregabalin, opioid, diphenhydramine, cannabis. Note muscle tension and review raw EEG, because pain and jaw-neck guarding can smear the high-frequency map into something that looks like anxiety or stimulant effect. Medication timing in chronic pain is often irregular. PRN opioids, rescue migraine medications, cannabis, and muscle relaxants follow symptom intensity, not clock. If the client took extra medication because of a flare, the QEEG should be labeled as a flare-treatment state.

Consequence if you get it wrong. OSA stays undiagnosed while the report scolds sedative polypharmacy. A post-attack map is frozen as neurofeedback baseline. Modafinil is credited with fixing sleep while fragmented sleep remains the driver. Pain beta is relabeled anxiety. Topiramate is asked to explain the entire posterior field without migraine timing on the page.

25.4 Sleep Deprivation and Circadian Disruption

Looks like a sedative hangover, stimulant rebound, or caffeine withdrawal. Acute sleep loss and drowsiness during the recording reproduce the entire sedative column: benzodiazepine, Z-drug, antihistamine, sedating antidepressant, antipsychotic, opioid, cannabis, and gabapentinoid signatures all become plausible when the real driver is state (Cajochen et al., 1995; De Gennaro et al., 2001; Santamaria & Chiappa, 1987; Strijkstra et al., 2003). Stimulants or caffeine can preserve behavioral alertness while theta and alpha dynamics still carry sleep pressure. Early-morning testing, shift work, or jet lag can shift apparent alpha peak so the map reads as trait underarousal or medication effect (Olbrich et al., 2009).

Here's why. Homeostatic sleep pressure increases low-frequency expression in wakefulness and lowers the threshold for drowsiness. Eyes-closed recording invites sleep-onset physiology before the client reports feeling asleep (Santamaria & Chiappa, 1987). Averaging across alert and drowsy epochs produces trait-like features from state mixture. Automated artifact rejection does not fix this. Drowsiness is a physiologic state, not line noise or electrode pop. ICA may remove ocular components, but it does not remove the cortical theta and alpha changes of declining vigilance.

How to tell. Document hours slept last night and over the prior 48 hours. Record habitual schedule, clock time of the visit, shift work, naps, and caffeine and meal timing. Ask subjective sleepiness at arrival.

In the raw EEG, look for alpha instability across the eyes-closed run, theta rising across the segment, slow rolling eye movements, and technician notes on drifting or head nods. If drowsiness dominates the latter half of eyes closed, treat the processed map as vigilance-contaminated.

Medicated clients need the same vigilance split. Clonazepam may deepen drowsiness, but the end product may still be a drowsy sample rather than a stable drug fingerprint. When a theta/beta ratio or slow alpha peak shows up in a sleep-restricted adolescent tested at 8 a.m., the sensible reading is "this is what the brain looks like at this clock time on this much sleep," not a trait label.

Circadian mismatch transforms phenotype meaning. Slow alpha in an early-morning recording after short sleep should not carry the same weight as slow alpha in a well-rested late-morning recording. Elevated theta after lunch may reflect state more than trait. A night-shift worker recorded at 9 a.m. after work is in a different physiologic context than a day worker at the same clock time. A baseline at 10 a.m. after adequate sleep and a follow-up at 4 p.m. after a short night is not a clean before-and-after; match time of day, sleep duration, caffeine, meals, and medication clock, or document the mismatch as a measured confound.

Consequence if you get it wrong. A theta/beta ratio or slow alpha frequency is frozen as an ADHD phenotype when the sample was sleep-restricted and early-drowsy. Longitudinal maps improve or worsen from sleep and clock changes rather than from training or dose adjustment. A sedating antidepressant or antihistamine takes the blame for diffuse slowing that was mostly microsleep in the segment. Adolescents on school-night sleep debt, night-shift workers tested at the wrong circadian phase, and older adults with fragmented sleep and stacked hypnotics are high-risk for trait labels that reflect clock and debt rather than stable endogenous physiology.

25.4.1 Drowsiness as a Pharmaco-EEG Confound

Drowsiness deserves a separate callout because it is the highest-frequency confound this chapter names and the one most likely to be missed by standard pipelines. Wake-to-N1 transition is gradual and subjectively invisible: many clients are unaware they have become drowsy, especially in eyes-closed paradigms that are by design low-arousal conditions. The spectral vector is consistent across the literature: theta increase, individual alpha peak frequency deceleration, beta decrease, and slow rolling eye movements (Cajochen et al., 1995; De Gennaro et al., 2001; Olbrich et al., 2009; Santamaria & Chiappa, 1987). None of those features look like artifact. Amplitude-threshold artifact rejection does not catch drowsiness because drowsiness does not produce high-amplitude signals. ICA does not catch it because drowsiness is not an artifact at all; it is a change in the neural activity the recording is meant to measure. The clinician who reads only the processed z-score report, without inspecting raw waveforms or vigilance trajectory, may never see it.

The phenotypes most vulnerable to drowsiness contamination are the ones whose features overlap the drowsiness vector directly: frontal theta elevation, theta / beta ratio elevation, slow individual alpha peak frequency, low global beta, diffuse slowing, and mixed fast / slow patterns. Any of these read off a recording with undetected drowsiness can produce a confidently labeled trait phenotype that is, in fact, a vigilance confound. The word artifact is wrong for it, for the reason given just above, and using it invites the reader to think a cleaning step will remove it. For an operational detection apparatus (within-recording iAPF first-vs-last-third deceleration, theta / alpha slope, slow-eye-movement bandpass, alpha amplitude coefficient of variation, and a composite vigilance score), and for a working prevalence estimate of undetected drowsiness in eyes-closed clinical recordings, see Hill 2026 (Hill, 2026). That paper is the operational counterpart to the qualitative guidance above; the two together cover both clinical recognition and pipeline-grade detection.

25.5 Case vignette

Mara is 44 years old. She played competitive volleyball through college, took multiple blows to the head over fifteen years, and describes one documented concussion at 23 that required two weeks of cognitive rest. She is currently on bupropion 300 mg (for depression and smoking cessation), gabapentin 300 mg at bedtime (for chronic neck pain and restless legs), and lorazepam 0.5 mg as needed for anxiety. She reports waking twice most nights, snoring, and morning grogginess. She used a quarter milligram of lorazepam the evening before the recording. Her coffee intake is two large cups before noon. The QEEG shows elevated posterior theta, reduced posterior alpha, mild frontal slowing, and variable beta excess.

Wrong report: "Findings are consistent with depression phenotype. Posterior theta and reduced alpha reactivity may reflect SSRI-class medication effect or mood-related hypoactivation. Beta excess may reflect anxiety or stimulant response in the context of bupropion's noradrenergic mechanism. Recommend alpha / theta neurofeedback protocol targeting posterior coherence."

Better report: "Recording was obtained in the context of: (1) post-concussive history with chronic cervical pain; (2) stable bupropion, for which direct resting-QEEG evidence is limited, so it is documented rather than assigned a band; (3) gabapentin residual from last evening, read through drowsiness and condition overlap rather than a compound-specific signature; (4) lorazepam residual from last evening, which can produce beta excess and reduce alpha reactivity; (5) possible untreated obstructive sleep apnea (snoring, morning grogginess, two-night-wake pattern); (6) sleep restriction; (7) caffeine exposure. The posterior theta, reduced alpha, and frontal slowing findings are consistent with multiple concurrent mechanisms. Phenotype confidence for depression, anxiety, or attention labeling is substantially reduced. The most important next clinical step is OSA screening, because undiagnosed sleep-disordered breathing in the presence of gabapentin, lorazepam, and bupropion represents a safety concern that takes interpretive precedence over phenotype assignment."

If you know Mara's bupropion dose but have not screened for apnea, you are not doing medication-QEEG work. You are doing brand-name storytelling.

This chapter is the counterweight to overconfident medication attribution. The Field Guide carries the full profile for each condition; this chapter just flags the conditions whose spectral fingerprints can be mistaken for the medication list when the bottle is not the only thing moving the trace.

QEEG does not direct prescribing, stopping, or switching drugs; that stays with the prescriber.

25.6 Evidence Summary

- **Spectral effect.** Chronic TBI associates with slow activity, alpha, and connectivity abnormalities (Haneef et al., 2013; Thatcher, 2010). Long COVID, ME/CFS, and fibromyalgia studies show heterogeneous but real resting EEG shifts (Cecchetti et al., 2022; Fallon et al., 2018; Kopanska et al., 2022; Vanneste et al., 2017; Zinn et al., 2018). OSA, migraine state, and chronic pain alter waking EEG through sleep fragmentation, sensory load, and medication burden (Perucca & Gilliam, 2012; D. Wang et al., 2015; W. W. Wang et al., 2003). Sleep loss and drowsiness shift theta, alpha stability, and alpha peak (Cajochen et al., 1995; De Gennaro et al., 2001; Olbrich et al., 2009; Santamaria & Chiappa, 1987; Strijkstra et al., 2003). Operational detection criteria and a working prevalence estimate for undetected drowsiness in clinical eyes-closed recordings are available in Hill 2026 (Hill, 2026).

- **Phenotype inference.** Each of these conditions can mimic, mask, or inflate apparent sedative, antipsychotic, antidepressant, stimulant, gabapentinoid, opioid, cannabis, and sleep-aid effects. Combined states are typical in real clients.
- **Workflow heuristic.** If history, symptom state, apnea screen, migraine calendar, exertion timeline, and recording vigilance are absent from the chart, treat medication attribution as provisional and name the non-drug alternatives explicitly in any text you hand to clients and prescribers.

25.7 Interpretation traps

- Blaming frontal theta on the sedative or antipsychotic list when apnea, post-viral state, or chronic post-concussive illness was never screened.
- Treating wake-promotion response (modafinil, stimulant, caffeine) as diagnostic of ADHD or as evidence that a sleep problem is solved.
- Comparing QEEG dates across different sleep durations, migraine phases, PEM crash versus stable week, or clock times without labeling the state shift.
- Writing one-sentence medication-effect verdicts when the client was in a flare, post-attack window, or when drowsiness contaminated the eyes-closed run.
- Ignoring CPAP adherence detail. "On CPAP" is not a clinical fact until you know nights used, mask leak, and symptom response.

25.8 Intake questions

- **Head injury and repetitive impact:** How many head injuries with confusion or loss of consciousness? Any hospitalization, imaging, or seizure? Current post-concussive symptoms?
- **Post-viral and fatigue illness:** Cognitive symptoms after COVID or other infection? Post-exertional malaise? Fibromyalgia or widespread pain? Severity today?

- **Sleep-disordered breathing:** Snoring, witnessed apneas, morning headache, unrefreshing sleep? CPAP or appliance use, including nights per week and use last night?
- **Migraine and pain:** Last severe headache or migraine? Rescue and preventive medications? Pain 0-10 today? Atypical PRN analgesic use?
- **Sleep and circadian state at test:** Hours slept last two nights? Shift work or jet lag? Caffeine and meal timing? Sleepiness now? Any drifting during eyes closed?

Ch 26: How to Read a Medicated Client QEEG: The Decision Framework

26.1 Why this class matters in NFB practice

This chapter is the practical center of the book. The earlier chapters describe what medications, substances, conditions, formulations, withdrawal states, pipelines, and comorbidities can do to QEEG. This chapter turns that information into a repeatable workflow for reading one medicated client's recording.

Strongest evidence	Multiple medication classes and recording / pipeline factors produce systematic EEG effects, but individual interpretation depends on state and context.
Biggest interpretation trap	Skipping raw EEG safety review: Quantitative maps do not replace clinical EEG review.
Default clinical action	Use the ten-step decision framework to assign confidence, write explicit caveats, and decide when to record as presenting, repeat, defer, or coordinate.

The decision framework has one purpose: prevent overconfident phenotype interpretation when an active medication, substance, condition, or pipeline factor can plausibly produce the same direction of finding. It is a clinical heuristic, not a validated diagnostic algorithm. It helps the clinician write clearer reports, ask better intake questions, and decide when a finding is strong enough to guide training.

The framework also protects scope. QEEG findings should not be used to recommend medication discontinuation, dose changes, or pharmacologic substitution. Those decisions rest with the prescriber. The neurofeedback clinician's role is to document exposure state, interpret

QEEG cautiously, flag safety concerns, and coordinate when medication context limits interpretation.

26.2 Mechanism (clinician-level pharmacology)

Medication interpretation begins before z-scores. Raw EEG safety review comes first. The ACNS reporting guideline requires structured documentation of background features, interictal discharges, and clinical correlation using standardized terminology (Tatum et al., 2016). A quantitative map does not substitute for that review. If the raw EEG suggests seizure risk, encephalopathy, nonconvulsive status, medication toxicity, or withdrawal complication, the next step is medical evaluation, not phenotype labeling.

After safety comes state. Was the client eyes closed, eyes open, task-engaged, drowsy, hyperventilating, photic-stimulated, caffeinated, sleep-deprived, in pain, anxious, or in withdrawal? IPEG guidelines emphasize standardized recording and evaluation for pharmaco-EEG because measurement context shapes interpretation (International Pharmaco-EEG Society, 2012).

Then comes exposure. Moore and Mattison show that psychiatric medication exposure is common enough that clinicians should expect it, not treat it as an exception (Moore & Mattison, 2017). Kerson's practitioner text remains the anchor for qualitative class-level drug effects (Kerson, 2023). This book extends that foundation with confounder, timing, pipeline, and decision-framework discipline.

26.3 Known spectral effects

The decision framework does not require the clinician to memorize every drug signature. It requires a structured question: can an active factor plausibly produce the same direction as the detected phenotype?

If frontal theta is elevated, active factors include antipsychotics, opioids, high sedative load, drowsiness, untreated OSA, TBI, Long COVID, ME/CFS, fibromyalgia, pain, and adolescent maturation. If beta is high, active factors include benzodiazepines, stimulants, caffeine, nicotine, withdrawal, anxiety, akathisia, and pipeline or muscle artifact. If iAPF is slow, active factors include age, antipsychotics, TCAs, opioids, cannabis, hormonal state, sleep deprivation, and pipeline choices.

The framework therefore weakens direct phenotype claims when overlap exists. The finding may still be real. It may still guide training. It should be described as lower-confidence and context-dependent.

26.4 Phenotype interaction effects

The framework applies the four interaction modes defined in Chapter 1 (masking, mimicry, exaggeration, and transformation) as a structured question at each step. For any finding, ask: could an active factor hide it (masking), create it (mimicry), amplify it (exaggeration), or change what it means (transformation)? A beta excess in a client on benzodiazepines is not the same as beta excess in an unmedicated anxious client. Slow alpha in a postmenopausal client on antipsychotics is not the same as slow alpha in an unmedicated adolescent.

26.5 The Ten-Step Workflow

This ten-step workflow integrates safety-review tradition (ACNS), pre-recording protocol (IPEG, 2012), exposure-inventory discipline (Moore and Kerson), the four interaction modes (Chapter 1 of this book), and the three claim types (Chapter 4) into a single repeatable clinical sequence. This is one of the first attempts to bring all five of those traditions into a unified decision structure.

Step 1: safety and raw EEG first. Look for epileptiform activity, severe slowing, asymmetry needing medical review, medication toxicity, withdrawal risk, delirium, encephalopathy, nonconvulsive status concern, or poor data quality. If safety is unresolved, do not proceed to confident phenotype interpretation.

Be precise about what this step is. It is screening for features that require someone else to look, not clinical EEG interpretation. The question being answered is whether this record needs a reader qualified to interpret clinical EEG, not what the record shows. A brief resting recording with a limited montage and no video cannot rule out epilepsy, intermittent events, or nonconvulsive status, so nothing found or missed at this step clears a client of anything. Know your referral routes before you need them, and match the response to the urgency ladder under Safety Overrides below.

Step 2: verify recording state against the governing rule (Appendix C). Was the recording obtained in the client's ordinary prescribed and

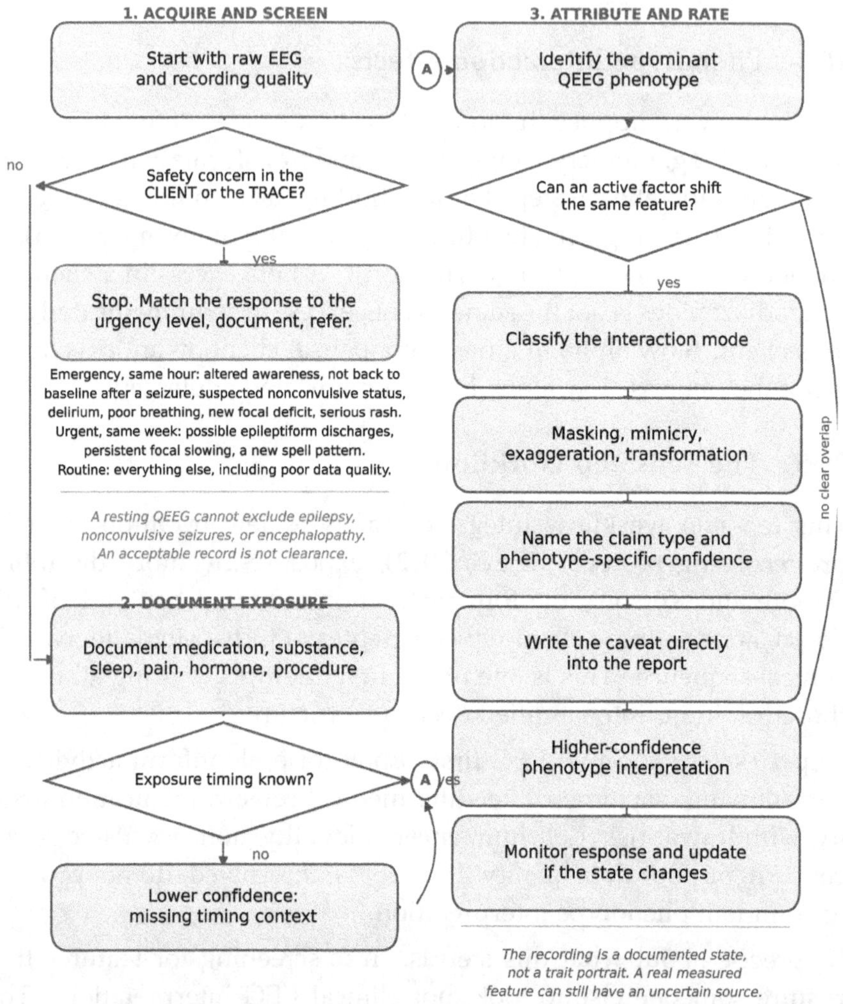

Figure 26.1: Ten-step medicated-client QEEG decision tree: from raw EEG review through medication inventory, interaction-mode classification, claim-type assignment, and report-caveat generation.

habitual functional state? If the state was deliberately altered for a clinical question, was that alteration initiated by the prescriber (for prescribed medications) or documented with a stated reason (for habitual substances)? Document caffeine timing, stimulant timing, cannabis timing, alcohol, nicotine, and whether each reflects habitual or atypical exposure. If any exposure is atypical, note the departure and its effect on interpretive confidence.

Step 3: define recording state. Label EC, EO, task, HV, photic, vigilance trajectory, drowsiness, pain, anxiety, fatigue, and sleepiness. A band-power finding without condition is incomplete.

Step 4: collect the full exposure inventory. Prescriptions, OTC medications, supplements, caffeine, nicotine, alcohol, cannabis, recreational substances, recent anesthesia, ketamine treatment, PRN medications, and recent discontinuations all count.

Step 5: document timing and formulation. Last dose, IR/XR, patch, nasal, sublingual, LAI cycle position, steady state, titration, discontinuation, holiday, generic switch, and pharmacogenetic context can all change interpretation.

Step 6: ask whether a known class effect points in the same direction as the finding. Use class-level evidence as a starting point, not as proof.

Step 7: screen non-drug confounders. Sleep deprivation, drowsiness, TBI, OSA, Long COVID, ME/CFS, fibromyalgia, migraine, chronic pain, pregnancy/postpartum/cycle/OCP, adolescence, aging, and pipeline factors must be considered.

Step 8: consider interaction mode. Is the active factor masking, mimicking, exaggerating, or transforming the phenotype? Treat the answer as a hypothesis about the recording rather than as something the recording measured. A single cross-sectional map rarely shows which mode operated, and more than one can run at once. Indeterminate is a legitimate answer, and so is naming two. Write it as possible mimicry, or as overlap consistent with masking, rather than assigning a mode as though it had been observed.

Step 9: assign confidence. High confidence requires clean data, stable state, no major overlapping medication/condition/pipeline alternative, and a finding consistent across relevant conditions. Moderate confidence allows some context but not a dominant alternative explanation. Low confidence applies when active factors plausibly produce the same direction.

Step 10: write the caveat directly. Do not hide uncertainty in vague prose. State the active factor and its interpretive consequence.

After the ten steps: the inverse-direction handoff. The ten steps above complete the forward-direction reading. Once forward-direction confidence has been established across Steps 1–10, the clinician may consult Part III to ask whether the identified phenotype carries treatment-response information. This handoff is conditional, not optional, because the quality of the inverse-direction inference depends entirely on the forward-direction work that precedes it. If forward-direction confidence is substantially reduced or low, the handoff should be deferred or explicitly flagged as premature. If forward-direction confidence is moderate or high, Part III entries provide hypothesis-generating context for the clinician-prescriber conversation.

When to consult Part III. Three conditions should be met before turning to a Chapter 21 entry: (1) the phenotype is reliably detected in clean data; (2) active medication, substance, condition, and state factors have been screened (Steps 5–7) and none produces a dominant confound for that phenotype; (3) the clinician has a specific clinical question the prescriber is also asking. If the prescriber has already chosen a medication and started it, the reverse question (what does this drug do to this phenotype?) is more useful than an inverse-direction prediction.

How to translate a Part III entry into prescriber-conversation language. A Chapter 21 entry is reference material for framing a question, not a prescription note. The correct translation moves through three steps:

1. Name the phenotype and its forward-direction confidence: "The recording shows elevated frontal theta with normal individual alpha peak frequency under documented stable conditions. I have moderate confidence this reflects a trait feature rather than stimulant timing or sleep debt."

2. State the inverse-direction association and its claim type: "Chapter 21 notes that this phenotype is associated at the group level with a stimulant response in ADHD samples, supported by the Arns (2008) work, rated as a phenotype inference. Individual-level prediction remains limited."

3. Frame it as a question, not a directive: "Does that association inform your treatment planning for this client, given the other factors you're weighing?"

This framing makes clear that the QEEG contributed a piece of the puzzle, not a prescription. It invites the prescriber to use the information or set it aside based on their clinical context. It does not imply that the QEEG has resolved the medication decision.

Worked example. A 34-year-old client referred for QEEG-guided neurofeedback presents with persistent inattention and poor response to two previous stimulant trials. The QEEG under stable no-medication conditions shows elevated frontal theta ($z > 2.0$ at Fz/F3/F4), normal iAPF (10.2 Hz), no prominent beta excess, and clean data. Sleep was adequate; no confounders dominate.
Forward direction: Moderate confidence. The phenotype is stable across the recording and is not explained by current medications (none), caffeine (documented mild), or condition factors on this recording day.

Inverse direction: The Slowed-Modality Composite in Chapter 21 does not apply (iAPF is normal). The Elevated TBR entry (Chapter 21) rates this pattern as a workflow heuristic for stimulant response, based on Suffin and Emory and Arns et al., but with the strong caveat that the 2026 Strzelczyk multiverse analysis has reduced confidence in TBR-based stimulant-response prediction significantly. The Elevated Frontal Theta entry (Chapter 21) notes group-level association with stimulant response as a phenotype inference, with modest effect sizes and incomplete replication.

Prescriber conversation: "The recording shows elevated frontal theta with a normal alpha peak, which in the literature is associated at the group level with a stimulant response, though individual-level prediction is limited. Given two failed stimulant trials, it may be worth asking whether a different stimulant class, a dose adjustment, or a non-stimulant pathway makes sense. I can track any changes against this recording as a baseline. The QEEG doesn't resolve the treatment question, but it may provide a monitoring frame."

Inverse-direction report language by claim type. All inverse-direction language in the report should reflect the claim type:

- *Phenotype inference:* "Elevated frontal theta with normal iAPF is associated at the group level with a stimulant response in ADHD samples (Arns et al., 2008), though individual-level prediction remains limited and recent methodological analyses have narrowed confidence in TBR-based prediction."
- *Workflow heuristic:* "The low-voltage fast phenotype has been associated with non-stimulant pathways in one prospective study; this is hypothesis-generating and should not direct prescribing."

Inverse-direction entries should never be framed as treatment recommendations. They inform the conversation; they do not replace clinical judgment or prescriber authority.

26.6 Confidence Table

Use these report-level categories. Each one compresses several separate judgments into a single word: how clean the data were, how representative the state was, how portable the pipeline is, how good the evidence is for the drug effect being invoked, and how many non-drug alternatives are live. Two careful clinicians can land on different labels for the same map. Name the inputs that moved yours, so a reader can disagree with a step rather than with the adjective.

High confidence: the finding is reliable, state-stable, pipeline-stable, and not plausibly explained by a known medication, substance, condition, or timing factor.

Moderate confidence: the finding is reliable but one or more active factors could contribute. The report should include a caveat and may still use the finding for cautious planning.

Reduced confidence: an active factor produces the same direction as the finding. The report should avoid strong phenotype claims and recommend matched-state follow-up if the finding matters clinically.

Substantially reduced confidence: multiple active factors point in the same direction, the medication state is unstable, the client is in withdrawal/discontinuation, or the pipeline changed. Defer phenotype interpretation or frame it as provisional.

Not interpretable for phenotype attribution: safety concerns, poor data quality, severe drowsiness, acute intoxication, acute withdrawal, delirium, or major pipeline mismatch prevent valid phenotype interpretation.

For a phenotype-by-phenotype confidence matrix that maps specific QEEG findings to the active factors most likely to reduce confidence, see the decision-aid appendix (Appendix B). That matrix provides recommended interaction-mode classifications, adjusted confidence levels, and report language templates for the most commonly encountered phenotype-exposure pairings.

26.7 Report Wording Examples

The pairs below range from single-phenotype attribution to follow-up language. The pattern in every stronger example is the same: name what you observed, name the active factors, assign confidence, and write the limit directly.

1. Frontal theta and stimulant timing - Weak: "The QEEG shows ADHD theta excess." - Stronger: "Frontal theta elevation is present (+1.8 SD at Fz / F3). Confidence in ADHD-specific phenotype interpretation is reduced by stimulant exposure within the recording window and by sleep restriction the night before. This recording documents the current medication state; a comparison recording under prescriber-coordinated conditions would increase phenotype confidence."

2. Beta excess in a medicated client - Weak: "Beta excess indicates anxiety." - Stronger: "Global beta elevation (+2.0 SD, 18–30 Hz) occurs in a client taking clonazepam (Klonopin) and using caffeine before recording. Benzodiazepine-associated beta and stimulant-substance contribution are plausible mechanisms. Endogenous anxiety beta cannot be confirmed in this context."

3. FAA as SSRI biomarker - Weak: "Frontal alpha asymmetry indicates SSRI-responder phenotype." - Stronger: "Frontal alpha asymmetry is present (right-greater-than-left). This finding has sex-dependent antidepressant-response associations in the literature (Bruder et al., 2001), but recent meta-analytic evidence does not support FAA as a general SSRI-response predictor. Interpretation should account for reproductive-hormone context, reference-montage sensitivity, and individual variability."

4. Neurofeedback change score - Weak: "Neurofeedback normalized the map." - Stronger: "Baseline and follow-up recordings differ in frontal theta amplitude. Interpretation of this change is limited because medication dose was adjusted between recordings and the normative database version differs between sessions. The spectral change is documented but is not interpretable as a pure neurofeedback effect under these conditions."

5. Washout recommendation - Weak: "Medication washout is needed to obtain a baseline QEEG." - Stronger: "QEEG can be recorded as clinically presenting if medication timing is documented. Recording under current medication conditions is often the more clinically relevant state. Any decision to modify medication timing for a comparison recording should be made by the prescribing clinician, not by the QEEG report."

6. Diffuse slowing in a polypharmacy client - Weak: "Diffuse slowing is consistent with cognitive dysregulation and mood disorder." - Stronger: "Diffuse slowing (elevated delta and theta, globally) is present. The client is taking quetiapine 200 mg QHS (10 hours post-dose) and lamotrigine 200 mg BID. Both compounds independently contribute to slow-wave elevation. Mood-disorder contribution cannot be separated from medication contribution in this recording; this is a medicated-state measurement, not a drug-free trait baseline."

Dyads 7–12 (slow iAPF in polypharmacy, post-viral attribution, withdrawal state, follow-up change, seizure-risk medication, and protocol deviation) are in Appendix H alongside the worked complete reports, where they can be read in operational context.

26.8 When to Record as Presenting

Recording as presenting is often the right choice. If the client lives, works, sleeps, learns, and trains while taking medication, the medicated state may be the clinically relevant state. The question becomes: what does this client's EEG look like in the state in which treatment will occur?

Record-as-presenting is appropriate when medication is stable, the purpose is training planning in the current clinical state, safety concerns are absent, and timing is documented. The report should not pretend the recording is a drug-free trait baseline.

26.9 When to Defer or Repeat

Defer strong interpretation when the client is acutely intoxicated, in unsafe withdrawal, severely sleep deprived, delirious, medically unstable, or unable to sustain wakefulness. Repeat when medication timing was unknown, PRN use changed the state, the pipeline failed, the recording was dominated by drowsiness, or a major clinical decision depends on the finding.

For anesthesia, do not use an unsupported long washout rule. In uncomplicated elective anesthesia, a wait of at least one week is a conservative practical heuristic; longer may be appropriate when older age, cardiac surgery, complicated recovery, POCD risk, delirium, or ongoing cognitive symptoms are present.

26.10 The Front-Table Version

The article version of this chapter can be reduced to a front-table with five columns: finding, active factor, interaction mode, confidence adjustment, and report language. The goal is not to make a full diagnostic engine. The goal is to put the confidence adjustment in front of the reader before they encounter the narrative sections.

Frontal theta elevated. Active factors include drowsiness, untreated OSA, TBI, antipsychotics, opioids, high sedative load, Long COVID, ME/CFS, fibromyalgia, and adolescent maturation. Interaction modes are mimicry or exaggeration. Confidence is reduced or substantially reduced. Report language: "Frontal theta is present, but medication/condition/state factors plausibly contribute."

Global beta elevated. Active factors include benzodiazepines, stimulants, caffeine, nicotine, withdrawal, akathisia, anxiety, muscle artifact, and reference/filter choices. Interaction modes are mimicry or transformation. Confidence depends on timing and artifact review. Report language: "Beta elevation should be interpreted in the context of active exposures and artifact/pipeline sensitivity."

Global beta reduced. Active factors include sedating medications, hypothyroidism and other systemic causes, sleep deprivation, post-concussive recovery, and drowsiness during the recording. Interaction modes are mimicry or exaggeration. Confidence is reduced when vigilance trajectory is not documented; global beta reduction is downstream of state and metabolism more often than it reflects a primary trait. See Hill 2026 (Hill, 2026) for operational drowsiness detection.

Slow iAPF. Active factors include antipsychotics, TCAs, opioids, age, hormonal state, cannabis, drowsiness, and recording condition. Interaction modes are mimicry or transformation. Confidence drops when state or cycle/hormonal context is unknown.

Diffuse slowing. Active factors include sedative load, antipsychotics, anticonvulsants, opioids, alcohol withdrawal/recovery, OSA, TBI, Long COVID, ME/CFS, fibromyalgia, pain, and drowsiness. Interaction mode is usually exaggeration. Confidence is often substantially reduced.

Mixed fast/slow patterns. Active factors include polypharmacy stacks (stimulant plus sedative), withdrawal states, drowsiness layered onto an aroused baseline, and pipeline-induced apparent mixtures from epoch averaging across alert and drowsy segments. Interaction mode is usually transformation. Confidence is reduced unless vigilance is split across the recording and segment-level review is performed.

Frontal alpha asymmetry. Active factors include depression state, sex-dependent antidepressant-response findings, SSRI/SNRI exposure, reference choice, artifact handling, and recording condition. Interaction mode is transformation. Confidence is reduced unless methods and sex/context are specified.

Connectivity or coherence abnormality. Active factors include reference, volume conduction, artifact pipeline, source model, medication state, and drowsiness. Interaction mode is transformation. Confidence is variable and often lower than power findings unless pipeline is stable.

Task or ERP abnormality. Active factors include benzodiazepines, alcohol, cannabis, stimulants, fatigue, task effort, comprehension, pain, sleep, and practice effects. Interaction mode is transformation. Confidence depends on behavioral data.

26.11 Safety Overrides

Some findings stop the phenotype workflow. Suspected nonconvulsive status, epileptiform activity in a high-risk withdrawal context, delirium, severe encephalopathy, acute intoxication, recent serious head injury, medication toxicity, or inability to stay awake should be handled as safety issues. So should the client's presentation, independent of what the trace looks like. A safety issue is not a single disposition, and suspected nonconvulsive status does not belong in the same channel as poor data quality. Match the response to the urgency level.

Emergency, same hour. Activate emergency services and stay with the client: ongoing altered awareness, failure to return to baseline after a seizure, suspected nonconvulsive status, acute encephalopathy or delirium, unresponsiveness, slow or shallow breathing, new focal deficit, or serious rash with fever or mucosal involvement.

Urgent, same week. Medical or neurology assessment with a formal clinical EEG: possible interictal epileptiform discharges, persistent focal slowing, a new episodic spell pattern, or new unexplained diffuse slowing.

Routine, coordinate with the prescriber. Everything else, including poor data quality, artifact burden, and drowsiness that clears on arousal.

A resting QEEG cannot exclude epilepsy, nonconvulsive seizures, or toxic-metabolic encephalopathy. A record that looks acceptable is not neurologic clearance.

Safety override language should be direct: "This recording contains findings or context that require medical review before neurofeedback phenotype interpretation." It should not be softened into a training recommendation.

Sedative-hypnotic withdrawal is the common example. If a client recently stopped benzodiazepines and has confusion, altered awareness, tremor, or seizure history, QEEG interpretation belongs behind medical safety. Alcohol withdrawal follows the same logic. Antiseizure-medication discontinuation in a seizure-history client also requires caution.

26.12 Intake Integration

The decision framework works only if intake captures the right variables. The intake form should be treated as part of the QEEG method, not as administrative paperwork.

Medication inventory should include drug, dose, formulation, route, last dose, duration, prescriber, indication, recent changes, PRN use, and missed doses. Substance inventory should include caffeine, nicotine, alcohol, cannabis, psychedelics, stimulants, opioids, kratom, and timing. Condition inventory should include sleep, pain,

TBI, OSA, migraine, Long COVID, ME/CFS, fibromyalgia, pregnancy/postpartum/cycle/OCP, adolescent developmental stage, and aging/cognitive status.

The intake form should also ask about paradoxical responses and discontinuation. "Do sedatives ever make you agitated?" "Do stimulants ever make you sleepy?" "Have you recently stopped, reduced, missed, or changed any medication?" These questions often explain maps that would otherwise look contradictory.

26.13 Matching and Repetition

A single QEEG can support a current-state interpretation. It is weaker as a trait claim when medication and condition load is high. Repetition improves confidence only if the state is matched or the change is intentionally studied.

For follow-up, match clock time, medication timing, formulation, caffeine, sleep, pain status, recording condition, pipeline, and database when possible. If the goal is to observe medication change, document the change explicitly and avoid attributing all differences to neurofeedback.

When a finding is important but low-confidence, repeat under a better-defined state. For example, if frontal theta was elevated during a drowsy EC recording after poor sleep, repeat when sleep is more typical and include EO/task data. If beta was high after caffeine and PRN benzodiazepine, repeat with documented stable exposure if clinically appropriate and prescriber-aligned.

26.14 How to Use Claim Types in Prose

The three claim types from Chapter 4 translate directly into report language. A spectral-effect statement might read: "Benzodiazepines are associated with increased beta in typical responders." A phenotype-inference statement: "Benzodiazepine-related beta can mimic beta-excess phenotypes." A workflow-heuristic statement: "Repeat the QEEG under matched stimulant timing if the theta finding will drive protocol selection."

The report does not need to label every sentence with a claim type. It does need to avoid presenting a workflow heuristic as if it were spectral-effect evidence. When in doubt, write "as a clinical heuristic" or "confidence is reduced."

26.15 Prescriber Coordination

Prescriber coordination is not the same as telling the prescriber what to prescribe. The QEEG report can say that findings are difficult to interpret because medication timing is unstable, sedative burden is high, withdrawal context is present, or paradoxical response is reported. It can recommend that medication questions be reviewed by the prescriber.

Good language: "If medication timing or formulation changes are clinically being considered, repeating QEEG after a stable prescriber-directed regimen may improve interpretability." Poor language: "Stop medication for a clean baseline."

Good language: "Current findings may reflect sedative load; prescriber review may be useful if sedation is clinically concerning." Poor language: "Reduce the sedative."

26.16 Training Implications

The decision framework does not forbid training when confidence is reduced. It changes what the clinician claims. Training may target symptoms, regulation, sleep, arousal stability, or functional goals while acknowledging that the QEEG phenotype is medication-contextual.

For high-confidence findings, QEEG-guided protocol selection can be more direct. For moderate-confidence findings, use QEEG plus symptoms and monitor carefully. For reduced-confidence findings, favor conservative protocols, state regulation, and reassessment. For not-interpretable findings, address safety, sleep, medication stability, or recording quality before protocol selection.

Conservative needs a definition, because a clinician can soften every sentence in the report and still train straight at the confounded number. When attribution is reduced, do not select a protocol whose only rationale is normalizing the feature you could not attribute. Take the target from the symptom picture, the raw record, functional assessment, and low-risk regulation goals instead, and write down which of those you used. Set the review point before the first session rather than after it: how many sessions until reassessment, what would count as a response, and what would count as an adverse response worth stopping for. Sleep disruption, agitation, headache, and rising anxiety are the ones clients report and clinicians talk themselves out of.

Medication changes during a training block are the other half of this. If a drug, dose, or timing changes mid-course, a comparison against the pre-training recording is no longer a training effect, and assigning any improvement to one input or the other becomes guesswork. Ask clients to tell you when a prescriber changes something, log the date against the session number, and say so in any progress note that reports a spectral change.

Clinical humility is a better map of uncertainty than false confidence.

26.17 Minimum Report Checklist

Every medicated-client QEEG report should answer seven questions. What was recorded? What was the raw EEG safety status? What was the recording state? What medications and substances were active? What non-drug confounders were present? What pipeline/database was used? How did those factors change confidence in each major phenotype claim?

If the report cannot answer those questions, it should not make strong medication or phenotype claims. A short caveat is not enough when the missing information is central. "Medication list unavailable" is a major limitation, not a footnote. "Last-dose timing unknown" is a major limitation for stimulants, benzodiazepines, caffeine, cannabis, sleep aids, ketamine, and PRN medications.

The final impression should contain at least one confidence sentence. Example: "Confidence in interpreting frontal theta as an ADHD-relevant phenotype is reduced by drowsiness, suspected OSA, and stimulant timing." Example: "Confidence in diffuse slowing as a stable trait is substantially reduced by antipsychotic plus opioid exposure and poor sleep." Example: "Because acquisition and processing were stable across sessions, confidence in within-person change is higher than cross-system comparison would allow."

26.18 What This Framework Does Not Do

It does not diagnose medication effects. It does not prove causation. It does not decide whether a medication should be started, stopped, raised, lowered, or substituted. It does not replace the prescriber, neurologist, sleep physician, or primary clinician. It does not make QEEG a medication-management tool.

It also does not reduce clinical practice to checkboxes. The framework organizes judgment. A skilled clinician still needs to inspect raw data, listen to the client, understand symptoms, recognize artifacts, and know when findings are outside the scope of neurofeedback.

What the framework does is make uncertainty visible. It gives the author, clinician, reviewer, and reader a shared language for why a phenotype interpretation is high-confidence, provisional, or not interpretable.

26.19 Quick Decision Rules

If the raw EEG is unsafe, stop and refer. If the client is acutely intoxicated or medically unstable, defer. If the client is drowsy, label the state before interpreting theta or alpha. If medication timing is unknown, lower confidence. If a drug or condition can produce the same direction as the phenotype, lower confidence. If the pipeline changed, do not compare z-scores directly. If the finding persists across matched states and no major alternative is active, confidence rises.

These rules are simple by design. The complexity lives in the chapters before this one; the framework turns that complexity into a usable clinical sequence.

26.20 Case vignette

A client presents with ADHD, anxiety, insomnia, stimulant treatment, SSRI treatment, caffeine use, and suspected OSA. The QEEG shows elevated frontal theta and elevated beta. A simplistic report would call this mixed ADHD/anxiety. The decision framework slows the interpretation down.

Raw screening shows no feature that requires referral, which is not the same as a clean neurologic record. Recording state shows drowsiness during late EC. Medication inventory shows methylphenidate

XR, sertraline (Zoloft), trazodone (Desyrel), caffeine, and occasional cannabis. Timing shows the stimulant was taken one hour before recording and caffeine 30 minutes before. Confounder screen flags poor sleep and OSA risk. Interaction mode is mixed: stimulant and caffeine may mask theta and exaggerate beta, while drowsiness and OSA may mimic theta.

The final wording: "Frontal theta and beta elevations are present, but phenotype confidence is reduced by drowsiness, suspected OSA, stimulant / caffeine timing, and SSRI / sedative context. Findings should be interpreted as the client's current treated presentation rather than a clean ADHD or anxiety phenotype."

26.21 Interpretation traps

- **Skipping raw EEG safety review.** Quantitative maps do not replace clinical EEG review.
- **Calling medicated state a baseline.** Say "recorded on current medication regimen."
- **Ignoring last-dose timing.** "On medication" is not a timing variable.
- **Treating drowsiness as phenotype.** Vigilance state must be documented.
- **Using class effects as proof.** They are starting points, not individual causation.
- **Comparing mismatched pipelines.** Cross-system z-score comparisons are low-confidence.
- **Hiding uncertainty.** Write confidence reductions directly.

26.22 Intake questions

When this chapter's topic appears on the intake form, ask:

- **What did you take, use, or stop in the last 72 hours?** Include prescriptions, OTC, supplements, caffeine, nicotine, alcohol, cannabis, and PRN medications.
- **When was each last dose?** Clock time, formulation, and whether this is steady-state, titration, taper, holiday, or missed dose.
- **What is your sleep and alertness state?** Sleep in last 48 hours, current sleepiness, OSA risk, pain, fatigue, headache, and caffeine timing.

- **What medical or developmental contexts apply?** TBI, Long COVID, ME/CFS, fibromyalgia, migraine, chronic pain, pregnancy/postpartum/cycle/OCP, adolescence, aging, developmental variants.
- **What recording conditions were collected?** EC, EO, task, HV, photic, and whether drowsiness occurred.
- **Were acquisition and processing settings stable?** Reference, filters, artifact handling, database, and source methods for comparisons.

26.23 Clinical recommendations

Use the decision framework for every medicated-client report. The framework is faster than repairing an overconfident interpretation later.

Record as presenting unless there is a clear reason not to. Stable medication use is not a flaw; undocumented medication use is the flaw.

Reserve strong phenotype claims for findings that survive medication, condition, state, and pipeline checks. If a factor plausibly produces the same direction, lower confidence.

When uncertain, write a better caveat rather than forcing a conclusion. The goal is not to eliminate clinical judgment; it is to make the judgment traceable.

The framework in this chapter is the operational core of the perturbation engine: the volume in a three-part clinical system (Field Guide / Brain on Drugs / Dynamic Brain) that answers the question "what changed the recording from the baseline state?" Every step in this workflow applies the perturbation-engine logic: identify the input forces, separate them from trait physiology, assign confidence, and write sentences that state what the recording supports. The baseline engine (Dynamic Brain) and the perception engine (Field Guide) handle the questions this book does not. This framework handles the middle one.

26.24 Evidence summary

- **Spectral effect:** Multiple medication classes and recording/pipeline factors produce systematic EEG effects, but individual interpretation depends on state and exposure context.

- **Phenotype inference:** Active medications, substances, conditions, and pipeline factors can mask, mimic, exaggerate, or transform QEEG phenotype interpretation.
- **Workflow heuristic:** Use the ten-step decision framework to assign confidence, write explicit caveats, and decide when to record as presenting, repeat, defer, or coordinate with the prescriber.

Part V

Time

Ch 27: Formulations, Kinetics, and Drug Holidays

27.1 Why this class matters in NFB practice

Medication status is not binary. A client is not labeled only as "on methylphenidate," "on paliperidone (Invega)," or "on lamotrigine (Lamictal)." The relevant question is what brain exposure was present during the EEG. Immediate-release, extended-release, delayed-release, transdermal, intranasal, sublingual, compounded, generic, and long-acting injectable products can produce different concentration-time curves even when the medication name looks familiar.

Strongest evidence	Pharmacokinetic exposure changes across formulation, route, steady state, and genotype are well established; direct QEEG mapping is strongest for stimulants.
Biggest interpretation trap	Writing "on medication" without timing: Document last dose, formulation, and recording block timing.
Default clinical action	Treat formulation and timing metadata as mandatory for medicated-client QEEG, and match timing across longitudinal recordings whenever possible.

For QEEG interpretation, formulation timing is not a pharmacology footnote. Peak, plateau, trough, and holiday states can change the same stimulant's appearance on the map. Antipsychotic recordings vary with position in an injection cycle. Lamotrigine maps can shift after a generic switch. Atomoxetine (Strattera) exposure at the same nominal dose can differ markedly between CYP2D6 poor metabolizers and normal metabolizers (Clinical Pharmacogenetics Implementation Consortium, 2019).

This chapter turns formulation and kinetics into recording metadata. Every medicated-client QEEG should document time since last dose, formulation, dose phase, recent changes, and for long-acting injectables, position within the injection cycle. Without those details, "medicated baseline" is too vague for clinical interpretation.

27.2 Mechanism (clinician-level pharmacology)

Pharmacokinetics describes what the body does to a drug: absorption, distribution, metabolism, and elimination. For EEG, the most useful simplified variables are onset, peak concentration, half-life, duration of action, and steady state. These variables determine when the drug's brain effect is likely to be rising, peaking, fading, or adapting.

Immediate-release products tend to produce faster rise and clearer peak-trough patterns. Extended-release products flatten the curve, but they do not eliminate timing effects. Delayed-release products may shift exposure later in the day. Transdermal systems add skin absorption and patch-wear time. Intranasal and sublingual routes can produce faster or more variable peaks. Long-acting injectables create slow cycles across weeks or months.

Steady state matters because acute EEG effects are not always the same as chronic EEG effects. A single-dose stimulant study captures an acute exposure window. A client taking the same drug daily for months has receptor adaptation, sleep effects, behavioral compensation, and illness-course changes layered onto the drug signature.

The half-life is also not the whole story. Some drugs leave the plasma quickly but produce longer behavioral or sleep consequences. Others have active metabolites. Some, such as atomoxetine, are strongly affected by pharmacogenetics (Clinical Pharmacogenetics Implementation Consortium, 2019). Formulation, metabolism, and clinical state must be interpreted together.

Another practical distinction is exposure phase. Acute phase means the first dose or a single challenge dose. Titration phase means the dose is being raised or lowered and the nervous system is adapting. Steady state means the dosing pattern has been stable long enough that day-to-day exposure is more predictable. Discontinuation phase means the drug is being reduced, stopped, or missed. These phases are not interchangeable for EEG.

The neurofeedback report does not need to model plasma concentration mathematically. It does need enough information to avoid false precision. "Recorded two hours after morning IR methylphenidate" is much stronger than "on stimulant." "Recorded week nine of a twelve-week paliperidone injection cycle" is much stronger than "on antipsychotic." "Recorded after two missed sertraline (Zoloft) doses" is much stronger than "on SSRI."

27.3 Known spectral effects

The literature search for this book found formulation-specific EEG data to be thin. Most pharmaco-EEG studies use immediate-release or single-dose designs, while clinical practice is full of extended-release stimulants, patches, LAIs, generic substitutions, compounded preparations, and intermittent holidays.

Stimulant data illustrate the problem. The familiar stimulant pattern, reduced excess slow activity with increased faster activity or improved task response, is usually studied near acute exposure or under broad "medicated" conditions. Immediate-release products should have sharper peak-trough visibility, while extended-release products should show smoother time courses. This is a pharmacokinetic inference, not a fully mapped QEEG result.

Drug-holiday studies in ADHD focus on symptoms, appetite, growth, and sleep rather than EEG. Ibrahim and Donyai reviewed drug holidays as a real-world ADHD practice (Ibrahim & Donyai, 2015). Martins and colleagues ran a randomized clinical trial of weekend methylphenidate holidays and found clinical tolerability advantages without EEG measures (Martins et al., 2004). For QEEG, the main point is that a holiday-day EEG is not equivalent to an on-day EEG.

Generic-switch evidence is strongest for antiepileptic clinical pharmacology rather than QEEG. Privitera and colleagues found bioequivalence between generic and branded lamotrigine in epilepsy (Privitera et al., 2017), and Ting and colleagues studied generic lamotrigine in generic-brittle patients (Ting et al., 2015). These data argue against broad fear of approved generics, but they still support documenting recent switches when EEG interpretation involves seizure threshold, cognition, or subtle medication attribution.

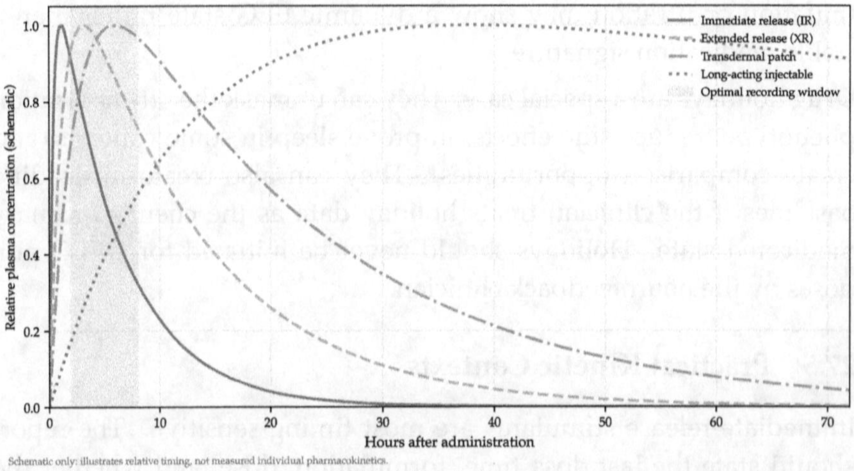

Figure 27.1: Formulation comparison: IR, XR, transdermal, and LAI concentration-time curves with QEEG recording windows. Schematic only.

27.4 Phenotype interaction effects

Formulation can mask a phenotype. A morning IR stimulant recorded near peak may suppress frontal theta enough to hide an underlying attention phenotype. The same client recorded before dosing or late in the day may look more impaired.

Formulation can mimic a phenotype. A sedating medication recorded near peak may create slow activity that resembles sleep deprivation, encephalopathy, or a slow-alpha phenotype. A late-cycle LAI antipsychotic recording may show less slowing than a mid-cycle recording, leading the clinician to underestimate medication contribution.

Formulation can exaggerate a phenotype. A CYP2D6 poor metabolizer taking atomoxetine may have higher and longer exposure than expected, making noradrenergic activation, sleep disruption, or task-state effects more visible than the nominal dose suggests (Clinical Pharmacogenetics Implementation Consortium, 2019).

Formulation can transform a phenotype over time. A client switching from IR to XR stimulant may show less dramatic peak activation but more consistent daytime vigilance. A client changing from oral antipsychotic to LAI may show fewer daily peaks and troughs but a more constant antipsychotic background. A client moving through discontinuation or titration may show a dynamic EEG state rather than a stable medication signature.

Drug holidays are a special case. They can unmask the off-medication phenotype, reduce side effects, improve sleep in some contexts, and create comparison opportunities. They can also create misleading baselines if the clinician treats holiday data as the client's ordinary medicated state. Holidays should never be initiated for QEEG purposes by the neurofeedback clinician.

27.5 Practical Kinetic Contexts

Immediate-release stimulants are most timing-sensitive. The report should state the last dose time, formulation, dose, and whether the recording occurred near expected onset, peak, plateau, or offset. If the EEG includes both resting and task blocks, timing by block matters.

Extended-release stimulants are often more clinically stable but still variable. Different products have different release technologies. A single label such as "XR" does not tell the clinician whether the product has early pulse, delayed pulse, late-day tail, or absorption variability. When the clinical question is medication response, record the product name, not only the molecule.

Transdermal systems introduce wear time, application site, adherence, skin irritation, and removal time. The same patch can produce different effective exposure if applied late, removed early, poorly adhered, or placed on irritated skin. This is especially relevant for stimulant patches and nicotine patches.

Long-acting injectables require cycle position. A paliperidone, risperidone (Risperdal), aripiprazole (Abilify), haloperidol (Haldol), or fluphenazine injection is not a single state across the whole dosing interval. Early-cycle, mid-cycle, and late-cycle recordings should not be compared without notation.

Generic, brand, and compounded products require recent-change history. Approved generic lamotrigine studies are reassuring (Privitera et al., 2017; Ting et al., 2015), but a recent switch can still coincide with symptom change, adherence change, or anxiety about equivalence. Compounded ketamine, hormones, low-dose naltrexone (Vivitrol), and other preparations add more variability because nominal dose may not predict exposure well.

Pharmacogenetics is most relevant when exposure is unexpectedly high or low for the dose. Atomoxetine and CYP2D6 are the clean example (Clinical Pharmacogenetics Implementation Consortium, 2019). The QEEG report should not diagnose metabolizer status, but it can say that unexpectedly strong or weak medication signatures may warrant prescriber review of pharmacokinetic factors.

27.6 Route and Formulation Notes

Oral immediate-release products are easiest to misunderstand because they feel familiar. Their clinical effects rise and fall over hours. If the EEG is collected near peak, the medication signature may look cleaner and stronger. If the EEG is collected before onset or after offset, the map may look closer to the underlying untreated phenotype. This is most relevant for stimulants, short-acting benzodiazepines, some sleep agents, caffeine, nicotine, and PRN medications.

Oral extended-release products reduce but do not remove timing problems. Different technologies create different curves: bead systems, osmotic pumps, delayed-release components, prodrugs, and multi-pulse products do not behave the same way. A client may say "Adderall" when the product is immediate-release, XR, or Mydayis. A client may say "methylphenidate" when the product is Ritalin, Concerta, Focalin XR, Quillivant XR, Cotempla XR-ODT, or Jornay PM. The molecule is not enough.

Transdermal delivery shifts attention from swallowing time to application time, wear time, adhesion, and removal. A methylphenidate patch applied late may not be at effective exposure when the EEG begins. A nicotine patch worn overnight can alter sleep, which may then alter a daytime EEG. A clonidine patch may produce steadier exposure than oral dosing but still contributes to sedation or arousal context.

Intranasal and sublingual products often create a sharper clinical timing issue. Intranasal esketamine has a monitored acute window. Intranasal benzodiazepines are seizure-rescue products with rapid effects. Sublingual or buccal ketamine, buprenorphine (Subutex), and asenapine can have variable absorption. If such a product was used recently, the recording should state route and time, not only drug name.

Compounded products deserve a separate line because they combine route variability with manufacturing variability. Ketamine troches, hormone preparations, low-dose naltrexone, and custom blends may have meaningful differences across pharmacies, batches, and use technique. This does not mean they are unsafe or ineffective. It means labeled dose is a weaker predictor of brain exposure than it is for standardized products.

27.7 Longitudinal Interpretation

The most common kinetic error in neurofeedback is comparing two EEGs as if medication exposure were constant. A baseline may be recorded on an IR stimulant at peak and a follow-up on an XR stimulant at trough. A baseline may be recorded early in SSRI titration and a follow-up after months of steady use. A baseline may be recorded shortly after a depot injection and a follow-up late in the cycle. The maps may differ for reasons unrelated to training.

The report should therefore include a medication-comparability sentence. For example: "Medication formulation and timing were comparable across recordings" or "Medication timing differed; baseline was recorded two hours after IR stimulant dosing, whereas follow-up was recorded before morning dose." This sentence protects the interpretation from pretending that a protocol change is a brain change.

When medication exposure differs, the clinician can still interpret the recording, but the inference changes. The report can say that EEG findings reflect the client in the sampled medication state. It should not claim that all changes are treatment effects unless medication timing, sleep, task condition, and pipeline were reasonably matched.

27.8 Drug Holidays

A drug holiday is an intentional break from medication under prescriber guidance. It is most commonly discussed for stimulant medication in ADHD. Ibrahim and Donyai describe holidays as common and clinically motivated by side effects, growth, appetite, and tolerance concerns (Ibrahim & Donyai, 2015). Martins and colleagues randomized children with ADHD to weekend methylphenidate holidays and focused on symptoms and side effects, not EEG (Martins et al., 2004).

For QEEG, the holiday is a state label. An on-day EEG answers one question. A holiday-day EEG answers another. A Monday-after-weekend EEG may answer a third because sleep, appetite, rebound symptoms, and re-dosing can all affect the recording. The report should not blend these states.

Stimulant holidays can be clinically useful comparison windows when they already exist in the treatment plan, but they should not be created by the neurofeedback clinician. Holidays for SSRIs, SNRIs, benzodiazepines, antipsychotics, anticonvulsants, lithium, and many other drugs carry discontinuation, relapse, seizure, or withdrawal risks. The book's recommendation is documentation and interpretation, not medication scheduling.

27.9 Report Language

Use plain, state-specific language. "The recording was obtained approximately 90 minutes after the client's morning IR methylphenidate dose, likely during the expected active window." "The client was recorded on a prescriber-approved stimulant holiday; findings should not be interpreted as the ordinary medicated state." "The client was near the end of a long-acting injectable antipsychotic cycle; medication exposure may be lower than at mid-cycle."

When timing is unknown, say so. "Last-dose timing was not available, reducing confidence in medication attribution." This is better than silently writing a medication interpretation that cannot be defended.

When pharmacogenetics is relevant, avoid overclaiming. "CYP2D6 status may affect atomoxetine exposure; if clinical response appears disproportionate to dose, prescriber review of pharmacokinetic factors may be useful." Do not write that QEEG has identified a metabolizer phenotype.

When generic switches are relevant, avoid both extremes. Do not dismiss all client concerns as placebo effect. Do not assume that any EEG change after a generic switch was caused by the switch. A balanced sentence is: "A recent lamotrigine product switch was reported; approved generic lamotrigine products have demonstrated bioequivalence in controlled epilepsy studies, but the switch is documented because seizure threshold and clinical symptoms are central to interpretation" (Privitera et al., 2017; Ting et al., 2015).

27.10 Case vignette

A 14-year-old is referred for QEEG because methylphenidate "does not work." The medication list says methylphenidate ER, 36 mg. The recording occurs at 8:15 a.m.; the dose was taken at 7:45 a.m. The eyes-closed map shows elevated theta and low beta engagement. During a later task block, after the medication has had more time to absorb, performance and engagement improve.

The interpretation changes when timing is known. The first block was not a full on-medication sample. The report should say that early recording may underestimate the ER stimulant effect and that follow-up comparison should match dose timing.

A second client receives a paliperidone LAI every three months. One QEEG is recorded two weeks after injection; the follow-up is recorded near the end of the cycle. The second map shows less slowing. Without cycle position, the clinician might infer improvement from training. With cycle position, a medication-exposure difference becomes a plausible contributor.

A third client with epilepsy switches lamotrigine generics between recordings. Approved products are expected to be bioequivalent, and the best evidence supports that expectation (Privitera et al., 2017; Ting et al., 2015). Still, the switch should be documented because seizure history and medication timing are central to interpretation.

27.11 Interpretation traps

- **Writing "on medication" without timing.** Document last dose, formulation, and recording block timing.
- **Treating XR products as interchangeable.** Different release technologies can create different exposure windows.
- **Ignoring LAI cycle position.** Record injection date, product, dose, and interval.
- **Overreading holiday recordings.** A holiday EEG is a state, not a universal baseline.
- **Assuming generic switches explain everything.** Approved generics often perform well, but recent switches still belong in the metadata.
- **Missing compounded variability.** Troches, creams, hormones, and LDN may have exposure variability not visible from the label.

- **Making medication-timing recommendations independently.** Timing changes are prescriber decisions when they affect treatment.

27.12 Intake questions

When this chapter's topic appears on the intake form, ask:

- **What is the exact formulation?** IR, SR, ER, XR, delayed-release, patch, nasal, sublingual, compounded, LAI, or other.
- **When was the last dose?** Record clock time and relation to each EEG block.
- **Is the client at steady state?** Note new starts, titration, dose increases, tapers, missed doses, and discontinuation.
- **For LAIs, when was the last injection?** Record product, dose, interval, and position in the injection cycle.
- **Any recent brand/generic/pharmacy switch?** Include date, product, and perceived clinical change.
- **Any planned or recent drug holiday?** Note on-day, off-day, weekend holiday, summer holiday, or accidental missed doses.
- **Any pharmacogenetic results?** Especially CYP2D6 or CYP2C19 results relevant to current medication.
- **Any compounded products?** Record pharmacy, route, dose, batch if known, and timing.

27.13 Clinical recommendations

Record medication timing before acquisition, not afterward. If the timing is unknown, interpretation should be qualified in the report.

For short-acting or timing-sensitive drugs, annotate the EEG by block. A long session can move from pre-peak to peak exposure. Resting and task data may therefore sample different drug states.

For longitudinal QEEG, match dose timing and formulation whenever possible. A baseline recorded at stimulant peak should not be compared casually with a follow-up recorded before dosing.

For LAIs, match cycle position when possible or explicitly state the difference. If matching is impossible, the report should say that cycle position may affect the comparison.

For recent switches, document rather than assume causation. Generic lamotrigine evidence is reassuring at the population level (Privitera et al., 2017; Ting et al., 2015), but individual symptom changes still require careful clinical context.

For drug holidays, the QEEG report should describe the state collected. If the client is on a prescriber-approved stimulant holiday, label the recording as holiday-state. Do not call it an ordinary medicated baseline.

27.14 Evidence summary

- **Spectral effect:** Pharmacokinetic exposure changes across formulation, route, steady state, and genotype are well established; direct QEEG mapping is strongest only in selected areas.
- **Phenotype inference:** Last-dose timing, formulation, LAI cycle position, generic switches, and holiday states can mask, mimic, exaggerate, or transform medication-related phenotype interpretation.
- **Workflow heuristic:** Treat formulation and timing metadata as mandatory for medicated-client QEEG, and match timing across longitudinal recordings whenever possible.

Ch 28: Withdrawal and Discontinuation as Distinct EEG Phenomena

28.1 Why this class matters in NFB practice

Withdrawal and discontinuation are not the absence of medication. They are active physiologic states. A client who stopped a benzodiazepine last week, skipped venlafaxine (Effexor) for three days, completed alcohol detox one month ago, or is tapering an anticonvulsant is not equivalent to a never-exposed client.

Strongest evidence	Sedative / alcohol withdrawal can involve hyperexcitability, epileptiform risk, and severe medical EEG abnormalities; methamphetamine abstinence shows persistent slowing.
Biggest interpretation trap	Calling post-discontinuation EEG a clean baseline: Previously medicated clients may carry persistent trait-like signatures.
Default clinical action	For most drug classes, QEEG should be treated as prognostic in discontinuation contexts, not diagnostic of withdrawal versus relapse. It can raise concern about a medical complication; it cannot exclude one.

This chapter has two defensive messages. First, a previously medicated client does not automatically return to a "pristine baseline." Alcohol, stimulant, and benzodiazepine literatures show that trait-like EEG signatures can persist after abstinence or discontinuation. Second, resting QEEG cannot reliably distinguish discontinuation syndrome from relapse of the underlying condition for most drug classes.

Its role is prognostic: relapse risk and recovery trajectory. It can raise concern about seizure risk, nonconvulsive status epilepticus, or encephalopathy, and it cannot exclude any of them. A resting QEEG of ordinary length is not a diagnostic EEG, and a clean-looking record in a withdrawing client is not evidence that nothing dangerous is happening.

The exception is safety-critical sedative withdrawal. Benzodiazepine, alcohol, and barbiturate withdrawal can produce epileptiform abnormalities, seizures, delirium, and nonconvulsive status patterns. In those settings, EEG may identify a medical withdrawal complication rather than anxiety, insomnia, or relapse. That distinction belongs in medical care, not neurofeedback interpretation alone.

28.2 Mechanism (clinician-level pharmacology)

On-drug effects, withdrawal effects, discontinuation effects, and relapse effects are different categories. On-drug effects reflect current exposure; withdrawal effects reflect neuroadaptation after reduction or cessation. Discontinuation syndrome describes the symptom cluster after stopping or reducing a medication, relapse is return of the underlying condition, and recovery is the longer process in which symptoms and physiology stabilize after exposure ends.

GABAergic withdrawal is the clearest EEG safety issue. Benzodiazepines and alcohol enhance inhibitory tone during exposure. Abrupt reduction can produce rebound excitability, insomnia, autonomic symptoms, tremor, seizures, and in severe cases status epilepticus. Ashton describes benzodiazepine withdrawal phenomenology and the need for gradual tapering (Ashton, 2002).

Stimulant discontinuation is different. Therapeutic stimulant holidays often show re-emergence of baseline ADHD symptoms rather than a unique EEG withdrawal signature. Stimulant-use-disorder abstinence, especially methamphetamine and cocaine, has clearer EEG recovery literature. Newton and colleagues reported abnormalities in recently abstinent methamphetamine-dependent participants (Kalechstein et al., 2009; Newton et al., 2003).

Antidepressant discontinuation is mostly clinical rather than EEG-defined. Brain zaps, disequilibrium, insomnia, nausea, hyperarousal, and flu-like symptoms are time-linked to dose reduction, but EEG does not reliably separate discontinuation from depression or anxiety relapse. Antipsychotic discontinuation raises relapse and supersensitivity questions, classically discussed by Chouinard and colleagues (Chouinard & Jones, 1980), but EEG does not provide a validated supersensitivity signature.

Anticonvulsant discontinuation sits between psychiatry and neurology. In epilepsy, EEG can help estimate seizure recurrence risk during antiseizure-medication withdrawal (Ruiz, 2018). In mood, pain, migraine, or anxiety uses of anticonvulsants, the evidence is far thinner.

28.3 Known spectral effects

Benzodiazepine withdrawal is clinically important but quantitatively under-studied. The strongest EEG signal is not a subtle spectral fingerprint; it is seizure-risk physiology. Abrupt withdrawal can be associated with spikes, spike-wave, paroxysmal activity, and nonconvulsive status patterns in vulnerable clients. Protracted symptoms may include sleep fragmentation and sensory hyperarousal, but there is no validated resting-QEEG pattern that distinguishes benzodiazepine withdrawal from anxiety relapse in ordinary outpatient cases (Ashton, 2002).

Alcohol withdrawal and abstinence have a stronger EEG literature. Early withdrawal can involve cortical hyperexcitability, beta excess, and seizure or delirium risk. Longer abstinence studies suggest that elevated fast activity and altered synchronization may persist and may relate to relapse vulnerability. The clinical implication is that "sober" does not always mean "normative baseline."

Methamphetamine abstinence shows clearer QEEG abnormalities than therapeutic stimulant discontinuation. Newton and colleagues found increased slow activity and conventional EEG abnormalities in recently abstinent methamphetamine-dependent participants (Newton et al., 2003). Kalechstein and colleagues linked QEEG abnormalities to neurocognitive performance (Kalechstein et al., 2009). These findings should not be generalized to prescribed stimulant holidays in ADHD.

Antidepressant discontinuation has little direct QEEG evidence. The chapter therefore treats SSRI/SNRI discontinuation as a clinical-

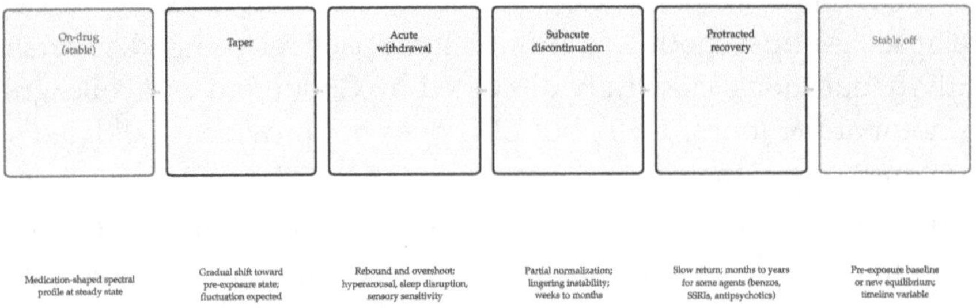

Figure 28.1: Discontinuation timeline: on-drug through taper, acute withdrawal, subacute discontinuation, protracted recovery, and stable off, with expected QEEG direction at each phase.

timeline phenomenon with EEG used mainly to exclude other problems if symptoms are severe or atypical.

Antipsychotic discontinuation has strong relapse literature and weak EEG-discontinuation literature. Chouinard's supersensitivity framework is clinically relevant (Chouinard & Jones, 1980), but QEEG cannot currently separate supersensitivity psychosis from ordinary psychotic relapse at the individual level.

Antiseizure medication withdrawal has the most defensible EEG role when seizure risk is the question. Abnormal EEG before withdrawal can predict recurrence in epilepsy populations (Ruiz, 2018). That does not mean a neurofeedback clinician should infer mood-stabilizer withdrawal status from QEEG.

28.4 Phenotype interaction effects

Withdrawal can mimic a phenotype. Benzodiazepine or alcohol withdrawal can create fast activity, irritative patterns, sleep disruption, and slow-wave instability that may be mistaken for anxiety, hyperarousal, or seizure vulnerability without medication history.

Discontinuation can mask a medication effect. A client who stops a sedating medication may show less slowing, creating the appearance of neurofeedback improvement if the recording timing is ignored.

Abstinence can exaggerate a trait. A client in early stimulant-use-disorder recovery may show slowing and cognitive fatigue that exaggerate an attention phenotype. A client in early caffeine withdrawal may show drowsiness and frontal theta that resemble sleep deprivation.

Relapse and discontinuation can transform each other. A client stopping an SSRI may have discontinuation symptoms, return of depression, sleep disruption, and anxiety in the same month. The EEG is unlikely to sort those into separate causal bins.

The practical solution is timeline discipline. The report should state the medication or substance stopped, dose and duration before stopping, taper or abrupt cessation, days / weeks since last dose, symptom onset timing, current symptoms, and medical risk factors.

28.5 Recovery Timelines

Withdrawal-state interpretation begins with the clock. The first hours to days after stopping alcohol, benzodiazepines, barbiturates, or short-acting sedatives are the danger period for acute medical withdrawal. In that window, the neurofeedback question is secondary to medical safety. Tremor, autonomic activation, confusion, seizure history, or altered awareness should move the client out of routine QEEG interpretation.

The first days to weeks after stopping antidepressants, stimulants, opioids, nicotine, caffeine, cannabis, or many sleep medications are more often discontinuation and rebound windows. Symptoms may be intense, but the EEG literature is thinner and less specific. Sleep disruption, drowsiness, autonomic arousal, pain, craving, nausea, irritability, and sensory symptoms can all change the EEG indirectly.

The first months after alcohol, cocaine, methamphetamine, benzodiazepine, or heavy cannabis cessation are recovery windows. Some clients improve clinically while their EEG still carries trait-like or recovery-related features. Others show persistent fatigue, sleep disruption, or cognitive slowing. In that context, the correct comparison is not "drug-free equals normative." It is "this is the client's current recovery-state EEG."

Stable-off status should be earned, not assumed. A client who stopped a medication three days ago, three weeks ago, three months ago, and three years ago occupies different interpretive categories. The report should say which one applies.

28.6 Differential Framing

Ask four questions before interpreting a withdrawal-state QEEG. What was stopped? How quickly was it stopped? How long ago? What symptoms appeared, and when?

Fast onset after dose reduction supports discontinuation or withdrawal. Gradual return of the original symptom pattern supports relapse, but overlap is common. Sensory disturbances, disequilibrium, brain zaps, tremor, autonomic activation, delirium, seizure, or confusion should raise medical concern rather than routine phenotype interpretation.

For most drug classes, QEEG cannot decide the differential diagnosis. It can show that the recording is abnormal, unstable, drowsy, hyperexcitable, or encephalopathic. It can suggest that a medical EEG or prescriber review is warranted. It cannot independently determine whether the client is experiencing SSRI discontinuation versus recurrent anxiety, or antipsychotic withdrawal versus psychotic relapse.

28.7 Class-Specific Practical Notes

Benzodiazepines require explicit safety language. Abrupt cessation after sustained use is a medical risk. Neurofeedback clinicians should document current use, taper plan if disclosed, last dose, prescriber involvement, alcohol co-use, seizure history, and current symptoms. A QEEG suggesting irritative activity, confusion, altered awareness, or seizure risk should prompt medical referral.

Alcohol withdrawal should be treated as a medical context. Early abstinence after heavy use, especially with tremor, autonomic symptoms, confusion, hallucinosis, or seizure history, is not a routine neurofeedback baseline. Persistent beta excess or altered arousal in abstinent clients may reflect trait vulnerability, withdrawal recovery, sleep disruption, or relapse risk rather than a simple medication effect.

Antidepressant discontinuation should be described with restraint. EEG may show nonspecific instability or sleep-related effects, but the syndrome is identified clinically. Short half-life agents and abrupt stopping create higher concern, but the report should not claim an EEG biomarker for "brain zaps" or discontinuation syndrome.

Antipsychotic discontinuation is relapse-sensitive. The EEG role is limited unless there is concern for seizures, encephalopathy, delirium, or medication toxicity. Supersensitivity psychosis is a clinical hypothesis, not a QEEG diagnosis (Chouinard & Jones, 1980).

Anticonvulsant withdrawal is different in epilepsy and non-epilepsy use. In epilepsy, EEG can inform seizure-risk decisions (Ruiz, 2018). In migraine, pain, mood, or anxiety use, EEG evidence does not support strong discontinuation claims.

Stimulant discontinuation must separate therapeutic stimulant holidays from stimulant-use-disorder abstinence. A weekend methylphenidate holiday is not methamphetamine recovery. Methamphetamine abstinence data support real slow-wave and cognitive recovery issues (Kalechstein et al., 2009; Newton et al., 2003), but those findings should not be mapped onto prescribed ADHD medication without caveat.

Opioid withdrawal is clinically dramatic but QEEG-poor. Autonomic activation, pain, insomnia, diarrhea, restless legs, craving, and agitation can all alter EEG state, but there is no clear opioid-specific resting-QEEG withdrawal fingerprint. Methadone (Dolophine) or buprenorphine (Subutex) taper states should be documented, especially because sleep, pain, depression, and polysubstance context often dominate interpretation.

Cannabis withdrawal is often sleep-centered. The client may have irritability, craving, vivid dreams, fragmented sleep, and rebound insomnia. If QEEG is collected during this window, posterior alpha, vigilance, and slow activity may reflect sleep disruption as much as cannabis recovery. Heavy-use histories also carry heterogeneous chronic findings, so early abstinence should be labeled explicitly.

Nicotine withdrawal often affects vigilance and task performance. A client who quit smoking or vaping two days before QEEG may be fatigued, irritable, headache-prone, and attentionally unstable. Nicotine replacement changes the state again. A patch, gum, pouch, cigarette lapse, or vape use shortly before testing should be recorded.

Caffeine withdrawal is common enough to deserve routine screening. Headache, drowsiness, and reduced alertness can appear after abrupt reduction. If a habitual high-caffeine client records after skipping morning caffeine, frontal theta or low engagement may be a withdrawal-state effect, not a stable phenotype.

Polypharmacy withdrawal is the ordinary hard case. A client may be tapering a benzodiazepine, missing SSRI doses, reducing cannabis, and increasing caffeine at the same time. No EEG pattern can cleanly attribute effects in that setting. The report should describe aggregate CNS instability and recommend matched-state follow-up after the taper stabilizes.

28.8 Report Language

Use state labels rather than causal certainty. "Recorded during benzodiazepine taper" is defensible. "The QEEG proves benzodiazepine withdrawal" is not. "Findings are compatible with a withdrawal/recovery state but nonspecific" is often the correct language.

For relapse-vs-discontinuation questions, write the limitation plainly: "Resting QEEG cannot reliably distinguish antidepressant discontinuation syndrome from recurrence of anxiety or depression. Symptom timing, taper history, and prescriber assessment are required." Similar language applies to antipsychotics, opioids, cannabis, nicotine, and most stimulant contexts.

For safety findings, be more direct. "Given recent benzodiazepine reduction and reported altered awareness, medical evaluation is indicated before interpreting these findings as a neurofeedback phenotype." "Recent alcohol detox and current confusion make this a medical-risk recording, not a routine training baseline."

For recovery tracking, emphasize repeated conditions. "If follow-up QEEG is used to monitor recovery, medication/substance state, sleep, caffeine, time of day, and recording condition should be matched." This is a workflow heuristic, but it prevents false attribution.

28.9 Case vignette

A client presents with insomnia, sensory sensitivity, anxiety, and intermittent derealization. The QEEG shows unstable vigilance and intermittent fast activity. The medication history reveals a long-term alprazolam (Xanax) taper that accelerated two weeks earlier. The wrong interpretation is "anxiety phenotype with beta excess." The safer interpretation is "recording obtained during benzodiazepine taper with symptoms consistent with withdrawal/discontinuation; EEG interpretation is limited, and medical taper coordination is essential."

A second client in alcohol recovery is recorded three weeks after detox. The map shows elevated fast activity and poor sleep history. This is not a neutral baseline. The report should identify early abstinence and relapse-risk physiology as context, not over-assign the finding to anxiety or neurofeedback target selection.

A third client stops venlafaxine abruptly and develops dizziness, brain zaps, insomnia, and crying spells within days. The EEG is nonspecific. The report should not decide between discontinuation and relapse. It should state that symptom timing strongly affects interpretation and that prescriber review is indicated. The QEEG here does not provide a verdict. It provides a measurement that says: the brain is not in a stable state, and the clinical conversation has not yet happened. Send this person back to their prescriber before the training protocol starts.

28.10 Interpretation traps

- **Calling post-discontinuation EEG a clean baseline.** Previously medicated clients may carry persistent trait-like signatures.
- **Using EEG to diagnose relapse versus discontinuation.** For most classes, EEG is not validated for that distinction.
- **Missing sedative-withdrawal safety risk.** Benzodiazepine, alcohol, and barbiturate withdrawal can be medically dangerous.
- **Generalizing substance-use-disorder abstinence to prescribed medication holidays.** Methamphetamine recovery is not the same as methylphenidate weekend holiday.
- **Ignoring taper speed.** Abrupt cessation and gradual taper are different brain states.
- **Treating symptom improvement as EEG normalization.** Clinical recovery and EEG recovery may occur on different timelines.

28.11 Intake questions

When this chapter's topic appears on the intake form, ask:

- **What medication or substance was stopped or reduced?** Include dose, duration, and indication.
- **When was the last dose or use?** Record date, time, and number of days/weeks since reduction.
- **Was the change abrupt or tapered?** Note prescriber involvement and planned taper schedule.
- **What symptoms appeared, and when?** Link symptom onset to dose change.

- **Any seizure, delirium, confusion, hallucination, tremor, or altered awareness?** These are medical red flags.
- **Any alcohol, benzodiazepine, barbiturate, Z-drug, or anticonvulsant withdrawal context?** Document carefully.
- **Any prior withdrawal complications?** Include seizures, hospitalization, detox, or reinstatement.
- **Is the recording intended as on-drug, taper, withdrawal, holiday, abstinent, or stable-off?** Label the state.

28.12 Clinical recommendations

Do not treat a withdrawal-state recording as a standard baseline. Label the phase explicitly: taper, acute withdrawal, discontinuation syndrome, early abstinence, protracted recovery, holiday state, or stable-off.

For sedative-hypnotic and alcohol withdrawal concerns, use medical-safety language. If there are seizures, altered awareness, delirium, confusion, or suspected nonconvulsive status, refer for medical evaluation rather than neurofeedback interpretation.

For antidepressants and antipsychotics, avoid EEG overclaiming. The report can say that discontinuation or relapse context limits interpretation. It should not claim to diagnose the cause of symptoms from resting QEEG.

For longitudinal comparisons, do not compare on-drug and withdrawal recordings as if they were treatment-response data. If medication state changed, that is a major confounder.

For previously medicated clients who are stable off medication, avoid the phrase "pristine baseline." Use "stable off medication as of [date]" and describe known exposure history.

Scope of practice. QEEG interpretation does not direct prescribing. Medication decisions, including discontinuation, dose changes, and substitution, rest with the prescriber.

Safety notice. Withdrawal from benzodiazepines, alcohol, barbiturates, and certain anticonvulsants can cause seizures and death. Opioid withdrawal is medically serious and carries overdose risk on resumption. SSRI discontinuation can cause prolonged neurological symptoms in some clients. None of these processes should be initiated, accelerated, or managed on the basis of a QEEG recording. If a client presents in active withdrawal or acute medical distress, prioritize referral to emergency medical services or their prescribing clinician before proceeding with a QEEG.

28.13 Evidence summary

- **Spectral effect:** Sedative / alcohol withdrawal can involve hyperexcitability, epileptiform risk, and severe medical EEG abnormalities; methamphetamine abstinence and antiseizure-medication withdrawal have class-specific evidence.
- **Phenotype inference:** Withdrawal, discontinuation, early abstinence, and stable-off states can mimic, mask, or exaggerate medication and phenotype interpretations.
- **Workflow heuristic:** For most drug classes, QEEG should be treated as prognostic in discontinuation contexts, not diagnostic of withdrawal versus relapse, and never as exclusionary.

Ch 29: Hormonal Timing, Pregnancy, and Exogenous Hormones (OCP, HT, Cycle-Linked Dosing)

29.1 Why this class matters in NFB practice

Hormonal state is a time-varying drug problem for QEEG because it changes pharmacokinetics, clearance, effective dose, and (when people change what they take by calendar) the actual molecules on board. The baseline you interpret is a brain under a given exposure profile; that profile moves with trimester, lactation, starting or stopping oral contraceptives, luteal-only antidepressant schedules, and menopause-related hormone or symptom-targeted drugs.

Strongest evidence	Pregnancy and postpartum change clearance, volume of distribution, and effective exposure to many psychotropics; a fixed dose is not a fixed exposure.
Biggest interpretation trap	Treating drug exposure as stable when luteal SSRI, OCP, trimester, or HT changed.
Default clinical action	Time-stamp drugs, doses, and schedules together with gestational week, postpartum month, OCP/HT, and luteal regimen before strong attributions.

The practical correction is to document when those shifts occur relative to the recording and to match medication timing in longitudinal comparisons. If two visits differ in pregnancy trimester, OCP type or recent start/stop, or luteal vs continuous SSRI exposure, a change in the map can reflect different drug delivery as much as training or a new psychotropic.

This chapter does not recapitulate cycle-phase or resting-spectral norms; those sit with Dynamic Brain. Here the subject line is substances and exposure: what was taken, when, and in which reproductive or endocrine-treatment context.

29.2 Mechanism (clinician-level pharmacology)

Pregnancy and postpartum increase plasma volume, alter protein binding, and change activity of many drug-metabolizing enzymes and transporters. Antiseizure drugs, many antidepressants, and other psychotropics often need dose or level monitoring; a stable milligram dose does not guarantee stable CNS exposure. The QEEG question is not abstract "hormone state" but whether brain exposure to the same prescription changed.

Hormonal contraceptives are exogenous hormones and possible interaction partners (enzyme effects, protein binding) for other drugs. Combined vs progestin-only methods and formulation changes are not interchangeable for interpreting exposure. Contraceptive status may also moderate how antidepressant or other responses show up in biomarker work; treat method and recency of change as drug-context fields.

Lactation matters for some agents' transfer into milk and for prescriber decisions; it is part of the same exposure story as oral doses.

Luteal or symptom-triggered SSRI dosing (e.g. PMDD) creates discontinuous exposure across the month. The same total diagnosis can mean "on SSRI that week" vs "off" at another visit; that is a drug-timing documentation problem.

Perimenopause and postmenopause often add hormone therapy, SSRIs/SNRIs, or gabapentin (Neurontin) for various indications. The chapter treats those as named drugs with their own kinetics and interactions, not as general endocrine pathophysiology without a medication list.

PCOS and related labels in intake usually imply OCP, metformin, or other prescribed drugs; those prescriptions are what belong in a medication-effects book. Endocrine pathophysiology without a drug on the list does not get its own story here.

Gender-affirming or replacement hormone therapy is exogenous hormone exposure and should be documented like any other ongoing drug.

29.3 Hormonal Contraceptives

Hormonal contraceptive status is not just yes/no. Ask about combined oral contraceptives, progestin-only pills, hormonal IUDs, implant, injection, ring, patch, recent start/stop, skipped placebo week, and breakthrough bleeding. Different methods create different exogenous hormone levels and can differ in drug interaction and adherence profiles.

Combined OCPs and progestin-only methods are not equivalent. OCPs add exogenous hormones and can flatten or reshape the cyclic variation in alpha power and related spectral features documented across the natural menstrual cycle (Becker et al., 1982; Solis-Ortiz et al., 2004); a client on combined OCPs may not show the same time-varying pattern of symptoms or concomitant drugs as a naturally cycling client. A client who recently started or stopped OCPs may be in a transition window for both hormones and any interacting medications.

For medication interpretation, contraceptive method and recency of change should be listed with the same seriousness as age, sleep, and last dose. Ignoring it weakens claims about antidepressant response, biomarker studies that stratified on contraception, and clean longitudinal drug comparisons.

29.4 Pregnancy and Postpartum

Pregnancy remodels brain gray matter over a time course that extends beyond delivery (Hoekzema et al., 2017), and it should be documented by trimester or gestational week. Pharmacokinetics (clearance, volume of distribution, protein binding, enzyme up- or down-regulation) and fetal safety are prescriber domains; the QEEG report's job is to note where in that trajectory the recording falls so exposure is not misread as a fixed trait. Antiseizure and many psychiatric drugs are classic examples of changing levels across gestation with a nominally "unchanged" dose.

Postpartum: document month since delivery, lactation when it affects drug choice or level, and medication changes (including switches driven by pregnancy vs breastfeeding). Sleep fragmentation and acute stress can add state noise; the chapter keeps those as confounds that stack on top of changing PK/PD after birth, not as a standalone "brain state" section.

Lamotrigine (Lamictal) is the clearest example of pregnancy-driven pharmacokinetic shift in this book. UGT1A4 glucuronidation of lamotrigine is induced by rising estrogen, increasing clearance two- to threefold across pregnancy; postpartum, clearance drops rapidly and can produce toxicity at the same dose. A QEEG recorded in the third trimester on a pregnancy-adjusted lamotrigine dose is not comparable to one recorded six weeks postpartum at the same nominal dose; the effective brain exposure may differ dramatically. If a pregnant client with epilepsy reports a breakthrough seizure, missed doses, or persistent vomiting, that is an urgent neurology and obstetric coordination problem and it comes before any elective recording. The QEEG clinic does not adjust or hold an antiseizure medication in pregnancy for any reason, including recording quality. See Chapter 11 for the corrected lamotrigine spectral direction and Appendix E for the full UGT1A4 pharmacogenomic discussion.

Valproate (Depakote) carries the highest teratogenic risk among commonly used antiseizure medications, with FDA boxed warnings for neural tube defects, other major malformations, and neurodevelopmental effects including reduced IQ in exposed children. Pregnancy or pregnancy potential in a valproate-treated client is therefore a coordination priority, not a routine intake detail; the QEEG clinician's role is documentation and referral to the prescriber and obstetric team, never dose adjustment or discontinuation.

Document trimester and postpartum month so gestational and postpartum drug-exposure are visible; two visits at different points along that arc are not the same comparison for medication or training attributions.

29.5 PMDD, Premenstrual Exacerbation, and Luteal Dosing

PMDD and premenstrual exacerbation create a special medication-timing problem. Some clients use SSRIs continuously. Others use luteal-phase dosing or symptom-onset dosing. That means the same client may be on SSRI during one QEEG and off SSRI during another, depending on cycle timing.

This matters for any interpretation that assumes stable drug exposure. A luteal recording on sertraline (Zoloft) is not directly comparable to a follicular recording off sertraline unless the report names the dosing schedule. A symptom-onset regimen adds variability because drug exposure can differ cycle to cycle.

Luteal-only versus continuous SSRI scheduling is a prescriber choice, not a QEEG readout. Document whether the recording occurred under luteal symptoms, SSRI exposure, sleep disruption, and distress.

29.6 Perimenopause and Menopause

Document menopausal status, use of hormone therapy, and use of SSRIs, SNRIs, or gabapentin (and other relevant psychotropics) with timing relative to the recording. Cycle irregularity in perimenopause can coincide with new or changed drugs; that is the main time-and-exposure point for this chapter. Where aging-specific norms matter, use the norms appropriate to the client's age band; here the focus is on which drugs are on board and whether they changed between visits.

29.7 PCOS and Other Endocrine Reproductive Conditions

Although a narrative review has linked PCOS to altered QEEG patterns (Pinto et al., 2024), in practice "PCOS" on a chart most often co-occurs with OCP, metformin, stimulants, antidepressants, or other prescriptions. List those drugs and any recent change. Endometriosis and hyperprolactinemia are reasons to expect analgesics, hormones, or dopamine-related drugs; hyperprolactinemia in particular is sometimes iatrogenic from antipsychotics, again a medication mechanism worth naming in the med list.

29.8 Longitudinal comparison rules (drug timing)

Ask: Was medication (name, dose, schedule) the same? Was luteal vs continuous SSRI exposure comparable? Was OCP method stable? Did pregnancy trimester or postpartum month change? Was hormone therapy or other endocrine-treatment drug added, stopped, or retitrated? Was recording time of day and sleep comparable enough that sedating drugs are not confounded by a single bad night?

If the answer is no, the report should name the exposure mismatch before attributing change to training or to a new psychotropic. A shift after titration is hard to read if OCP or gestational week changed the underlying PK. Baseline and follow-up are most comparable for drug questions when cycle phase and scheduled drugs are aligned, or the mismatch is explicit.

29.9 Case vignette

A 32-year-old woman with ADHD and PMDD takes lisdexamfetamine (Vyvanse) daily and uses luteal-phase sertraline. Her baseline QEEG is recorded mid-luteal, on sertraline, after poor sleep. Follow-up is recorded early follicular, off sertraline, after better sleep. Band powers and common ratios shift.

A simplistic report might call this a neurofeedback effect or stimulant inconsistency. A better report documents cycle phase, luteal SSRI exposure, sleep, and stimulant timing. The comparison is valid but confounded: what changed between recordings was the hormonal context in which the drug operates, not the drug alone. An unmedicated depressed woman, a woman on an SSRI, a woman on oral contraceptives, and a postmenopausal woman should not be treated as the same clinical object even when the surface alpha measure looks similar. Cycle phase belongs in the measurement, not in a footnote.

A second client with PCOS, anxiety, and OCP use shows a pattern that could be read as anxiety or ADHD. The list belongs in the interpretation: OCP and other current drugs, not a lecture on androgen profiles.

29.10 Report language examples

Use language that makes drug exposure and schedule visible:

- "SSRIs were taken in a luteal-only schedule; exposure differs from follicular or continuous use."
- "Baseline and follow-up differ in pregnancy trimester; PK and prescribing context may differ even if the dose in milligrams is unchanged."
- "Hormonal contraceptive method changed between visits; interpret medication effects cautiously."

- "Postpartum month, lactation, and psychotropic changes are documented; longitudinal comparison is state- and exposure-heavy."
- "Menopause-related hormone therapy and/or gabapentin/SSRI use is documented for this recording."

Avoid over-causal wording:

- "The medication changed the map" when exposure or schedule changed.
- "The QEEG proves PMDD."
- "OCP alone caused the pattern."
- "Pregnancy explains all findings" without separate PK/PD and state notes.

The report can describe reduced confidence without dismissing the QEEG. A single careful sentence often suffices: "Findings can still guide protocol planning, but medication attribution is limited by exposure and schedule differences across visits."

29.11 Interpretation traps

- **Treating drug exposure as stable** when luteal SSRI, OCP, trimester, or HT changed.
- **Ignoring OCP type or recent start/stop** for exposure and interaction context.
- **Comparing different cycle phases** as if they were the same drug-on state when the schedule is luteal or symptom-triggered.
- **Omitting gestational week or postpartum month** when PK is non-stationary.
- **Forgetting** that an antipsychotic may be the cause of both prolactin-related endocrine labels and the EEG-relevant drug on board.

29.12 Intake questions

When this chapter's topic appears on the intake form, ask:

- **Menstrual status:** cycling, irregular, amenorrheic, perimenopausal, postmenopausal, pregnant, postpartum, lactating, or not applicable.

- **Cycle timing (when drug schedules tie to it):** first day of last period, current cycle day, estimated phase, and whether the visit reflects usual timing for any luteal drug.
- **Hormonal contraception:** method, formulation if known, start/stop date, placebo week, skipped cycles, breakthrough bleeding.
- **Pregnancy/postpartum:** gestational week or postpartum month, lactation, psychotropic and antiseizure changes relevant to the recording.
- **Endocrine labels:** PCOS, endometriosis, hyperprolactinemia, premature ovarian insufficiency, menopause; hormone therapy and other drugs used for those contexts.
- **Medication timing:** SSRIs/SNRIs (continuous vs luteal), stimulants, benzodiazepines, sleep aids, anticonvulsants, gabapentin, hormone therapy, and any calendar-driven dosing.

29.13 Clinical recommendations

Document reproductive and hormonal-treatment context when interpreting maps that are used to judge medication or training effects. If state is unknown, say so rather than omitting it.

For naturally cycling clients who use cycle-linked dosing, try to match baseline and follow-up to comparable on-drug windows when the question is about a specific drug or stable exposure. If matching is not possible, document the mismatch.

For hormonal contraceptive users, document method and recent changes. A new start, discontinuation, or formulation change is a transition for both hormones and any interacting medications.

For pregnancy and postpartum, dose, level, and safety follow prescriber and obstetric care (see Clinical recommendations for scope on QEEG and prescribing).

For PCOS and related labels, lead with prescriptions (OCP, metformin, stimulants, etc.) and recent changes. Interpret "attention" or "mood" maps as sharing variance with those drugs and with sleep, not with a standalone endocrine monograph.

Do not force disclosure beyond clinical relevance. Intake language should be professional, optional where appropriate, and inclusive.

The goal is to document variables that affect exposure and timing, not to police identity or reproductive choices.

When a client cannot or does not want to provide details, record "not available" and lower certainty. Missing data should reduce strength of claims, not block care.

For databases and team communication, reproductive and contraceptive fields are modifiers to exposure and timing, not deterministic diagnoses. The lookup should flag when medication comparisons are shaky, not when a QEEG "type" is implied.

For research, pooling people who take time-varying or luteal-scheduled drugs without logging schedule and OCP will muddy drug effects. Pharmaco-EEG work should record these exposure variables as standard columns.

QEEG findings should not be used to recommend medication discontinuation, unsupervised titration, or substitution; those decisions rest with the prescriber.

29.14 Evidence summary

- **Spectral effect:** Resting alpha frequency and alpha power shift with menstrual cycle phase and with oral-contraceptive use (Becker et al., 1982; Brötzner et al., 2014; Solis-Ortiz et al., 2004); hormonal state is a genuine source of spectral variation across visits.
- **Phenotype inference:** Visits that differ in trimester, OCP, luteal drug window, or new menopause-related SSRI/HT/gabapentin are easy to misread as trait change or a single new drug when several exposure dimensions moved.
- **Workflow heuristic:** Time-stamp drugs, doses, and schedules together with gestational week, postpartum month, OCP/HT, and luteal regimen before strong medication attributions; pair with Dynamic Brain for resting-spectral and cycle norms.

Part VI

Substances

Ch 30: Caffeine

30.1 Why this class matters in NFB practice

Caffeine is the most common psychoactive substance in many QEEG clinics. Clients may not list it as a drug because it arrives as coffee, espresso, tea, matcha, yerba mate, soda, energy drinks, pre-workout powder, caffeine pills, chocolate, or headache medication. Yet caffeine can change vigilance, anxiety, sleep, withdrawal state, and the apparent arousal phenotype.

Strongest evidence	Acute caffeine can shift waking EEG toward activation, but simple alpha-enhancement claims are not supported by the available evidence.
Biggest interpretation trap	Treating caffeine as irrelevant: It is a psychoactive recording-state variable.
Default clinical action	Document usual daily amount, last dose, skipped-dose state, energy drink / pre-workout use, sleep, and withdrawal symptoms before assigning a phenotype.

The practical issue is timing. A client recorded after two coffees, an energy drink, and poor sleep is not the same client recorded in caffeine withdrawal after skipping a usual morning dose. Caffeine can push the map toward activation, while withdrawal and sleep debt can push it toward slowing, headache, fatigue, and poor attention.

This chapter treats caffeine as a recording-state variable, not a moral issue or a trivial lifestyle detail. The intake form should capture ordinary daily amount, last-dose timing, missed-dose state, energy drink use, and sleep.

30.2 Mechanism (clinician-level pharmacology)

Caffeine is primarily an adenosine receptor antagonist at ordinary doses. By blocking adenosine signaling, it promotes wakefulness, reduces perceived fatigue, and can increase alertness, anxiety, tremor, gastrointestinal symptoms, and sleep disruption. Individual response varies with tolerance, sleep debt, anxiety vulnerability, CYP1A2 metabolism, ADORA2A-related sensitivity, pregnancy, medications, and time of day.

The same dose can have different clinical meaning. A habitual morning coffee may normalize a client's usual wake state. A late-afternoon energy drink may disrupt sleep and produce next-day slowing. A skipped morning dose in a heavy user may produce withdrawal headache, fatigue, irritability, and reduced vigilance.

Caffeine often appears with other compounds. L-theanine in tea or supplements may alter subjective focus and alpha / task dynamics. Energy drinks add sugar, taurine, guarana, B vitamins, yohimbine-like pre-workout ingredients, or other stimulants. The QEEG clinician should document the product, not only the word caffeine.

30.3 Known spectral effects

Barry and colleagues provide a useful caffeine EEG anchor, but the chapter does not invent a single magnitude from it (Barry et al., 2005). The safe clinical phrasing is that acute caffeine tends to promote an activated waking state, with effects depending on dose, task, baseline arousal, and tolerance.

Keane and colleagues matter here: their findings do not support a simple caffeine-to-alpha claim (Keane & James, 2008). This chapter therefore avoids writing caffeine as a generic alpha-raising substance. If alpha changes appear, timing, task, eyes-open / eyes-closed condition, withdrawal, and baseline arousal matter.

L-theanine evidence is relevant because caffeine is often consumed in tea or supplement combinations. Nobre and colleagues support alpha-related attention findings for L-theanine (Nobre et al., 2008), while Gomez-Ramirez and colleagues support the idea that theanine may reduce tonic alpha while enhancing task-related modulation (Gomez-Ramirez et al., 2009). That does not mean every tea drinker has elevated resting alpha.

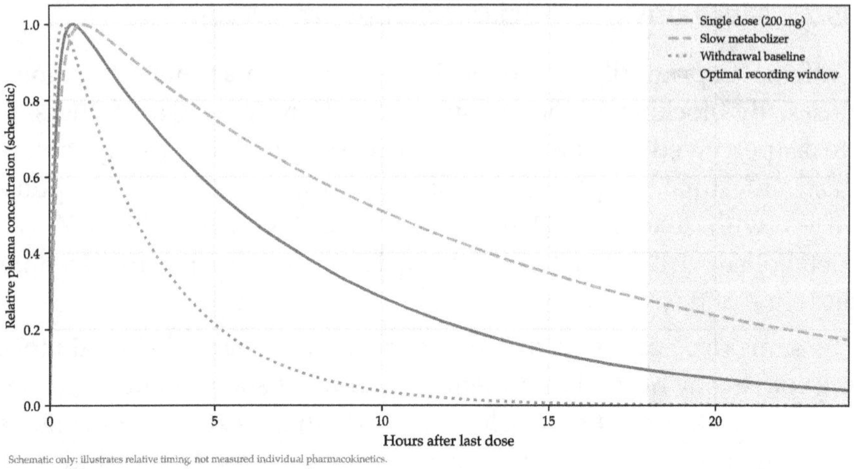

Figure 30.1: Caffeine timing: single-dose and slow-metabolizer curves with withdrawal baseline. Schematic only.

Withdrawal is messier in the QEEG literature than acute dose, but the physiology is obvious. Document it. A heavy caffeine user who skips caffeine before the test may be in a withdrawal state with headache, fatigue, low mood, and poor vigilance. That state can mimic underarousal or sleep deprivation.

30.4 Phenotype interaction effects

Caffeine can mimic hyperarousal, beta activation, anxiety, tremor, and muscle artifact. In sleep-deprived clients, it can mask fatigue temporarily while leaving unstable vigilance. In heavy users, withdrawal can mimic underarousal, frontal theta, cognitive fog, or depression-like fatigue.

It can exaggerate stimulant effects. A client taking methylphenidate, amphetamine, modafinil (Provigil), bupropion (Wellbutrin), or high-dose thyroid medication and also using energy drinks may look more activated than expected. It can also exaggerate anxiety and panic symptoms.

Caffeine can transform interpretation when it is used to self-medicate low arousal, ADHD symptoms, shift-work fatigue, or sleep apnea. A "normal" map after caffeine may be a compensated state. A slow map without caffeine may be withdrawal or sleep debt, not trait underarousal.

Paradoxical calming is sometimes reported, especially in ADHD or low-arousal clients, but QEEG-paired evidence is limited. Treat it as self-report plus mechanism plausibility, not as a validated phenotype marker.

30.5 Case vignette

A client with ADHD and anxiety arrives for QEEG after skipping his usual three morning coffees because he thought caffeine would "contaminate" the recording. He has a headache, slept six hours, and feels foggy. The QEEG shows frontal theta, diffuse slowing late in the recording, and reduced task engagement.

A simplistic report might describe an endogenous underarousal pattern. A better report identifies a caffeine-withdrawal and sleep-debt state. The map may still be useful as a current-state recording, but it is not the client's ordinary functioning state.

The defensible plan is to repeat under the client's typical morning routine if the goal is neurofeedback planning under ordinary conditions, or to label the current recording explicitly as caffeine-withdrawal state.

30.6 Interpretation traps

- **Treating caffeine as irrelevant.** It is a psychoactive recording-state variable.
- **Ignoring caffeine timing without documenting it.** Caffeine is a recording-state variable. Document last dose, usual daily amount, and whether the recording reflects habitual or atypical intake. If a habitual user was recorded after unusual abstinence, label the recording as a withdrawal-risk state (see Appendix C).
- **Calling caffeine a generic alpha-raising substance.** That simple claim is not supported by the evidence.
- **Ignoring energy drinks.** Products may contain multiple stimulants and high doses.
- **Missing late-day sleep effects.** Caffeine can affect tomorrow's QEEG through tonight's sleep.
- **Ignoring caffeine rescue.** A client may use caffeine to compensate for OSA, insomnia, or stimulant rebound.

30.7 Intake questions

When caffeine appears on the intake form, ask:

- **How much caffeine do you usually use per day?** Coffee, tea, soda, energy drinks, pills, pre-workout, headache medications.
- **When was the last dose today?** Record time and product.
- **Did you skip or reduce your usual caffeine today?** Withdrawal changes interpretation.
- **Do you use caffeine after noon or for shift work?** Sleep effects may matter more than acute effects.
- **Any jitters, anxiety, tremor, headache, fatigue, or paradoxical calming?** These symptoms guide phenotype confidence.

30.8 Pre-Recording Protocol

The default is to record the client in the habitual caffeine state (see the governing rule in Appendix C). For a daily coffee drinker, the caffeinated state is the functional baseline. Manufacturing withdrawal by enforcing abstinence substitutes one confound for a worse one: a heavy daily user who skips caffeine will arrive in a withdrawal state with headache, fatigue, slowed processing, and poor vigilance, none of which represent the person's ordinary physiology.

Caffeine half-life is approximately 5 hours in healthy adults. Five half-lives (~25 hours) is the conservative pharmacokinetic clearance window. These numbers are useful for interpretation, not for imposing a timing rule. A recording obtained 2 hours after a large coffee sits near peak caffeine exposure; a recording 18 hours after the last dose reflects minimal residual. Document the timing and read accordingly. The same timing logic applies to coffee, tea, energy drinks, soft drinks, chocolate, pre-workout products, caffeine pills, matcha, yerba mate, and caffeine-containing headache medications. Decaf still contains 2 to 15 mg per cup.

For occasional caffeine users, abstaining before a recording does not produce withdrawal and may reduce a confound the clinician would otherwise need to document. For habitual users, the habitual state is the representative state.

30.9 Clinical recommendations

For routine clinical QEEG, record the client in the habitual caffeine state and document the timing (see Appendix C). If the client arrives under usual caffeine conditions, the recording captures the functional state and should be labeled with last-dose timing for interpretation.

If caffeine timing is atypical for any reason, such as an unusually large dose, a skipped usual dose, or a new product, decide whether to proceed as current-state assessment or reschedule for a representative morning. Document the departure.

When sleep apnea, insomnia, anxiety, stimulant dosing, pregnancy, cardiovascular issues, or other medication problems are in play, they need appropriate medical follow-up. The map does not replace that.

30.10 Tolerance and Habitual Use

For habitual users, day-to-day arousal is entangled with caffeine. A morning coffee may restore their expected alertness rather than create obvious overactivation. A non-user given the same dose may feel anxious, tremulous, or overactivated. The QEEG effect therefore depends on baseline use and tolerance.

Tolerance does not make caffeine irrelevant. It changes the comparison. The key question is whether the recording reflects the client's usual functional state. If a client drinks coffee every morning and will train after coffee, the typical caffeinated state may be clinically relevant. If the client doubles intake on the morning of the QEEG because of poor sleep, that state should be labeled as atypical.

The report should avoid both extremes: ignoring caffeine because it is common, or enforcing abstinence in a habitual user and manufacturing withdrawal. Document caffeine timing; note whether the recording reflects the client's typical exposure state.

30.11 Withdrawal

Caffeine withdrawal is one of the easiest ways to create a misleading "clean" recording. Heavy users who skip caffeine may develop headache, fatigue, low mood, irritability, slowed processing, reduced motivation, and poor attention. That state can look like underarousal, depression, sleep deprivation, or frontal theta.

Withdrawal timing varies, but the practical rule is simple: ask whether the client had their usual caffeine. If not, ask why and whether symptoms are present. A withdrawal-state QEEG should be labeled as such.

Withdrawal can also interact with medications. A client taking stimulants who skips caffeine may look different from the same client on an ordinary day. A migraine client may use caffeine-containing analgesics and then present in headache rebound or withdrawal.

30.12 Energy Drinks and Pre-Workout Products

Energy drinks and pre-workout powders require product-level documentation. They may include caffeine, guarana, taurine, sugar, artificial sweeteners, B vitamins, amino acids, yohimbine-like stimulants, creatine, beta-alanine, or undisclosed proprietary blends. A client may consume one before the gym and arrive for QEEG in a highly atypical state.

Adolescents and young adults often use energy drinks during sleep restriction, with emerging evidence that habitual adolescent caffeine use alters sleep EEG architecture (Lunsford-Avery et al., 2022). The QEEG may reflect caffeine, sleep deprivation, developmental EEG features, ADHD medication, anxiety, and academic stress together.

The intake should ask about cans, shots, scoops, and timing. "One coffee" and "two energy drinks plus pre-workout" should not be treated the same.

30.13 Sleep and Circadian Effects

Caffeine can affect tomorrow's QEEG by disrupting tonight's sleep. Late-day caffeine may reduce sleep duration or sleep quality even if the client feels alert during the evening. The next-day recording may show slowing or poor vigilance from sleep loss, not acute caffeine activation.

Shift workers create a special case. Caffeine may be used to manage circadian misalignment, and "morning" may not mean the same thing. Record the client's sleep / wake schedule, work shift, and caffeine relative to their biological day.

30.14 Individual Differences

CYP1A2 metabolism can influence how long caffeine remains active. ADORA2A-related sensitivity may influence anxiety, sleep disruption, and subjective response. Pregnancy, oral contraceptives, smoking, liver function, and some medications can alter caffeine kinetics. The book does not require genetic testing for caffeine interpretation, but it does recommend listening to the client's actual response.

If a client reports paradoxical calming, severe anxiety from tiny amounts, or long-lasting insomnia from afternoon caffeine, record it. Self-report is useful when the physiology is individualized.

30.15 Report Language Examples

Weak language: "The beta excess is endogenous anxiety."

Better language: "Beta / fast activity is present after recent caffeine and poor sleep; caffeine timing and sleep state reduce confidence in interpreting the finding as stable anxiety-related hyperarousal."

Weak language: "The theta excess is ADHD."

Better language: "Frontal theta was recorded after skipped usual caffeine with headache and fatigue; withdrawal state reduces confidence in assigning a stable ADHD-like theta phenotype."

Weak language: "The client should avoid caffeine before QEEG" without asking about habitual use or documenting timing.

Better language: "Record the client in the habitual caffeine state and document last-dose timing (see Appendix C). A habitual user's caffeinated state is the functional baseline; enforcing abstinence in that user manufactures withdrawal."

Weak language: "Tea caused alpha elevation."

Better language: "Caffeine-theanine products may affect attention and alpha dynamics depending on task and state; simple resting-alpha claims should be avoided."

30.16 Training Implications

Neurofeedback should be planned around the client's real caffeine pattern. If the client always trains after morning coffee, a caffeine-free map may be less useful than a representative caffeinated map. If the client uses energy drinks unpredictably, training response may vary by session. Outcome tracking should record caffeine at each QEEG and ideally at training sessions when arousal is unstable, since apparent protocol effects may reflect caffeine timing, sleep, or withdrawal. If a client uses caffeine to compensate for OSA, insomnia, depression, ADHD medication rebound, or sedative medications, the report should point to the compensation pattern rather than treating caffeine as an isolated exposure.

30.17 Evidence summary

- **Spectral effect:** Acute caffeine can shift waking EEG toward activation, but simple alpha-enhancement claims are not supported by the available evidence.
- **Phenotype inference:** Acute caffeine, withdrawal, tolerance, sleep disruption, and energy-drink combinations can alter confidence in arousal, beta, theta, and underarousal interpretations.
- **Workflow heuristic:** Document usual daily amount, last dose, skipped-dose state, energy drink/pre-workout use, sleep, and withdrawal symptoms before assigning phenotype meaning.

Ch 31: Alcohol

31.1 Why this class matters in NFB practice

Alcohol matters in QEEG practice because it is common, underreported, physiologically powerful, and clinically state-dependent. A client may arrive after a glass of wine the previous night, a weekend binge, early withdrawal, long-term sobriety, or a history of alcohol use disorder. These are not equivalent states.

Strongest evidence	Acute alcohol and chronic alcohol-use / familial-risk literatures support state- and trait-like EEG effects, including beta-related findings.
Biggest interpretation trap	Treating abstinence as never-exposed baseline: Prior heavy alcohol exposure may leave persistent signatures.
Default clinical action	Document last drink, typical use, withdrawal history, abstinence duration, sedative co-use, and sleep before assigning phenotype meaning.

Alcohol can acutely alter arousal and EEG rhythms, disrupt sleep, interact with benzodiazepines and other sedatives, increase seizure risk during withdrawal, and leave persistent EEG signatures in some abstinent alcohol-use populations. The report should not treat alcohol only as a lifestyle footnote.

This chapter separates acute intoxication, hangover / recovery, withdrawal, chronic alcohol-use disorder, and long-term abstinence. The separation matters because an alcohol-free recording is not automatically a never-exposed baseline. In previously heavy drinkers, persistent trait-like signatures may remain months or years after abstinence.

31.2 Mechanism (clinician-level pharmacology)

Alcohol has broad effects across GABAergic, glutamatergic, dopaminergic, opioid, sleep, autonomic, inflammatory, and metabolic systems. Acutely it can be sedating, disinhibiting, anxiolytic, impairing, and sleep-disrupting. With chronic heavy exposure, the brain adapts. During withdrawal, reduced GABAergic tone and glutamatergic hyperexcitability can produce tremor, anxiety, insomnia, seizures, delirium, and autonomic instability.

Kindling is a key clinical concept: repeated withdrawals may increase withdrawal severity and seizure risk. A client with a history of multiple withdrawals is not the same as a client who rarely drinks.

Alcohol also interacts with other exposures. Benzodiazepines, opioids, antihistamines, Z-drugs, cannabis, gabapentinoids, and antidepressants can all change the clinical and QEEG context.

31.3 Known spectral effects

Acute alcohol EEG findings vary by dose, timing, state, and study design. Lukas and colleagues provide an acute alcohol reference point for low-to-moderate exposure (Lukas et al., 1986). The chapter uses qualitative language and does not invent clean clinical magnitudes.

Chronic alcohol-use and familial-risk literature supports beta-related signatures in alcohol-use disorder and risk populations. Ehlers and colleagues and Rangaswamy and colleagues report increased beta and persistent EEG differences in alcohol-use disorder and family-risk contexts (Ehlers et al., 2010; Rangaswamy et al., 2002). Related work by Bauer ties elevated fast beta to relapse risk and premorbid vulnerability across substance-dependent populations rather than to alcohol alone (Bauer, 2001).

The correction is the pristine-baseline problem. A QEEG recorded during abstinence after heavy alcohol exposure is not equivalent to a never-exposed baseline. Persistent EEG findings may reflect risk, neuroadaptation, recovery, sleep, comorbidity, medication, or abstinence duration.

Withdrawal is a distinct state. Unlike many medication discontinuation states, alcohol withdrawal can carry clear seizure, epileptiform, delirium, and nonconvulsive-status risk. QEEG is not a detox tool, but withdrawal context is safety-relevant.

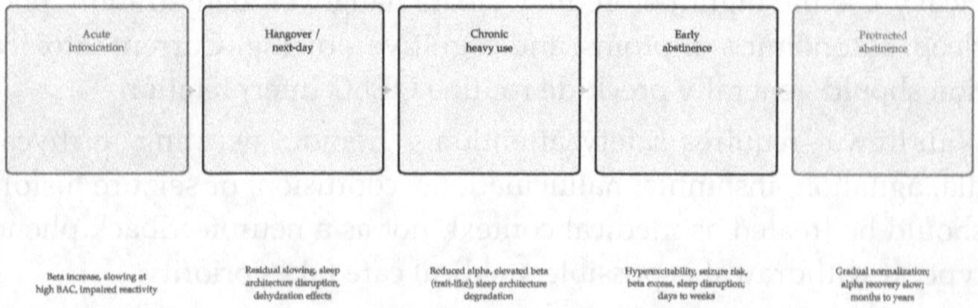

Figure 31.1: Alcohol state ladder: acute intoxication through hangover, chronic heavy use, early abstinence, and protracted abstinence, with dominant QEEG patterns.

31.4 Phenotype interaction effects

Acute alcohol can mimic sedation, reduced vigilance, slowed processing, and poor reactivity. Hangover can mimic sleep deprivation, autonomic strain, headache, fatigue, and underarousal. Withdrawal can mimic severe anxiety, insomnia, beta activation, tremor, artifact, and seizure-risk states.

Chronic alcohol-use disorder can transform beta interpretation. Elevated beta in a person with alcohol-use disorder or family history does not mean the same thing as beta in a caffeine-anxious client. It may reflect trait risk, neuroadaptation, medication, withdrawal, or current stress.

Alcohol can exaggerate sedative stacking. Alcohol plus benzodiazepines, opioids, Z-drugs, antihistamines, cannabis, or gabapentinoids is a different risk context from alcohol alone. It can also worsen sleep-disordered breathing and next-day fatigue.

Masking occurs when a client is abstinent but still carries persistent signatures. The absence of current alcohol does not erase exposure history.

31.5 Acute, Hangover, and Withdrawal States

The first intake question is timing: when was the last drink, how much, and was it typical? A drink the evening before may mainly affect sleep.

Heavy use the night before may create hangover, dehydration, poor sleep, autonomic symptoms, and cognitive slowing. Current intoxication should generally preclude routine QEEG interpretation.

Withdrawal requires safety attention. Tremor, sweating, tachycardia, agitation, insomnia, hallucinations, confusion, or seizure history should be treated as medical context, not as a neurofeedback phenotype. If withdrawal is possible, medical care takes priority.

Repeated withdrawal episodes raise kindling concerns. The report should document detox history, withdrawal seizures, delirium, and emergency care history when disclosed.

31.6 Persistent Abstinence and AUD Trait Signatures

For clients with a history of heavy alcohol use, "sober today" is not the same as never exposed. Persistent beta or other EEG differences may remain during abstinence and may reflect familial risk, chronic neuroadaptation, recovery stage, or comorbid conditions.

This matters for neurofeedback reports because a clinician may otherwise label persistent beta as anxiety, trauma hyperarousal, stimulant effect, or muscle artifact. Those remain possible, but alcohol-use history should be in the differential.

The report should use language such as: "Findings are interpreted in the context of prior alcohol-use disorder and current abstinence; prior exposure can carry persistent EEG signatures and reduces confidence in treating this as a never-exposed baseline."

31.7 Case vignette

A client in recovery from alcohol use disorder presents for QEEG-guided neurofeedback for anxiety and sleep instability. He has been abstinent for eight months, reports several prior withdrawals, and takes trazodone (Desyrel) for sleep. The QEEG shows elevated beta, intermittent tremor artifact, and poor alpha reactivity after a short sleep night.

A simplistic report might call the beta anxiety or trauma hyperarousal. A better report includes recovery history, prior withdrawal/kindling risk, sleep medication, poor sleep, and possible persistent alcohol-related beta trait. The QEEG is useful, but it is not a never-exposed baseline.

The defensible interpretation says: "Fast activity is interpreted in the context of alcohol-use disorder history, current abstinence, prior withdrawal episodes, poor sleep, and trazodone use. Stable phenotype assignment should consider persistent alcohol-related EEG signatures." The clinician should ask neutrally. Shame reduces accuracy, and inaccurate alcohol history weakens QEEG interpretation. A direct but nonjudgmental intake question ("how often do you drink, and when was your last drink?") improves both safety and science.

31.8 Interpretation traps

- **Treating abstinence as never-exposed baseline.** Prior heavy alcohol exposure may leave persistent signatures.
- **Ignoring withdrawal safety.** Alcohol withdrawal is medically significant and can include seizure risk.
- **Calling all beta anxiety.** AUD and familial-risk literature changes beta interpretation.
- **Ignoring last-drink timing.** Acute, hangover, and stable-abstinence states differ.
- **Missing sedative stacking.** Alcohol plus benzodiazepines, opioids, hypnotics, or antihistamines changes risk.
- **Ignoring sleep.** Alcohol may fragment sleep even when it initially feels sedating.

31.9 Intake questions

When alcohol appears on the intake form, ask:

- **When was the last drink, and how much?** Record timing, amount, and whether it was typical.
- **Any history of heavy use, alcohol-use disorder, detox, withdrawal, seizures, or delirium?** Safety and baseline interpretation depend on this.
- **Any current withdrawal or hangover symptoms?** Tremor, sweating, agitation, headache, insomnia, nausea, confusion.
- **Any sedative co-use?** Benzodiazepines, opioids, sleep medications, antihistamines, cannabis, gabapentinoids.
- **How was sleep after drinking or during abstinence?** Alcohol often changes the next-day QEEG through sleep.

31.10 Pre-Recording Protocol

The default is the governing rule in Appendix C: record the client in the ordinary habitual state and document it. For a routine drinker, that ordinary pattern is the functional baseline, and asking a dependent drinker to abstain is a medical decision rather than a recording preference, because alcohol withdrawal can produce seizures and delirium.

What the timing buys you is interpretation, not a cleaner client. A drink the night before shortens sleep latency and fragments the second half of the night, so a recording the next morning carries sleep-disruption physiology whether or not any alcohol remains. In someone who does not drink regularly, measurable pharmacology is gone within roughly a day, so a recording beyond that window reflects sleep and recovery rather than alcohol itself. Document last-drink timing and quantity and read the record accordingly.

Two limits stand apart from all of this. Do not record a client who is acutely intoxicated. Do not proceed when withdrawal is suspected. Both mean deferring the session and involving medical care.

Heavier prior-night drinking fragments sleep and introduces hangover physiology that confounds spectral interpretation independently of any direct alcohol pharmacology in the recording window.

31.11 Clinical recommendations

Do not perform routine phenotype interpretation during intoxication or suspected withdrawal. Medical safety comes first. If withdrawal symptoms, confusion, seizure history, or severe autonomic signs are present, refer for medical care rather than neurofeedback interpretation.

For stable abstinent clients, document alcohol-use history and abstinence duration. Do not call the recording a never-exposed baseline. Use persistent-signature language when interpreting beta, arousal, sleep, and recovery patterns.

For social drinkers, record the ordinary pattern and document last-drink timing, quantity, and sleep quality. A recording after poor sleep or hangover should be labeled as current state.

31.12 Acute Alcohol

Acute alcohol exposure is a poor condition for routine QEEG phenotype assessment. Even when the client is not visibly intoxicated, recent use can change sleep, arousal, reaction time, attention, hydration, headache, and autonomic state. Low-to-moderate exposure may have different EEG effects than heavy intoxication, and timing relative to peak blood alcohol level matters.

If alcohol was consumed the same day, the safest approach is usually to reschedule unless the goal is explicitly to document an alcohol-exposure state. If alcohol was consumed the prior evening, ask about amount, bedtime, awakenings, hangover symptoms, hydration, and sleep quality. The map may be shaped more by sleep fragmentation than by direct alcohol pharmacology.

Alcohol also alters artifact risk. Tremor, sweating, restlessness, nausea, jaw tension, or discomfort can contaminate high-frequency ranges. Technician notes should document whether the client appeared flushed, sleepy, tremulous, anxious, or ill.

31.13 Hangover and Recovery

Hangover is a recovery-state recording that can involve sleep loss, inflammation, dehydration, headache, autonomic symptoms, mood change, gastrointestinal distress, and cognitive slowing even after alcohol has cleared. A QEEG recorded during hangover documents that state, not baseline physiology.

This is clinically important because clients may minimize prior-night drinking if they are embarrassed or if they consider it normal. The intake should ask neutrally: "Any alcohol in the last 24-48 hours?" and "Was last night typical for you?"

The report should not overinterpret a hangover map. Slowing, poor alpha reactivity, unstable vigilance, and beta from tension can all be current-state features.

31.14 Alcohol Withdrawal

Alcohol withdrawal is a medical safety problem first, not a neurofeedback problem. Symptoms may include tremor, sweating, agitation, insomnia, anxiety, tachycardia, nausea, hallucinations, confusion, seizures, or delirium. The QEEG clinician should not attempt to distinguish anxiety relapse from alcohol withdrawal by map reading alone when symptoms suggest withdrawal.

Withdrawal can produce hyperexcitability and seizure risk. Benzodiazepines may be used medically for detox, which then adds its own EEG effects. A client recently discharged from detox, newly abstinent, or in early withdrawal should be interpreted as a transition-state recording.

Repeated withdrawals can worsen risk through kindling. A history of multiple detox episodes or withdrawal seizures should reduce confidence in routine phenotype interpretation and increase safety attention.

31.15 Long-Term Abstinence

Long-term abstinence is not one state. A client at two weeks, two months, two years, and twenty years may differ by sleep recovery, nutrition, liver health, medications, psychiatric comorbidity, seizure history, cognitive recovery, and relapse risk. Persistent EEG findings may reflect enduring risk, recovery, or vulnerability rather than active alcohol effect.

The report should use time-anchored language: "recorded during early abstinence," "recorded after eight months of sobriety," or "recorded with remote AUD history." That is more useful than "no alcohol present."

Persistent beta or arousal findings should be interpreted with AUD history in mind. This does not mean every beta finding in a sober person is alcohol-related. It means exposure history belongs in the differential.

31.16 Alcohol and Sleep

Alcohol often feels sedating but fragments sleep later in the night. It can reduce sleep quality, worsen snoring or sleep-disordered breathing, increase awakenings, and produce next-day fatigue. A client who drinks at night may show waking slowing because sleep was poor, not because alcohol is acutely present.

Alcohol also interacts with insomnia treatment. Trazodone, Z-drugs, benzodiazepines, antihistamines, cannabis, and alcohol can appear in the same sleep history. This combination is clinically important and can reduce interpretive confidence.

The intake should ask not only "how much alcohol" but "how did you sleep after drinking?"

31.17 Report Language Examples

Weak language: "The beta pattern shows anxiety."

Better language: "Fast activity is present in a client with alcohol-use disorder history and current abstinence; AUD / familial-risk literature and recovery state reduce confidence in interpreting beta as ordinary anxiety alone."

Weak language: "The client is sober, so this is a clean baseline."

Better language: "The recording occurred during abstinence after prior heavy alcohol exposure; this should not be treated as a never-exposed baseline."

Weak language: "The slowing is medication effect."

Better language: "Slowing is present after poor sleep and recent alcohol exposure; hangover / recovery state, sleep disruption, and medication use all reduce specificity."

Weak language: "Withdrawal looks like anxiety."

Better language: "Withdrawal symptoms and seizure-risk history are safety context; QEEG should not be used to manage or diagnose alcohol withdrawal outside medical care."

31.18 Training Implications

Neurofeedback can be useful in recovery contexts, but timing and safety matter. Stable abstinence with documented sleep and medication state is different from early withdrawal, hangover, or unstable recovery. If relapse risk, withdrawal symptoms, or detox history is active, medical and addiction-treatment coordination comes first.

For stable recovery clients, neurofeedback targets may address sleep, arousal regulation, attention, craving-related states, or anxiety. The report should not promise that training reverses alcohol-related EEG signatures. It should frame the QEEG as current physiology within a recovery history.

Outcome tracking should document abstinence duration, relapse episodes, sleep, medications, and withdrawal history at each QEEG. A change in beta or slowing may reflect recovery, relapse, sleep, medication, or training.

31.19 Practical Confidence Levels

High-confidence interpretation is possible when the client has no recent alcohol exposure, no withdrawal symptoms, stable sleep, stable medications, and either no significant alcohol-use history or a well-documented stable recovery state.

Moderate confidence applies when alcohol-use history is present but stable, abstinence duration is known, sleep is adequate, and no acute withdrawal or hangover symptoms are present. Persistent beta or arousal findings should carry AUD-history caveats.

Low confidence applies during intoxication, hangover, early withdrawal, recent detox, relapse, severe insomnia, sedative stacking, confusion, tremor, or seizure-risk symptoms. In these cases, the recording is a state/safety document, not a stable phenotype baseline.

31.20 Documentation Standard

Minimum documentation includes last drink timing, amount, typical use pattern, abstinence duration if applicable, alcohol-use disorder history, detox/withdrawal/seizure history, family history when relevant, sedative co-use, sleep quality, and current symptoms.

The clinician should ask neutrally. Shame reduces accuracy, and inaccurate alcohol history weakens QEEG interpretation. A direct but nonjudgmental intake improves both safety and science.

31.21 What Not to Claim

Six overclaims are specific to alcohol interpretation:

- Do not treat sober as never-exposed.
- Do not label withdrawal-pattern beta as anxiety without confirming the medical context.
- Do not call all beta patterns trauma or anxiety in clients with AUD history.

- Do not interpret intoxication or hangover recordings as ordinary phenotype maps.
- Do not ignore alcohol-plus-sedative combinations as co-drivers of the picture.
- Do not use QEEG findings to recommend medication discontinuation, dose changes, or pharmacologic substitution; those calls belong with the prescriber.

The stronger claim is conditional: alcohol shapes QEEG interpretation through acute state, sleep, withdrawal, kindling, chronic exposure, abstinence duration, familial risk, and sedative co-use.

31.22 Medication-Assisted Recovery and Comorbidity

Alcohol recovery often occurs alongside medication treatment. A client may take naltrexone (Vivitrol), acamprosate, disulfiram, gabapentin (Neurontin), topiramate (Topamax), benzodiazepines during detox, SSRIs/SNRIs, sleep medications, antipsychotics, stimulants, or beta-blockers. Each medication changes the QEEG context. Naltrexone itself has limited direct resting-QEEG evidence, while gabapentin, topiramate, benzodiazepines, and sleep medications have more obvious interpretive consequences.

Early recovery may also involve depression, anxiety, trauma symptoms, insomnia, pain, nutritional deficiency, liver problems, or cognitive fog. The QEEG clinician should not treat these as background noise. They are often the reason the client is referred.

When alcohol-use history and medication treatment coexist, the report should name both. "Recorded during stable abstinence on naltrexone and trazodone" is more useful than "no current alcohol." "Recorded after recent detox with gabapentin and poor sleep" tells the reader that the map is still a recovery-state measurement.

31.23 Relapse and State Change

Relapse or return to heavy drinking can change interpretation quickly. A follow-up QEEG after relapse should not be compared to a sober baseline as if only neurofeedback changed. The same applies after detox, medication-assisted recovery changes, or new sleep treatment.

For clients in recovery, the QEEG report can respectfully ask for current status because it matters physiologically. The question should be clinical, not moral. "Any alcohol use since the last recording?" is as relevant as asking about medication changes or sleep.

If the client does not disclose alcohol use until after the QEEG, update the interpretation rather than treating the map as invalid. The recording may still be useful as a state marker.

31.24 Evidence summary

- **Spectral effect:** Acute alcohol and chronic alcohol-use/familial-risk literatures support state- and trait-like EEG effects, including beta-related findings in AUD/risk populations.
- **Phenotype inference:** Alcohol state reduces confidence in beta, arousal, slowing, sleep, and anxiety interpretations unless timing, withdrawal, and exposure history are documented.
- **Workflow heuristic:** Document last drink, typical use, withdrawal history, abstinence duration, sedative co-use, and sleep before assigning phenotype meaning.

Ch 32: Nicotine and Tobacco

32.1 Why this class matters in NFB practice

Nicotine matters because it is common, fast acting, route-dependent, and often used to regulate attention, anxiety, appetite, stress, or withdrawal. Clients may smoke cigarettes, vape, use nicotine pouches, chew tobacco, use gum or lozenges, or wear patches. They may not report nicotine unless asked directly.

Strongest evidence	Acute smoking/nicotine and transdermal nicotine evidence support arousal-related EEG effects, but route-specific evidence for vaping and pouches is sparse.
Biggest interpretation trap	Applying one nicotine policy to all users. A dependent smoker's nicotine-maintained state is their functional baseline, and abstaining before a session manufactures withdrawal; an occasional user abstaining does not (see Appendix C).
Default clinical action	Document route, last use, usual pattern, abstinence/withdrawal symptoms, caffeine/stimulant pairing, and sleep before assigning a phenotype.

Nicotine can acutely increase arousal and attention while withdrawal can create fatigue, irritability, poor concentration, anxiety, headache, and slowing. A smoker who abstains before QEEG may be in withdrawal rather than in a clean baseline state. A vaper who uses nicotine immediately before recording may be in an acute activation state.

This chapter separates nicotine from tobacco smoke, route, and withdrawal. Cigarette evidence cannot be transferred automatically to vaping or pouches. When route-specific evidence is absent, the report should label the gap.

32.2 Mechanism (clinician-level pharmacology)

Nicotine is a nicotinic acetylcholine receptor agonist with fast effects on attention, arousal, reward, autonomic state, and withdrawal relief. Combustible smoking delivers nicotine rapidly along with carbon monoxide, particulates, and many non-nicotine compounds. Vaping delivers aerosolized nicotine with device, liquid, and dose variability. Patches provide slower transdermal delivery. Gum, lozenges, and pouches create buccal/oral absorption with different kinetics.

Route matters because QEEG timing matters. A cigarette just before the recording, a nicotine patch worn all day, and a pouch used during the drive to the clinic are different exposures.

Withdrawal matters as much as dosing. Nicotine-dependent clients can develop withdrawal quickly enough that a clinic abstinence rule may create a withdrawal map.

32.3 Known spectral effects

Knott's cigarette-smoking dose-response work provides a verified QEEG anchor for acute smoking effects (V. J. Knott, 1989). The safe clinical phrasing is that acute nicotine/smoking can shift the waking EEG toward activation and arousal, depending on dose, baseline state, and dependence.

Pickworth and colleagues provide an additional early nicotine/smoking reference point (Pickworth et al., 1986). These older combustible-smoking studies are useful but should not be treated as complete evidence for modern vaping, pouches, or high-concentration products.

Transdermal nicotine has separate evidence. Knott's nicotine-patch work and later patch literature support route-specific arousal and sleep effects (Choi et al., 2017; V. J. Knott et al., 1999). Patch exposure is slower and more sustained than smoking.

Vape-specific resting-QEEG evidence is sparse. The chapter does not invent a vaping signature. It treats vaping as nicotine exposure with route-specific uncertainties.

32.4 Phenotype interaction effects

Nicotine can mimic activation, beta/arousal, attention improvement, anxiety, tremor, and autonomic arousal. Withdrawal can mimic underarousal, depression, irritability, poor attention, slowing, or sleep deprivation.

Nicotine can mask low arousal. A client who smokes before every cognitively demanding task may present a compensated state. If the same client abstains before QEEG, frontal theta or slowing may appear because withdrawal has changed the state.

It can exaggerate stimulant and caffeine effects. Nicotine plus caffeine plus ADHD medication can produce a different recording than any one exposure alone.

It can also transform adolescent interpretation. Vaping in adolescents occurs against a background of developmental EEG maturation, sleep restriction, caffeine/energy drinks, cannabis, and ADHD medication. Route-specific EEG evidence is limited, so documentation matters more than claims.

32.5 Case vignette

A client with ADHD and anxiety usually vapes nicotine throughout the morning. The clinic asks for no nicotine before QEEG, so he abstains for six hours. He arrives irritable, foggy, craving nicotine, and drinking coffee. The map shows frontal theta, reduced vigilance late in the recording, and intermittent beta from tension.

A simplistic report might call this ADHD plus anxiety. A better report identifies nicotine withdrawal, caffeine compensation, and atypical recording state. The client's ordinary functional state includes nicotine exposure, while this recording reflects withdrawal.

The defensible report says: "QEEG was recorded after atypical nicotine abstinence with withdrawal symptoms and caffeine compensation; phenotype confidence is reduced for stable attention and arousal labels."

32.6 Interpretation traps

- **Applying one nicotine policy to all users.** Light or occasional users are not dependent, so same-day abstinence before the session avoids an acute arousal shift without creating withdrawal. Dependent users face a genuine withdrawal-vs-substance trade-off; their habitual nicotine state is the functional baseline, and enforcing abstinence manufactures withdrawal (see Appendix C).
- **Treating vaping as cigarette smoking.** Route-specific EEG evidence is limited.
- **Ignoring nicotine replacement.** Patches, gum, lozenges, and pouches matter.
- **Missing caffeine pairing.** Nicotine and caffeine often travel together.
- **Calling withdrawal theta ADHD.** Atypical abstinence can mimic attention phenotypes.
- **Ignoring sleep.** Nicotine can alter sleep, especially with patches or late use.

32.7 Intake questions

When nicotine appears on the intake form, ask:

- **Which route?** Cigarettes, vaping, pouches, gum, lozenges, patch, chewing tobacco, or mixed.
- **When was the last nicotine use?** Record timing and whether it was typical.
- **Did you abstain or reduce today?** Ask about cravings, headache, irritability, fatigue, and poor concentration.
- **Any caffeine, stimulant, cannabis, or alcohol pairing?** Co-use changes arousal interpretation.
- **Any patch use overnight?** Sleep effects may matter.

32.8 Clinical recommendations

For light or occasional nicotine users, no nicotine on recording day before the session is reasonable (see Appendix C). Acute nicotine shifts arousal measures, and in non-dependent users, same-day abstinence does not create withdrawal.

For habitual dependent users, the nicotine-maintained state is the functional baseline (see the governing rule in Appendix C). Enforcing abstinence produces a withdrawal-state recording that is more confounding than the nicotine itself. Record the client's representative nicotine state, document the decision, and label the recording accordingly.

Treat vaping and pouches as nicotine exposures with route-specific evidence gaps. Use cigarette and patch studies as context, not as direct proof of every modern product's QEEG signature.

If nicotine cessation treatment is underway, label the recording as a transition state. Patch, gum, lozenge, varenicline, bupropion (Wellbutrin), and withdrawal symptoms may all shape the map.

32.9 Route-Specific Timing

Combustible cigarettes deliver nicotine rapidly and are often used in predictable cycles: first cigarette of the day, breaks, driving, stress, meals, and before appointments. A client may smoke immediately before walking into the clinic. That timing can create acute arousal and autonomic effects.

Vaping can be more continuous. Clients may take small doses throughout the day and may not know the total nicotine amount. High-concentration products and frequent use can produce exposure patterns unlike cigarettes. The QEEG report should document device type, nicotine strength if known, frequency, and last use.

Pouches, gum, and lozenges produce oral absorption and may be used during a commute or even shortly before the recording. Patches create sustained exposure and may be worn overnight. Overnight patch use can affect sleep in some clients, so sleep quality and vivid dreams should be documented.

32.10 Cessation Aids

Nicotine cessation often involves more than stopping nicotine. Clients may use patches, gum, lozenges, varenicline, bupropion, counseling, or abrupt abstinence. Varenicline and bupropion have their own neuropsychiatric and seizure-threshold context. Withdrawal symptoms may be strongest during the same period.

A QEEG recorded during cessation should be labeled as a transition-state recording. That does not make it useless. It may document the client's current state during quitting. But it should not be treated as a stable baseline for trait phenotype assignment.

32.11 Adolescents and Vaping

Adolescent nicotine exposure deserves separate caution because developmental EEG maturation, sleep restriction, caffeine/energy drinks, cannabis, ADHD medication, and vaping often overlap. No strong adolescent vape-specific resting-QEEG evidence base has been identified. That absence should be written as a gap, not filled with cigarette data.

For adolescents, ask specifically about vaping, disposable devices, pouches, social use, school-day timing, and caffeine/energy drink pairing. Many teens will not use the word nicotine unless asked about products.

32.12 Nicotine, Cognition, and Compensation

Nicotine can feel cognitive-enhancing, especially when it relieves withdrawal. A dependent smoker may experience a cigarette as improved focus because it reverses withdrawal-related attention decline. That is not the same as a pure cognitive enhancer effect in a nondependent person.

This distinction matters for QEEG interpretation. A stable smoker recorded after ordinary nicotine may look more organized than the same smoker in withdrawal. The ordinary-state map may be more relevant for neurofeedback if the client is not quitting. If the client is actively quitting, the withdrawal-state map may be clinically relevant but should be labeled as such.

32.13 Sleep Effects

Nicotine can affect sleep, and sleep affects the QEEG. Late vaping, overnight patch use, withdrawal insomnia, and early-morning craving can all alter next-day vigilance. A slow map in a nicotine user may reflect sleep disruption rather than direct nicotine effect. A beta-heavy map may reflect withdrawal restlessness, caffeine compensation, or recent nicotine.

Ask about sleep quality, patch use overnight, nighttime vaping, morning craving, and caffeine rescue. These questions often explain the map better than route alone.

32.14 Report Language Examples

Weak language: "The beta pattern is anxiety."

Better language: "Fast activity is present after recent nicotine and caffeine use; route and timing reduce confidence in interpreting beta as stable anxiety-related hyperarousal."

Weak language: "The client did not use nicotine today, so this is baseline."

Better language: "The client is nicotine-dependent and abstained atypically before recording with withdrawal symptoms; the QEEG should be interpreted as a withdrawal-state recording."

Weak language: "Vaping has the same EEG signature as cigarettes."

Better language: "Vaping is documented as nicotine exposure, but route-specific resting-QEEG evidence is limited; cigarette findings should not be transferred without caveat."

Weak language: "The patch is irrelevant."

Better language: "Transdermal nicotine provides sustained exposure and may affect arousal or sleep depending on timing; patch use should be documented."

32.15 Training Implications

Neurofeedback should be planned around the client's real nicotine state. If the client smokes before every session, training response may differ from a nicotine-abstinent QEEG. If the client is quitting, session-to-session physiology may change as withdrawal, replacement therapy, caffeine use, and sleep shift. Outcome tracking should record nicotine route and timing at each QEEG, especially when arousal instability is a major target. If nicotine is being used to compensate for ADHD symptoms, low arousal, medication sedation, or sleep deprivation, the report should name that compensation pattern.

32.16 Practical Confidence Levels

High confidence is possible when nicotine route and timing are typical, no withdrawal symptoms are present, sleep is stable, and caffeine/stimulant co-use is documented. Moderate confidence applies when recent nicotine, caffeine, or mild withdrawal is present but documented. Low confidence applies during atypical abstinence, severe craving, active cessation transition, heavy vaping with unknown dose, major sleep disruption, or strong stimulant/caffeine stacking; phenotype labels should carry explicit caveats in those cases.

32.17 What Not to Claim

Do not treat nicotine abstinence as a clean baseline in dependent clients. Do not transfer cigarette QEEG findings directly to vaping, pouches, or high-dose modern products. Do not ignore replacement therapy. Do not label withdrawal theta as ADHD without context. Do not ignore caffeine pairing. Do not use QEEG findings to recommend medication discontinuation, dose changes, or pharmacologic substitution. Those calls belong with the prescriber.

The stronger claim is conditional: nicotine shapes QEEG interpretation through route, timing, dependence, withdrawal, sleep, replacement therapy, and co-use with caffeine, stimulants, cannabis, or alcohol.

32.18 Documentation Standard

Minimum documentation includes route, product, nicotine strength if known, frequency, last use, whether use was typical, withdrawal symptoms, cessation aids, caffeine pairing, cannabis/alcohol pairing, and sleep quality. For patches, record whether the patch was worn overnight. For vaping or pouches, record approximate frequency rather than relying on number of cigarettes. The goal is not to police nicotine use but to keep arousal interpretation tied to the recorded state.

32.19 Evidence summary

- **Spectral effect:** Acute smoking/nicotine and transdermal nicotine evidence support arousal-related EEG effects, but route-specific evidence for vaping and pouches is limited.
- **Phenotype inference:** Nicotine exposure and withdrawal can reduce confidence in beta/arousal, attention, theta, and underarousal interpretations.

- **Workflow heuristic:** Document route, last use, usual pattern, abstinence/withdrawal symptoms, caffeine/stimulant pairing, and sleep before assigning phenotype meaning.

Ch 33: Cannabis, THC, and CBD

33.1 Why this class matters in NFB practice

Cannabis matters because clients may use it for sleep, anxiety, pain, trauma symptoms, appetite, nausea, recreation, or seizure-related indications. Products vary widely: smoked flower, vapes, concentrates, edibles, tinctures, high-THC products, CBD-dominant products, balanced THC/CBD products, and prescription cannabidiol. A single intake checkbox for "marijuana" is not enough.

Strongest evidence	Chronic cannabis findings are heterogeneous; evidence supports reduced slow activity and increased beta/gamma in some cohorts plus regional alpha effects.
Biggest interpretation trap	Claiming uniform chronic alpha elevation: The chronic literature is heterogeneous and regional.
Default clinical action	Document product, route, potency, last use, abstinence/withdrawal state, adolescent exposure, sleep, and polysubstance use before assigning a phenotype.

For QEEG interpretation, cannabis raises three problems. Acute intoxication changes state. Chronic use may leave heterogeneous resting-state findings that vary by cohort, abstinence duration, route, potency, and age of onset. CBD is not THC, and wellness-dose CBD has little direct resting-QEEG evidence.

Chronic cannabis should not be described as producing one consistent alpha direction. The findings are heterogeneous, with reduced delta/theta and elevated beta/gamma reported in some work, plus elevated frontal alpha power and coherence (with reduced alpha frequency) in long-term users.

33.2 Mechanism (clinician-level pharmacology)

THC acts primarily through CB1 receptor signaling and can alter attention, perception, memory, anxiety, sleep, reward, and autonomic state. CBD has different pharmacology and should not be treated as a non-intoxicating version of THC. Product ratios matter because a high-THC concentrate, a balanced edible, and prescription cannabidiol are different exposures.

Route matters. Inhaled cannabis has rapid onset. Edibles have slower onset, longer duration, and easier overconsumption. Vapes and concentrates can deliver high THC. Tinctures vary. Chronic daily use differs from occasional social use.

Age of exposure matters. Adolescent cannabis use intersects with developmental EEG maturation, sleep, nicotine/vape use, caffeine/energy drinks, ADHD medication, anxiety, and school schedules. Adult cannabis frameworks should not be transferred casually to adolescents.

33.3 Known spectral effects

Ilan and colleagues do not support an acute resting-alpha claim (Ilan et al., 2004). The study should not be cited for that purpose.

Struve and colleagues reported elevated alpha power and coherence over bilateral frontal cortex, together with a reduced alpha frequency, in long-term users in the non-intoxicated state (Struve et al., 1999). This supports careful regional language, because the effect was frontal rather than a single global alpha story.

Prashad and colleagues' earlier work found a different chronic-cannabis pattern at the group level: increased beta/gamma and reduced slow activity in users versus controls (Prashad et al., 2018). Their later study did not replicate that group-level difference; the reduced-slow and increased-beta/gamma relationships appeared only as within-person correlations with craving, days of use, and age of onset (Prashad et al., 2026). That non-replication from the same group is itself the case for heterogeneity, not one canonical signature.

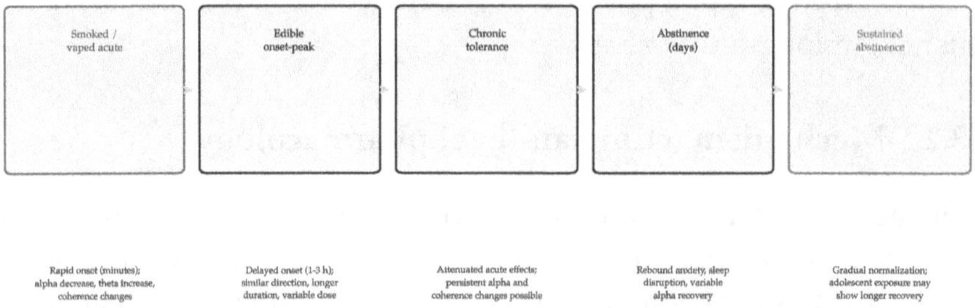

Figure 33.1: Cannabis product and state map: smoked / vaped acute, edible, chronic tolerance, and abstinence phases with expected QEEG direction.

CBD evidence must be separated. Prescription cannabidiol in epilepsy has EEG relevance through seizure / IED contexts, while wellness-dose CBD does not have a reliable resting-QEEG signature. Solowij and related CBD work can inform CBD / THC distinction, but the chapter avoids claiming a clean wellness-dose CBD map (Solowij et al., 2018).

33.4 Phenotype interaction effects

Acute THC can mimic altered vigilance, anxiety, dissociation, slowed processing, impaired attention, or panic. It can also reduce anxiety in some clients, which may mask baseline arousal. A QEEG recorded while intoxicated is a state recording, not a stable phenotype map.

Chronic cannabis can transform beta, gamma, alpha, and slowing interpretations because the literature is heterogeneous. A fast-activity finding may not mean ordinary anxiety. A regional alpha finding may not mean a stable alpha phenotype. Abstinence duration and cohort matter.

Withdrawal can mimic insomnia, irritability, anxiety, poor appetite, restlessness, and sleep disruption. It can also produce next-day slowing through poor sleep. Withdrawal should not be treated as a clean cannabis-free baseline.

CBD can create false reassurance. A product labeled CBD may contain THC, variable dose, contaminants, or other cannabinoids. Pure wellness-dose CBD is a gap category for resting QEEG, not an EEG-neutral guarantee.

33.5 Product-Specific Notes

Smoked flower has rapid onset and route-related respiratory context. Document strain if known, THC/CBD ratio if known, last use, and frequency.

Vapes and concentrates can deliver high THC. Route-specific and potency-specific QEEG evidence is limited, so the report should document high-potency exposure without inventing a signature.

Edibles have slower onset and longer duration. A client may be impaired the next morning after a high-dose edible, especially if sleep was disrupted.

CBD-dominant wellness products are pure-gap or near-gap for resting-QEEG claims. Document product, dose, certificate/testing if known, and whether THC contamination is possible.

Prescription cannabidiol belongs in a different evidence frame because it is used for epilepsy and seizure/IED contexts. Do not generalize Epidiolex findings to store-bought CBD gummies.

33.6 Case vignette

A client with anxiety, insomnia, and chronic pain uses high-THC vape cartridges nightly and CBD gummies during the day. She stops cannabis for two days before QEEG because she wants a clean baseline. She sleeps poorly, feels irritable, and drinks extra caffeine. The QEEG shows intermittent beta, poor alpha reactivity, and late-session drowsiness.

A simplistic report might call this anxiety with underarousal. A better report calls it cannabis-withdrawal/sleep-disruption state layered with caffeine compensation and chronic pain. The CBD gummies do not resolve the interpretive problem because product content and dose are unclear.

The defensible report states: "Findings were recorded during atypical cannabis abstinence with withdrawal symptoms, poor sleep, chronic pain, CBD-product use, and increased caffeine. Stable phenotype assignment should be reduced-confidence."

33.7 Interpretation traps

- **Claiming uniform chronic alpha elevation.** The chronic literature is heterogeneous and regional.
- **Citing acute cannabis as resting-alpha increase.** The available evidence does not support that claim.
- **Treating CBD as THC-free by default.** Product content varies unless verified.
- **Generalizing Epidiolex to wellness CBD.** Prescription epilepsy data do not equal wellness-dose resting-QEEG evidence.
- **Ignoring withdrawal.** Abstinence can create insomnia and arousal symptoms.
- **Ignoring adolescent exposure.** Developmental context changes interpretation.

33.8 Intake questions

When cannabis or CBD appears on the intake form, ask:

- **Which product and route?** Flower, vape, concentrate, edible, tincture, CBD, balanced product, prescription cannabidiol.
- **THC/CBD ratio and potency if known?** High-THC concentrates and CBD-dominant products differ.
- **When was the last use, and was it typical?** Acute use, abstinence, and withdrawal change the map.
- **Any withdrawal symptoms?** Insomnia, irritability, anxiety, appetite change, restlessness, vivid dreams.
- **Any nicotine, caffeine, alcohol, psychedelics, or sleep-medication co-use?** Polysubstance context is common.

33.9 Pre-Recording Protocol

The default is to record the client in the habitual cannabis state (see the governing rule in Appendix C). For heavy daily users, the habitual exposure is the functional state, and enforcing abstinence introduces withdrawal-state confounds (insomnia, irritability, anxiety, appetite changes) that are more misleading than the residual substance effect. First-pass hepatic conversion of THC to 11-OH-THC produces longer-acting effects from edibles than from inhalation, so edible timing context extends further. These intervals are useful for interpreting what a recording captured, not for imposing a client instruction.

Acute intoxication is a separate matter. A client who is actively impaired by recent cannabis use is not in a representative functional state. Deferral is appropriate when the client is visibly intoxicated, cognitively impaired, or unable to sustain engagement with the recording task.

33.10 Clinical recommendations

For routine clinical QEEG, record the client's habitual cannabis state and document product, route, last use, and frequency (see Appendix C). Do not perform stable phenotype interpretation during acute intoxication. If cannabis was recently used or abruptly stopped, label the recording as current state, intoxication-adjacent, or withdrawal-state as appropriate.

For heavy daily users where the clinician elected to allow representative cannabis state, document the decision. If the goal is specifically to study withdrawal or recovery, label the recording as a withdrawal-transition map.

Use gap language for wellness CBD and high-THC/vape-specific claims. Document product type and potency rather than inventing signatures.

33.11 Acute Use

Acute THC exposure is a state variable. It can change attention, time perception, anxiety, sensory processing, memory, motivation, and vigilance. Some clients become relaxed; others become panicky, dissociated, paranoid, or cognitively slowed. The QEEG meaning depends on dose, route, tolerance, product, and time since use.

If cannabis was used immediately before the recording, routine phenotype interpretation should usually be deferred. If the purpose is to document an intoxication state, label it that way. If the client used cannabis the prior night, ask whether sleep, dreaming, anxiety, pain, or morning grogginess changed.

Edibles require special timing. A client may still be affected the next morning after a high-dose edible, especially if sleep was disrupted. Vapes and concentrates require potency questions. A single "hit" may not mean the same thing across products.

33.12 Chronic Use and Abstinence Duration

Chronic cannabis findings depend on use pattern, abstinence duration, age of onset, product potency, route, and comorbidity. Long-term abstinent users can differ from daily users recorded soon after last use. A chronic user who stops for a few days may be in withdrawal rather than stable abstinence.

The report should document daily versus occasional use, years of use, age of first regular use, last use, abstinence duration, and withdrawal symptoms. If possible, note whether the product is high THC, balanced, CBD-dominant, or unknown.

The chronic-cannabis synthesis should stay cautious: some studies report reduced slow activity and elevated faster activity, others show elevated frontal alpha without a global pattern, and alpha is not a single global story. That language protects the report from overclaiming.

33.13 Withdrawal

Cannabis withdrawal can include insomnia, vivid dreams, irritability, anxiety, appetite change, restlessness, low mood, and craving. Sleep disruption is often the pathway into QEEG change. A client who stops nightly cannabis before the test may sleep poorly, drink more caffeine, and arrive anxious or foggy.

Withdrawal should not be treated as a cannabis-free baseline. It is a transition state. For heavy users, a representative-use QEEG may be more clinically useful for neurofeedback planning than an artificially abstinent recording, unless the goal is to study withdrawal or recovery.

33.14 CBD and Prescription Cannabidiol

CBD is not one exposure. Prescription cannabidiol used for epilepsy belongs in a medical and seizure-monitoring context. It may reduce interictal epileptiform discharges in some epilepsy contexts, but that is not a general wellness-dose resting-QEEG signature.

Wellness CBD products vary widely in dose, purity, labeling accuracy, and THC contamination. Some contain other cannabinoids or terpenes. A client may say "CBD" while using a product with enough THC to affect cognition or sleep.

The report should ask whether the product is prescription, dispensary, hemp-derived, full-spectrum, broad-spectrum, isolate, or unknown. If the product is not verified, write that uncertainty into the interpretation.

33.15 High-THC Concentrates and Vaping

High-THC concentrates, dabs, wax, vape pens, and cartridges are common enough to require separate documentation. They may produce stronger acute effects than lower-potency flower, but route-specific QEEG evidence remains limited. The report should not invent a "dab signature."

For adolescents and emerging adults, high-potency THC intersects with developmental EEG trajectories, sleep, anxiety, ADHD medication, nicotine vaping, caffeine, and school schedules. This is a high-uncertainty context and should be labeled as such.

33.16 Polysubstance Context

Cannabis often travels with nicotine, caffeine, alcohol, psychedelics, benzodiazepines, sleep medications, stimulants, and pain medications. The QEEG clinician should document co-use because the map may reflect a stack rather than cannabis alone.

Common patterns include cannabis for sleep with trazodone (Desyrel) or melatonin, cannabis for anxiety with SSRIs, cannabis for pain with gabapentin (Neurontin) or opioids, and cannabis plus nicotine vaping. Each pattern changes the interpretation.

33.17 Report Language Examples

Weak language: "Cannabis caused alpha elevation."

Better language: "Chronic cannabis findings are heterogeneous; this recording should be interpreted with route, product potency, last use, abstinence duration, and withdrawal / sleep context."

Weak language: "CBD has no EEG effect."

Better language: "Wellness-dose CBD lacks a reliable resting-QEEG signature in the available evidence; product content and THC contamination remain relevant."

Weak language: "The client stopped cannabis, so this is baseline."

Better language: "The recording occurred during atypical cannabis abstinence with insomnia and irritability; interpretation should treat this as a withdrawal-transition state."

Weak language: "Cannabis explains the beta."

Better language: "Fast activity is interpreted in the context of cannabis product history, caffeine, nicotine, anxiety, sleep, and possible withdrawal; cannabis alone cannot be assigned from the map."

33.18 Training Implications

Neurofeedback can proceed in cannabis users, but the recording state should match the clinical goal. If the client uses cannabis nightly and will continue, a representative current-state map may be relevant. If the client is reducing or stopping cannabis, the map may change as sleep and withdrawal change.

Protocol decisions should avoid overreacting to acute intoxication or withdrawal findings. A beta-heavy or drowsy map after recent cannabis change may not be durable. A repeat recording after stable sleep and stable use / reduction may be more informative.

Outcome tracking should document cannabis state every time. Changes in product potency, route, abstinence, sleep, or co-use can look like neurofeedback effects if not recorded.

33.19 Practical Confidence Levels

High-confidence interpretation is possible when product, route, last use, sleep, and co-use are documented, use pattern is stable, and the client is neither acutely intoxicated nor withdrawing.

Moderate confidence applies when chronic use is present but stable and sleep is adequate, or when CBD product details are partially known. Caveats are still needed.

Low confidence applies during acute intoxication, high-dose edible hangover, abrupt abstinence, withdrawal insomnia, unknown high-potency product use, adolescent high-THC use, or heavy polysubstance stacking.

33.20 What Not to Claim

Do not write chronic cannabis as one global alpha direction. Do not cite acute THC as a simple resting-alpha effect from the rejected source.

Do not generalize prescription CBD epilepsy findings to wellness CBD. Do not invent vape or concentrate signatures. Do not call cannabis withdrawal a clean baseline. Do not use QEEG findings to recommend medication discontinuation, dose changes, or pharmacologic substitution. Those calls belong with the prescriber.

The stronger claim is conditional: cannabis and cannabinoid products shape QEEG interpretation through THC/CBD ratio, route, potency, timing, chronicity, abstinence duration, withdrawal, sleep, age of exposure, and polysubstance context.

33.21 Adolescents and Emerging Adults

Adolescent cannabis exposure is a separate interpretive problem, not a smaller adult problem: myelination and synaptic pruning run through adolescence into early adulthood, and it is unclear how far adult findings translate (Jacobus & Tapert, 2014). Resting EEG changes across adolescence include alpha-frequency maturation, theta decline, aperiodic changes, and prefrontal-network development. Cannabis, nicotine vaping, caffeine/energy drinks, sleep restriction, ADHD medication, anxiety, and school schedules often overlap.

For this age group, the report should document age of first regular use, current frequency, product potency, route, vaping, concentrates, co-use with nicotine, and sleep. If the QEEG shows theta, beta/gamma, alpha changes, or poor vigilance, interpretation should explicitly acknowledge developmental uncertainty.

The chapter does not claim a validated adolescent cannabis QEEG signature. It states that cannabis exposure is a major confounder and research gap for adolescent QEEG interpretation.

33.22 Medical Cannabis and Pain

Medical cannabis is often used for chronic pain, migraine, sleep, PTSD symptoms, nausea, appetite, muscle spasm, or anxiety. The indication matters. A chronic pain client using THC at night and gabapentin during the day is not a pure cannabis case. A cancer client using THC/CBD for appetite and sleep has medical context that may dominate the map.

Pain, sleep, inflammation, opioids, gabapentinoids, antidepressants, and cannabis can all point in overlapping directions. The report should say "cannabis use in chronic pain context" rather than "cannabis effect."

If the client uses cannabis primarily for sleep, Chapter 15 logic also applies. Last night's product, sleep duration, awakenings, morning grogginess, and withdrawal/rebound sleep disruption may matter more than chronic-use labels.

33.23 Product Uncertainty

Cannabis product labels are not always reliable. Dispensary products may list THC/CBD percentage, but actual dose depends on amount used, route, tolerance, and absorption. Unregulated products may contain unexpected THC, synthetic cannabinoids, contaminants, or inaccurate CBD claims.

The QEEG clinician does not need forensic product testing. The report can document uncertainty: "product potency unknown" or "client reports CBD-dominant product, but THC content not verified." That is better than assuming the product is EEG-neutral.

Synthetic cannabinoids deserve particular caution because they can produce stronger and less predictable effects than cannabis. If suspected, they should be documented separately and treated as high-uncertainty exposure.

33.24 Synthetic Cannabinoids and Grey-Market Products

Delta-8 THC, delta-10 THC, HHC, THC-O, synthetic cannabinoids, and grey-market products are increasingly common. Direct resting-QEEG evidence is limited. These products may have different potency, contaminants, or legal labeling than clients expect.

The practical rule is gap-aware documentation. Ask about product source, label, route, frequency, last use, adverse reactions, panic, dissociation, and sleep. Do not import standard cannabis findings without caveat.

33.25 Raw EEG and State Review

Cannabis-related states can change artifact and vigilance. Acute intoxication may produce drowsiness, poor engagement, eye movement, or anxiety. Withdrawal can produce restlessness, muscle tension, and poor sleep. High-THC exposure may increase panic or dissociation in susceptible clients.

Raw EEG review and technician notes should document alertness, odor or reported use, red eyes if observed, anxiety, restlessness, drowsiness, and whether the client appeared intoxicated or withdrawn. These observations do not diagnose use, but they help interpret the map.

33.26 Documentation Standard

Minimum documentation includes product type, route, THC/CBD ratio if known, potency if known, last use, usual frequency, age of first regular use, abstinence duration, withdrawal symptoms, sleep quality, indication, and co-use with nicotine, caffeine, alcohol, psychedelics, opioids, benzodiazepines, or sleep medications.

For repeat QEEGs, document the same variables each time. Switching from flower to high-THC vape, stopping nightly cannabis, starting CBD, or adding nicotine can all change the comparison.

33.27 Scheduling the Recording

Routine phenotype interpretation should avoid acute intoxication and acute withdrawal. For occasional users, schedule away from recent use and document sleep. For daily users, decide whether the clinical goal is representative current-state mapping or abstinence/recovery tracking. Those are different questions.

If a client arrives after recent use, the recording may still be useful as a state marker, but the report should say so. If a client arrives after abrupt abstinence with insomnia, craving, or irritability, the recording should be labeled as withdrawal-transition state.

The goal is not to force one cannabis policy for every clinic. The goal is to prevent hidden product timing from masquerading as a durable neurofeedback phenotype.

33.28 Evidence summary

- **Spectral effect:** Chronic cannabis findings are heterogeneous; evidence supports reduced slow activity and increased beta/gamma in some cohorts plus elevated frontal alpha power and coherence (with reduced alpha frequency) in long-term users.

- **Phenotype inference:** Acute THC, chronic use, withdrawal, sleep disruption, product potency, and CBD / THC ratio can reduce confidence in alpha, beta / gamma, vigilance, anxiety, and underarousal interpretations.
- **Workflow heuristic:** Document product, route, potency, last use, abstinence / withdrawal state, adolescent exposure, sleep, and polysubstance use before assigning phenotype meaning.

Ch 34: Recreational Psychedelics and Empathogens

34.1 Why this class matters in NFB practice

Psychedelics and empathogens now appear in neurofeedback intakes because clients attend psilocybin retreats, ayahuasca ceremonies, MDMA-assisted underground sessions, ketamine experiences, microdosing regimens, and recreational events. Some use these substances for healing, spirituality, depression, trauma, creativity, or recreation. Others present after difficult experiences, sleep disruption, panic, derealization, or symptom worsening.

Strongest evidence	Acute psilocybin, DMT, ayahuasca, MDMA, and ketamine studies support strong state-dependent EEG/network effects; post-acute evidence is much thinner.
Biggest interpretation trap	Treating acute effects as trait phenotypes: Psychedelic-state EEG is not baseline EEG.
Default clinical action	Document substance, timing, setting, sleep, adverse effects, integration state, microdosing, co-medications, and polysubstance use before interpreting.

The QEEG problem is timing and context. Acute psychedelic EEG findings are often dramatic, but they do not automatically define a stable post-acute phenotype. A client recorded during a retreat, the morning after a ceremony, two weeks after psilocybin, or years after MDMA use represents different questions.

This chapter covers recreational and ceremonial use. Outpatient therapeutic ketamine and esketamine are handled in Chapter 13. Anesthetic ketamine is handled in Chapter 12. Cannabis is handled in Chapter 33.

34.2 Mechanism (clinician-level pharmacology)

Classic psychedelics such as psilocybin, LSD, DMT, ayahuasca, and 5-MeO-DMT act mainly through serotonergic 5-HT2A-related mechanisms, with effects on sensory processing, network dynamics, self-referential processing, emotion, perception, and meaning-making. MDMA is an empathogen with serotonergic, noradrenergic, dopaminergic, oxytocin-related, autonomic, and sleep effects. Recreational ketamine is an NMDA antagonist and dissociative.

The clinical context matters as much as the molecule. A supervised psilocybin research session is not the same as a festival dose, a multi-night retreat, or microdosing with unknown product. Ayahuasca ceremonies may involve fasting, sleep deprivation, vomiting, emotional intensity, travel, group ritual, and other substances or medications.

The QEEG clinician should document substance, dose if known, route, date, setting, adverse reactions, sleep, integration period, medication interactions, and current symptoms.

34.3 Known spectral effects

Psilocybin has strong acute EEG evidence. Carhart-Harris and colleagues, Muthukumaraswamy and colleagues, and related work support broadband desynchronization, altered complexity, and network-state changes during acute psychedelic states (Carhart-Harris et al., 2014; Muthukumaraswamy et al., 2013). Skosnik and colleagues provide rare post-acute evidence, including sub-acute changes in an evoked plasticity measure after psilocybin (Skosnik et al., 2023). The chapter treats these as timing-specific, not universal long-term phenotype signatures.

LSD has acute neuroimaging and EEG-relevant work showing altered perception and network dynamics, but controlled post-acute resting-QEEG evidence is limited. DMT has acute EEG evidence from Timmermann and colleagues, including rapid changes during the intense DMT state (Timmermann et al., 2019).

Ayahuasca has EEG evidence in ceremonial or acute contexts, including Schenberg and colleagues (Schenberg et al., 2015). These data should not be generalized to every retreat participant's later resting QEEG.

MDMA has LORETA / EEG evidence from Frei and colleagues (Frei et al., 2001). No controlled long-term post-abstinence resting-QEEG data sufficient for stable phenotype claims have been identified.

Recreational ketamine should not be collapsed with clinic ketamine. It may share NMDA-antagonist mechanisms, but dose, route, pattern, polysubstance context, and chronicity differ.

34.4 Phenotype interaction effects

Acute psychedelics can transform nearly every ordinary phenotype interpretation. Alpha, complexity, broadband power, connectivity, and sensory rhythms during an acute psychedelic state are not trait QEEG findings. They are drug-state findings.

Post-acute interpretation is more difficult. A client may report improved depression, worsened anxiety, altered sleep, emotional openness, derealization, or spiritual meaning after a session. The QEEG may reflect symptom change, sleep, medication changes, integration stress, or substance effects.

Microdosing is a pure-gap or near-gap category for routine QEEG. Subjective reports may be strong, but controlled EEG evidence for subperceptual repeated dosing is limited. Do not invent microdosing signatures.

MDMA can complicate arousal, sleep, autonomic state, mood, and serotonergic medication interactions. Recreational settings often include sleep deprivation, dancing, dehydration, overheating, alcohol, cannabis, stimulants, or psychedelics.

34.5 Substance-Specific Notes

Psilocybin has the strongest acute and some post-acute EEG support in this group. Still, a research dose with preparation and integration is not the same as recreational mushrooms of unknown dose.

LSD has long duration and can affect sleep and next-day state. Post-acute resting-QEEG evidence remains limited, so timing language is essential.

DMT and ayahuasca can produce intense acute states. Ayahuasca may include MAOI-containing brew components and medication-interaction concerns. Document retreat/ceremony setting, sleep, fasting, vomiting, and psychiatric aftereffects.

MDMA is an empathogen with stimulant and serotonergic features, not a classic psychedelic. Sleep loss and polysubstance use may be more QEEG-relevant than the compound alone.

Recreational ketamine differs from therapeutic ketamine. Chronic heavy use, bladder toxicity, dissociation, and polysubstance context belong in the history.

5-MeO-DMT and microdosing should be treated with gap-aware language unless direct evidence is available.

34.6 Case vignette

A client schedules QEEG five days after a psilocybin retreat. He slept poorly during travel, stopped cannabis for the retreat, took no antidepressants, and reports both emotional relief and derealization. The QEEG shows altered alpha reactivity, increased beta from tension, and unstable vigilance.

A simplistic report might assign a new alpha phenotype. A better report treats the recording as post-retreat integration state with sleep disruption, cannabis withdrawal, emotional activation, and recent psychedelic exposure.

The defensible report states: "QEEG was recorded five days after psilocybin retreat with sleep disruption and cannabis abstinence; findings should be interpreted as post-acute/integration-state physiology rather than stable baseline phenotype."

34.7 Interpretation traps

- **Treating acute effects as trait phenotypes.** Psychedelic-state EEG is not baseline EEG.
- **Ignoring retreat context.** Sleep, fasting, travel, ceremony, and integration matter.
- **Inventing microdosing signatures.** Evidence remains sparse.
- **Merging recreational and therapeutic ketamine.** Context and dose differ.

- **Ignoring medication interactions.** SSRIs, MAOIs, stimulants, lithium, antipsychotics, and benzodiazepines may matter.
- **Ignoring difficult experiences.** Panic, derealization, insomnia, and destabilization are clinical state variables.

34.8 Intake questions

When psychedelic, empathogen, or recreational ketamine use appears on the intake form, ask:

- **Which substance, dose, route, and date?** Include psilocybin, LSD, DMT, ayahuasca, MDMA, ketamine, 5-MeO-DMT, and microdosing.
- **What was the setting?** Research, therapy, retreat, ceremony, festival, private use, or unknown source.
- **Any adverse or lingering effects?** Panic, derealization, insomnia, mood change, flashbacks, suicidality, or psychosis symptoms.
- **Any medication or substance co-use?** SSRIs/SNRIs, lithium, antipsychotics, stimulants, benzodiazepines, cannabis, alcohol, MAOIs.
- **What was sleep like before and after?** Sleep disruption can dominate QEEG state.

34.9 Clinical recommendations

Do not use acute or immediate post-session QEEG as a stable baseline. Label timing explicitly. If the goal is neurofeedback planning, wait until sleep, mood, and acute integration state stabilize. For recording-state guidance applicable to all Part VI exposures, see Appendix C.

Use gap language for microdosing, 5-MeO-DMT, long-term MDMA abstinence, and post-acute LSD/DMT/ayahuasca unless direct evidence is available. Do not invent signatures.

If the client reports psychosis, mania, suicidality, severe derealization, seizure, or dangerous medication interactions, medical or psychiatric evaluation takes priority.

34.10 Acute, Post-Acute, and Integration Windows

The acute window is the least appropriate time for routine phenotype interpretation. During an acute psychedelic or empathogen state, the

EEG is part of the drug state. It may be useful for research, but it should not be compared to resting clinical norms as if it were baseline.

The immediate post-acute window can also be unstable. Clients may be sleep deprived, emotionally activated, nauseated, dehydrated, jet-lagged, overstimulated, or still integrating difficult material. A next-day QEEG after a ceremony or festival is usually a recovery-state recording.

The integration window is clinically meaningful but variable. Some clients feel improved mood and openness. Others experience anxiety, insomnia, derealization, resurfaced trauma, or confusion. A QEEG during this period should document symptoms and sleep carefully.

Later follow-up may be more suitable for neurofeedback planning, but only if sleep, mood, substance use, and medications have stabilized. There is no single universal waiting period because substances, doses, settings, and reactions differ.

34.11 Therapeutic-Dose Psilocybin and QEEG Timing

As psilocybin-assisted therapy moves toward FDA consideration and state-level access programs, the QEEG clinician will increasingly see clients who have undergone supervised high-dose psilocybin sessions for depression, end-of-life distress, or substance-use disorders. This is distinct from recreational use in setting, dose precision, therapeutic framing, and follow-up expectations.

The most relevant EEG finding comes from Skosnik and colleagues, who studied 19 adults with major depressive disorder in a double-blind, placebo-controlled within-subject design, placebo first and psilocybin 0.3 mg/kg four weeks later (Skosnik et al., 2023). Auditory evoked theta power in a tetanus-induced long-term potentiation paradigm doubled in amplitude two weeks after the single psilocybin dose, but not after placebo, and the theta increase correlated with improvement in depression symptoms rather than with mystical-experience intensity. Note what that measure is: evoked theta in an LTP paradigm, not resting theta. A routine resting QEEG would not show it. Companion fMRI data from psilocybin therapy trials suggest that functional connectivity changes may begin normalizing by three months, though EEG-specific longitudinal data are sparse.

For QEEG recording timing, a conservative recommendation is to wait at least six to eight weeks after a supervised psilocybin session before interpreting a resting-state recording as representative of a stable post-treatment phenotype. Recordings obtained within the first two to four weeks may show residual treatment effects rather than a stable endogenous trait. If the clinical question specifically concerns early treatment response, a recording at two to four weeks can be informative but should be labeled as a post-treatment state recording, not a trait baseline.

The recording context should document: date of psilocybin session, dose, setting (clinical trial, state-legal therapy center, retreat), number of sessions, concomitant psychotherapy, concurrent medications (especially SSRIs, which can attenuate psilocybin effects), sleep quality since the session, and any adverse psychological reactions. A client who underwent psilocybin therapy while on an SSRI may show attenuated theta changes; a client who had a difficult experience may present with insomnia and anxiety that dominate the recording.

34.12 Microdosing

Microdosing is common in referrals, but the QEEG evidence base is thin. Clients may microdose psilocybin or LSD while also using caffeine, cannabis, antidepressants, stimulants, or supplements. Products may be mislabeled, inconsistent, or placebo-influenced.

The report should not claim a microdosing EEG signature. It should document compound, schedule, dose if known, day-on/day-off cycle, last dose, subjective effects, sleep, mood, and co-use. If the client is on a repeating microdose cycle, the QEEG timing within that cycle should be stated.

Microdosing can also mask or mimic medication effects. A client may attribute mood or attention changes to microdosing while simultaneously changing caffeine, cannabis, sleep, or antidepressants.

34.13 Medication Interaction Context

Psychedelic and empathogen use can interact with prescribed medications. SSRIs/SNRIs may alter subjective psychedelic effects. Lithium has been associated clinically with elevated risk in some psychedelic contexts. MAOIs are relevant to ayahuasca. Stimulants, antipsychotics, benzodiazepines, and sleep medications may shape both the experience and the post-experience QEEG.

You do not manage these interactions from the QEEG chair alone. Document them in the report and point to medical or psychiatric consultation when safety is in question.

34.14 Recreational Ketamine

Recreational ketamine deserves its own paragraph because many clients distinguish it poorly from therapeutic ketamine. Recreational use may involve unknown dose, intranasal or other routes, repeated redosing, polysubstance use, dissociation, bladder symptoms, and variable abstinence. Therapeutic ketamine has monitoring and dosing structure. The QEEG interpretation should follow the actual context.

If a client reports frequent recreational ketamine, ask about frequency, last use, route, memory/cognition, urinary symptoms, dissociation, mood effects, and co-use. Do not transfer clinic ketamine timing assumptions directly.

34.15 Adverse Experiences

Some clients seek neurofeedback after a difficult psychedelic experience. They may report panic, derealization, depersonalization, insomnia, intrusive imagery, emotional flooding, mania-like symptoms, psychosis-like symptoms, or fear that their brain has changed permanently. The QEEG report should be careful and non-alarming.

The map may be useful, but it should not be used to validate catastrophic interpretations. If severe psychiatric symptoms are present, referral and coordination are essential.

34.16 Report Language Examples

Weak language: "Psilocybin changed the client's alpha phenotype."

Better language: "The QEEG was recorded during the post-psilocybin integration period with sleep disruption; alpha findings should be interpreted as post-acute state features until stability is documented."

Weak language: "Microdosing improves attention on QEEG."

Better language: "The client is microdosing on a repeating schedule, but direct resting-QEEG evidence for microdosing is limited; interpretation should document timing, sleep, mood, and co-exposures."

Weak language: "MDMA caused the beta finding."

Better language: "Fast activity is interpreted in the context of recent MDMA, sleep deprivation, autonomic activation, caffeine, and festival-related polysubstance exposure."

Weak language: "This is a psychedelic damage pattern."

Better language: "The recording reflects current physiology after a difficult experience; QEEG should be interpreted with psychiatric symptoms, sleep, and recovery context, not as proof of irreversible injury."

34.17 Training Implications

Neurofeedback can be part of care after psychedelic or empathogen use, but timing matters. If the client is acutely destabilized, sleep deprived, or psychiatrically unsafe, stabilization and clinical care come first. If the client is in a stable integration period, neurofeedback targets may focus on sleep, arousal regulation, grounding, and attention.

Protocol decisions should avoid overinterpreting recent psychedelic-state carryover. A post-retreat QEEG may change as sleep normalizes, cannabis resumes or stops, antidepressants stabilize, or emotional arousal settles.

Longitudinal tracking should document substance timing every time. A baseline before a retreat, a recording one week after, and a recording two months later are three different state questions.

34.18 Practical Confidence Levels

High-confidence interpretation is possible when the client is not acutely intoxicated, sleep is stable, no severe adverse symptoms are present, and the psychedelic/empathogen exposure is remote or explicitly documented.

Moderate confidence applies during stable integration with known timing and stable sleep/medications. Caveats remain appropriate.

Low confidence applies during acute use, next-day recovery, severe insomnia, adverse psychiatric symptoms, polysubstance recovery, unknown products, repeated microdosing with unclear dose, or recreational ketamine instability.

34.19 Documentation Standard

Minimum documentation includes substance, dose if known, route, date, setting, number of sessions / doses, acute adverse effects, lingering symptoms, sleep before and after, medications stopped or continued, and co-use with cannabis, alcohol, stimulants, benzodiazepines, or other substances.

For retreat or ceremony use, add travel, fasting, sleep deprivation, vomiting / purging, group context, and integration support. For MDMA / festival use, add heat, hydration, sleep loss, and pill / source uncertainty.

34.20 What Not to Claim

Do not turn acute psychedelic EEG into stable phenotype language. Do not invent microdosing signatures. Do not collapse recreational and therapeutic ketamine. Do not ignore retreat, ceremony, or festival context. Do not use QEEG to reassure or alarm clients about adverse experiences without broader clinical assessment. Do not use QEEG findings to recommend medication discontinuation, dose changes, or pharmacologic substitution. Those calls belong with the prescriber.

The stronger claim is conditional: psychedelics and empathogens can powerfully alter acute EEG and subjective state, while post-acute QEEG interpretation depends on timing, sleep, setting, medication interactions, adverse effects, and polysubstance context.

34.21 Scheduling the Recording

For routine phenotype work, avoid recording during acute use, the next-day recovery window, or severe integration distress. If the client recently returned from a retreat or festival, ask whether sleep and mood have returned to ordinary levels. If not, either reschedule or label the recording as a recovery-state map.

For clients using microdosing schedules, record the day in the cycle. A dose day, off day, and washout period are not interchangeable. If the product or dose is unknown, that uncertainty should appear in the report.

For clients seeking help after a difficult experience, the QEEG may be useful as part of a stabilization plan, but the interpretation should emphasize current state and clinical support rather than causal certainty about the substance experience.

34.22 Evidence summary

- **Spectral effect:** Acute psilocybin, DMT, ayahuasca, MDMA, and ketamine studies support strong state-dependent EEG/network effects; post-acute evidence is much thinner.
- **Phenotype inference:** Recent psychedelic/empathogen use can reduce confidence in alpha, broadband, complexity, connectivity, arousal, and mood-phenotype interpretations.
- **Workflow heuristic:** Document substance, timing, setting, sleep, adverse effects, integration state, microdosing, co-medications, and polysubstance use before assigning phenotype meaning.

Limitations and Future Directions

Why this class matters in NFB practice

This book is intentionally practical, but it should not be read as a finished map. Pharmaco-EEG has strong anchors in some areas and striking gaps in others. Kerson's practitioner text remains the essential class-level reference for drug effects on EEG (Kerson, 2023). IPEG guidelines show how carefully pharmaco-EEG should be recorded and evaluated when it is used as a pharmacodynamic measure (International Pharmaco-EEG Society, 2012). Yet ordinary neurofeedback practice is messier than most studies: polypharmacy, comorbidity, sleep problems, substances, chronic illness, developmental stage, aging, pipeline differences, and incomplete medication timing.

The limitation is not that QEEG is useless in medicated clients. The limitation is that unqualified phenotype interpretation is too easy. This book argues for a middle path: record as presenting when clinically appropriate, document exposure state, lower confidence when active factors overlap, and avoid medication-management claims outside scope.

Mechanism (clinician-level pharmacology)

The central mechanism of limitation is mismatch. Research studies often isolate one drug, one condition, one dose, one time window, and one pipeline. Clinical practice combines many drugs, conditions, states, and pipelines. Evidence becomes weaker each time interpretation moves away from the studied context.

Another limitation is metric mismatch. Traditional bands remain useful, but newer metrics such as aperiodic exponent and excitation-inhibition balance may help distinguish band-power change from background spectral shape. Donoghue and colleagues' FOOOF framework is important because it separates periodic oscillations from aperiodic spectral structure (Donoghue et al., 2020). Future pharmaco-QEEG will likely need both conventional bands and aperiodic metrics.

The third limitation is time. Acute dose, steady state, discontinuation, recovery, and long-term exposure are not the same. Many studies capture a single time point, then the discussion overgeneralizes.

Known spectral effects

The best-supported class effects are useful but incomplete. Benzodiazepines, stimulants, antipsychotics, anticonvulsants, opioids, caffeine, alcohol, cannabis, and anesthetics have recognizable patterns in at least some contexts. Those patterns do not automatically solve individual interpretation.

Several categories remain pure or near-pure gaps for human resting QEEG. This book has repeatedly flagged GLP-1 agonists, SGLT-2 inhibitors, PDE-5 inhibitors, beta-blockers in many contexts, low-dose naltrexone (Vivitrol), naltrexone for many routine psychiatric interpretations, pure CBD at wellness doses, and newer antipsychotics such as lurasidone (Latuda), lumateperone (Caplyta), brexpiprazole (Rexulti), pimavanserin (Nuplazid), and cariprazine (Vraylar). These should not receive invented signatures.

Reactivity, formulation, withdrawal, paradoxical response, comorbidity, and pipeline chapters are also gap-heavy. The correct response to a gap is explicit tiering, not silence or speculation disguised as fact.

Phenotype interaction effects

The largest open question is medication-aware phenotype validation. Research still needs studies that ask whether common QEEG phenotypes remain stable, change, or become misleading under medication exposure.

Stimulant studies should track resting and task phenotypes across dose timing, formulation, and adolescent-to-adult development. Antidepressant studies should separate sex, hormonal state, FAA, alpha, sleep, activation, and discontinuation. Antipsychotic studies should separate drug-naive illness, monotherapy, LAI cycle, and polypharmacy. Substance studies should separate acute use, withdrawal, persistent abstinence, and relapse risk.

We also need medication-aware normative databases or at least medication-tagged reference datasets, so a clinician can eventually

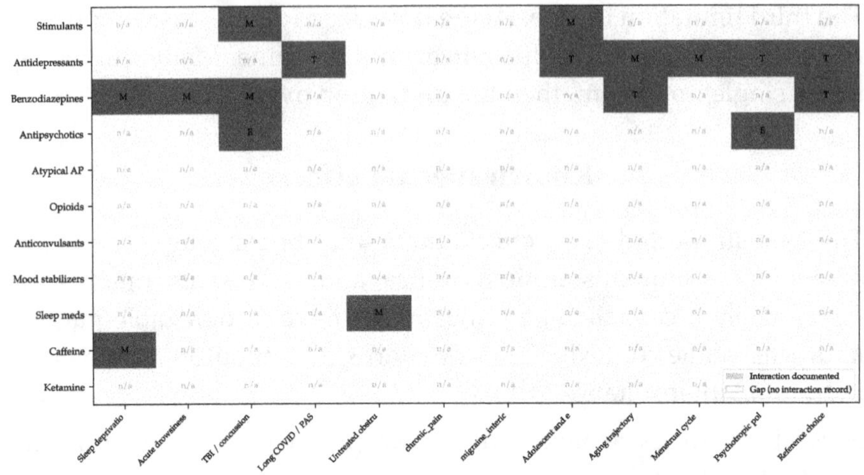

Figure BM.1: Evidence coverage: drug classes mapped against clinical confounders, showing where interaction records exist and where evidence gaps remain.

ask: how unusual is this EEG for age, sex, state, pipeline, and medication exposure?

What Should Not Be Built

Do not build overconfident medication detectors from routine QEEG. A classifier that says "benzodiazepine present" or "SSRI effect present" without timing, dose, state, comorbidity, and pipeline context would likely mislead clinicians.

Do not create washout dogma. Some research questions require controlled medication conditions. Many clinical questions are better answered by recording the client as they present. Medication changes for QEEG convenience are prescriber decisions and may be unsafe.

Do not turn every gap into a mechanism story. Mechanistic plausibility is useful for hypothesis generation, not proof.

What Should Be Built

First, an open medication-aware QEEG registry. It should store de-identified EEG metrics, raw-data availability when possible, medication inventory, dose timing, formulation, recording condition, sleep, caffeine, substances, comorbidities, and pipeline settings.

Second, prospective within-person studies. These should compare stable on-medication, off-medication when clinically appropriate, dose timing, formulation changes, and follow-up after prescriber-directed changes. The same raw data should be processed through locked pipelines.

Third, cross-pipeline benchmarks. The same raw data should be analyzed with different references, filters, ICA choices, and databases so clinicians can see how much medication signatures move.

Fourth, aperiodic and E/I-aware pharmaco-QEEG. FOOOF-style approaches (Donoghue et al., 2020) may help clarify whether a drug changes a true oscillation, the aperiodic background, or both.

Fifth, living evidence tables. A print book freezes at publication. A database can update as evidence changes.

Priority Study Designs

The first priority is within-person medication timing studies. A stimulant study should not compare medicated and unmedicated groups in isolation. It should record the same person at pre-dose, near expected peak, later in the day, and under task conditions, while documenting sleep and caffeine. Similar timing designs are needed for benzodiazepines, caffeine, cannabis, ketamine, sleep medications, and PRN drugs.

The second priority is formulation studies. Immediate-release, extended-release, patch, intranasal, sublingual, LAI, and compounded products should not be treated as interchangeable. QEEG studies should record dose timing and formulation explicitly, and should model concentration-time curves when possible.

The third priority is discontinuation and recovery studies. We still need time-course data for taper, acute withdrawal, subacute discontinuation, early abstinence, protracted recovery, and stable-off states. These studies should be careful not to confuse relapse, withdrawal, recovery, and trait vulnerability.

The fourth priority is comorbidity and polypharmacy. Studies should intentionally enroll the clients clinicians see in practice: ADHD plus anxiety, depression plus chronic pain, PTSD plus TBI, bipolar plus SUD history, and older adults with multiple medications. Excluding complexity creates clean papers and weak clinical generalization.

The fifth priority is paradoxical responders. A registry could identify people who reliably report opposite medication effects, then compare their QEEG and pharmacogenomic profiles with typical responders. This would turn a clinical nuisance into a researchable phenotype.

Publication and Update Process

The print book should be treated as version 1 of the framework. The live database should carry row-level update dates, claim type, source type, clinical portability, and whether the row is direct evidence, extrapolation, or gap.

Quarterly literature updates are enough for v1. Each quarter can focus on several classes: stimulants and caffeine; antidepressants and benzodiazepines; antipsychotics and mood stabilizers; substances and withdrawal; medical confounders and pipeline methods. Rows that change should receive an "Updated YYYY-MM" note.

A print revision should be triggered when enough rows change to alter clinical guidance, not every time a single paper appears. A practical threshold is when a major drug class, confounder category, or decision-framework table changes materially.

Reader submissions should be structured. A useful observation includes medication list, dose timing, formulation, indication, recording condition, sleep, caffeine / substance timing, pipeline, phenotype finding, and clinical outcome. An anecdote without those fields is a lead, not evidence.

Ethical Limits

The future of medication-aware QEEG should not drift into medication advice by non-prescribers. Better data can improve interpretation, but it does not change scope. A QEEG report can state that medication context reduces confidence, that findings may be compatible with sedative burden, or that prescriber review may be useful. It should not instruct the client to start, stop, or change medication.

We also need to protect clients from overclassification. A medication-aware database should not make a person feel reduced to a drug signature, genotype, diagnosis, or developmental variant. It should help clinicians avoid mistakes, not create new labels.

What Success Looks Like

Success, in this book's terms, is a clinician who sees elevated theta and asks about sleep, OSA, stimulant timing, antipsychotic exposure, pain, and recording state before calling it ADHD; a report that says "confidence reduced" when the evidence demands it; and a database row that says "no human resting QEEG evidence identified" instead of inventing a signature.

Success is also cumulative: each careful recording, if structured and ethically handled, can contribute to better evidence. The book provides the vocabulary. The database provides the update mechanism. Future studies provide the validation.

Case vignette

A clinician reads this book and looks up a client taking a newer antipsychotic, a GLP-1 agonist, caffeine, cannabis, and an SSRI. The database has no direct human resting-QEEG row for two of the drugs. The correct action is not to invent signatures. The report should say which parts are supported, which are extrapolated, and which are unknown.

Two years later, a new controlled study appears for one pure-gap agent. The database row is updated, the claim type changes, and the next print revision can incorporate it. This is the right relationship between book and database: the book teaches the framework; the database keeps the evidence current.

Interpretation traps

- **Filling gaps with confident prose.** If no human QEEG evidence exists, say so.
- **Treating class effects as individual causation.** A class pattern is not proof in one client.
- **Ignoring pipeline limits.** Cross-system comparisons require caution or raw reprocessing.
- **Overusing washout language.** Recording as presenting is often clinically appropriate.
- **Forgetting aperiodic structure.** Band-power changes may reflect background spectral shifts.

- **Letting the book become static.** A live update process is part of the project design.

Intake questions

When this chapter's topic appears on the intake form, ask:

- **Is the evidence for this drug or stack direct, extrapolated, or absent?** Use the claim type.
- **Is the finding conventional band power, aperiodic, source-localized, ERP, or connectivity?** Metrics differ in maturity.
- **Can the recording be compared to prior data?** Check pipeline, timing, state, and medication stability.
- **Does the database have an updated row?** The live resource may supersede the print snapshot.
- **Would a safer conclusion be "unknown"?** Unknown is sometimes the most accurate answer.

Clinical recommendations

Use claim types consistently. Do not inflate workflow heuristics into spectral-effect claims.

Maintain a living bibliography and database. Every new drug row should separate spectral effect, phenotype interpretation consequence, and clinical recommendation.

When a category is pure gap, write "no human resting QEEG evidence identified" rather than extrapolating a signature.

For future editions, prioritize updates in areas with the largest clinical burden: polypharmacy, adolescent/emerging adult pharmaco-EEG, aging, Long COVID/ME-CFS/fibromyalgia, OSA, withdrawal, and newer psychiatric medications. Invite readers to contribute structured observations, but do not treat anecdotes as evidence until aggregated and reviewed.

Evidence summary

- **Spectral effect:** Selected medication classes have well-supported EEG effects, but many modern agents, stacks, and states remain under-studied.

- **Phenotype inference:** Medication-aware phenotype validation, pipeline benchmarking, and aperiodic metrics are needed before strong individualized claims can be made.
- **Workflow heuristic:** Maintain a living database, label gaps honestly, update claim types over time, and treat the print book as a framework rather than a final catalog.

Unified Reference Membership

Purchase of a paperback, Kindle edition, or direct EPUB from any book in this clinical QEEG series qualifies the purchaser for one year of unified membership beginning when membership is activated. Membership includes Literature Chat and the searchable medication-EEG database, with ongoing evidence updates during active access.

Literature Chat helps readers find and summarize source-linked literature. Its answers are navigation aids, not evidence by themselves or case-specific clinical conclusions. Readers must open and verify the cited sources and check current labels, regulatory information, and professional guidance.

The database organizes the medication–EEG evidence in this book as research and regulatory information change. Its workflow is deliberately narrow:

1. The practitioner selects the drugs, brand/generic identity, formulations, routes, and other exposures documented for a recording. Each item retains a timestamped provenance status: client reported, label/photo verified, EHR or pharmacy verified, or unknown.
2. The database returns possible EEG associations reported in relevant sources. Each row identifies the studied population, dose or exposure state when available, recording method, claim type, source type and regulatory date when relevant, important limits or a direct-evidence gap, last review date, and citation.
3. Direct-evidence gaps remain visible. The database does not create a spectral direction for a drug or combination when the literature does not support one.
4. The practitioner may export an editable medication-evidence attachment containing the selected rows and a citation backlist. The practitioner supplies the observed EEG findings and decides whether each row belongs in the case report.

Neither membership tool determines which drug caused a person's finding, adds single-drug effects into a predicted polypharmacy signature, diagnoses a condition, infers a neurotransmitter deficit, predicts individual treatment response, or recommends a drug, dose, hold, taper, substitution, augmentation, or challenge.

Every exported attachment must retain per-item exposure provenance, claim type, source type, evidence limits or gaps, last review date, source citations, and the statement that medication-associated EEG changes are nonspecific. It should never replace raw-EEG review, recording-state documentation, medical evaluation, or professional judgment.

Current activation instructions, renewal terms, privacy terms, support details, service address, and operational update policy are supplied with the released membership. Access to these tools does not establish clinical validation or expand any reader's professional scope.

Online Book Index and Errata

The public reader-resources page at **brainondrugs.org** provides an alphabetical index of generic names, brand names, drug classes, formulations, and substances covered in this edition, with chapter and print-page locators. It also carries confirmed errata and edition updates. The index and errata do not require membership access.

Scan to activate one year of database access

or visit **brainondrugs.org**

Appendix A: Medication × Phenotype × Confounder: Quick Reference

This is a confidence-adjustment tool, not a diagnostic algorithm. Each entry names a medication or substance, the QEEG phenotype it can affect, and the confounder that compounds the interpretive problem. All entries are workflow heuristics (mechanistic reasoning; no controlled prediction trials). Interaction modes (masking, mimicry, exaggeration, transformation) are defined in Chapter 1. Confidence key: **Reduced** = one plausible overlapping factor; **Substantially reduced** = multiple converging factors.

Methylphenidate + adolescent maturation → TBR elevated (masking + mimicry, substantially reduced). TBR in ages 16–20 can reflect maturation rather than ADHD pathology; stimulant exposure may simultaneously mask maturation-related elevation. Document age and developmental context.

Methylphenidate + unknown last-dose timing → spectral pattern (masking, substantially reduced). IR, XR, patch, and delayed-release formulations create different recording windows. Undocumented timing makes any stimulant effect interpretation unreliable.

Methylphenidate + paradoxical response → sedation/arousal (transformation, substantially reduced). Stimulant-induced sedation is documented; do not assume stimulant exposure always increases arousal or reduces slow activity.

Benzodiazepines + sleep deprivation → beta excess (mimicry, reduced). Benzo-induced beta and sleep-loss slow-band confounds can occur simultaneously, pulling interpretation in opposite directions.

Benzodiazepines + acute drowsiness → frontal theta (mimicry, substantially reduced). Drowsiness mimics and amplifies apparent sedative effects on slow-band activity.

Benzodiazepines + withdrawal → hyperexcitability (exaggeration, substantially reduced). Benzodiazepine withdrawal carries medical seizure risk; the recording may reflect a medically significant state, not a stable phenotype.

Benzodiazepines + paradoxical response → activation/arousal (transformation, substantially reduced). Disinhibition or activation after benzodiazepine exposure invalidates ordinary sedative class-level expectations.

SSRIs + Long COVID/PASC → alpha disruption (transformation, substantially reduced). Long COVID alpha and theta findings can overlap with antidepressant-associated state changes; neither source can be isolated from a single recording.

SSRIs + menstrual cycle phase → iAPF shift (mimicry, reduced). Cycle-phase alpha-frequency variation can be mistaken for medication effects in women; document reproductive hormone context.

SSRIs + aging trajectory → alpha decline (mimicry, reduced). Late-life alpha changes can be mistaken for antidepressant effects unless age and cognitive status are documented.

SSRIs + discontinuation → state change (mimicry, substantially reduced). QEEG cannot separate SSRI / SNRI discontinuation syndrome from symptom relapse; document taper schedule and symptom state.

Antipsychotics + TBI/concussion history → frontal theta elevated (exaggeration, substantially reduced). Antipsychotic slowing and post-concussive frontal slowing are difficult to separate from a single resting QEEG.

Anticonvulsants + fibromyalgia → pain-network pattern (exaggeration, substantially reduced). Gabapentinoid / sedative burden and fibromyalgia pain-network abnormalities can compound; treated condition shapes the recording as much as the drug.

Z-drugs + untreated OSA → daytime slowing (mimicry, substantially reduced). Untreated OSA produces daytime slowing that can mimic residual sleep-aid effect; document OSA risk and sleep quality.

Topiramate + migraine state → interictal pattern (transformation, reduced). Migraine interictal state and topiramate exposure both alter the recording; document headache timing.

Opioids + chronic pain → arousal pattern (exaggeration, substantially reduced). Opioids, gabapentinoids, cannabis, and sleep disruption produce composite arousal states that cannot be attributed to any single factor.

Caffeine + sleep deprivation → low beta (masking, reduced). Caffeine can mask subjective sleepiness while sleep-loss physiology continues to suppress beta activity.

Lamotrigine + generic/brand switch → spectral shift (mimicry, reduced). Recent formulation switches should be documented; bioequivalence data are generally reassuring but timing changes matter.

This list covers the highest-frequency clinical encounters. Additional confounder overlays and citation keys are in the shared data files included with this book.

Appendix B: Medication-Aware QEEG Decision Aid

This is a clinical heuristic, not a validated algorithm. It makes confidence adjustment explicit when an active medication, substance, condition, recording state, or pipeline factor can plausibly produce the same direction of QEEG finding.

Ten-Step Decision Workflow

1. **Review raw EEG first.** Safety-relevant patterns, drowsiness, muscle artifact, movement, electrode noise, and paroxysmal activity take priority over phenotype labeling.

2. **Verify recording state.** Was the recording obtained in the client's ordinary prescribed and habitual functional state (Appendix C)? If any substance or medication timing was atypical, document the departure and note whether confidence is affected.

3. **Document recording state.** Eyes open or closed, task condition, vigilance, drowsiness, pain, anxiety, sleep loss, caffeine, nicotine, recent exertion, acute illness, time of day.

4. **Build the full medication and substance inventory.** Prescriptions, OTC agents, supplements, recreational substances, procedural sedation, outpatient ketamine, recent starts / stops, missed doses, formulation changes.

5. **Document timing.** Last dose, formulation, duration on medication, steady state vs. taper vs. withdrawal, drug holiday, LAI cycle position, unknown timing.

6. **Ask whether a known class effect points in the same direction as the finding.** Use class-level evidence as a starting point, not as proof. If a medication class is known to push the finding in the direction observed, the phenotype claim weakens even when the finding itself is real.

7. **Screen non-drug confounders.** Sleep deprivation, drowsiness, TBI, OSA, Long COVID, ME / CFS, fibromyalgia, migraine, chronic pain, pregnancy / postpartum / cycle / OCP, adolescence, aging, and pipeline factors can each produce the same direction of finding and must be considered before attribution.

8. **Consider the interaction mode.** Masking, mimicry, exaggeration, or transformation (see Chapter 1). One recording rarely shows which one operated, and more than one can be active at once, so indeterminate and multiple are both legitimate answers. Word it as possible, or as consistent with, rather than as measured.

9. **Assign confidence.** High confidence requires clean data, a stable state, no dominant overlapping medication / condition / pipeline alternative, and a finding consistent across relevant conditions. Moderate confidence allows some context but no dominant alternative explanation. Low confidence applies when active factors plausibly produce the same direction.

10. **Write the caveat and decide on next steps.** State the uncertainty directly in the report. Decide whether repeat recording after clinical stabilization would improve confidence.

Common Phenotype Confidence Adjustments

Frontal theta elevated. Antipsychotics, opioids, TCAs, high-dose mood stabilizers, untreated OSA, TBI, and Long COVID can all produce or amplify frontal slowing. Confidence is reduced to substantially reduced when any of these are active. Avoid treating frontal theta as a single-cause attention marker without ruling out these contributors.

TBR elevated. Antipsychotics, opioids, adolescent maturation, drowsiness, and sleep loss can all mimic or inflate TBR. Check age, sleep, medication timing, and recording state before treating elevated TBR as ADHD-specific.

Slow iAPF. Antipsychotics, TCAs, mood stabilizers, opioids, chronic cannabis, aging, and reproductive hormone state can all shift iAPF downward. Confirm age, reproductive context, vigilance, and medication timing; treat iAPF as one data point, not a fixed trait in isolation.

Global beta elevated. Benzodiazepines, stimulants, caffeine, withdrawal states, and muscle artifact can all produce or amplify fast-activity findings. Verify last-dose timing and artifact burden; document stimulant, caffeine, and benzodiazepine context.

Posterior alpha elevated. SSRIs / SNRIs, drowsiness, and eyes-closed state effects can all elevate posterior alpha. Cannabis stays on the list for a different reason: its alpha findings are regional and heterogeneous, the reported chronic effect is frontal rather than posterior, and no acute resting-alpha direction is established (Chapter 33). Document use and abstinence rather than assigning a direction. Compare EO / EC reactivity where available and qualify medication and state contributions.

Diffuse slowing. Antipsychotic plus opioid, high-dose anticonvulsant, sedative stacking, OSA, TBI, chronic pain, ME / CFS, and Long COVID can converge to produce diffuse slow activity. When multiple contributors are present, treat medication and condition burden as the primary explanation before assigning a phenotype.

Frontal alpha asymmetry. Depression state, SSRI response context, sex-dependent biomarker effects, and reference scheme all transform FAA interpretation. Document sex, hormone context, medication, and reference montage; avoid unqualified FAA biomarker claims.

SMR low at central sites. Drowsiness, sedative exposure, antipsychotic exposure, and filter or pipeline choices can all reduce apparent SMR power. Note medication and vigilance state before using SMR as a protocol rationale.

Confidence Levels

Higher confidence. No major active factor plausibly produces the same direction of finding, data quality is acceptable, and state and timing are documented. *Report language:* "Findings are interpreted with relatively higher confidence in the documented recording state."

Reduced confidence. A medication, substance, condition, or state could contribute to the same direction of finding. *Report language:* "Interpretive confidence is reduced because [factor] can contribute to [finding]."

Substantially reduced. Multiple active factors converge on the same finding, timing is uncertain, or the phenotype is highly confounded. *Report language:* "This finding should be interpreted as a composite state marker rather than a stable phenotype attribution."

Not interpretable for phenotype attribution. Safety issue, severe artifact, missing medication inventory, active withdrawal, acute intoxication, or unstable recording state dominates. *Report language:* "The recording is not suitable for confident phenotype attribution under the current conditions."

Report Caveat Templates

1. "The recording shows [finding]. Interpretive confidence is reduced because [medication / substance / state] can produce a similar direction of change."
2. "This QEEG should be read as a recording of the client's current treated state, not as an unmedicated baseline."
3. "Because medication timing was not available, phenotype attribution is limited and should be revisited if a repeat recording is obtained under documented conditions."
4. "The finding remains clinically relevant, but its source cannot be assigned to a stable trait without considering medication, sleep, pain, and recording-state context."
5. "Medication questions should be coordinated with the prescribing clinician; QEEG findings alone do not justify dose changes or discontinuation."

Five-Minute Triage Card

For the clinician with a stack of reports and five minutes. Five questions. Each a confidence gate.

Q1: Safety. Does the raw EEG show anything requiring medical review? (Epileptiform activity, severe symmetric slowing, unilateral asymmetry, paroxysmal event, severe drowsiness, encephalopathic pattern.) Ask the same question about the client in the room, not only about the trace. If yes on either: stop, document, and match the response to the urgency level below. Do not proceed to phenotype interpretation.

Emergency, same hour, activate emergency services. Ongoing altered awareness, failure to return to baseline after a seizure, suspected nonconvulsive status, acute encephalopathy or delirium, unresponsiveness, slow or shallow breathing, new focal deficit, or serious rash with fever or mucosal involvement. Stay with the client.

Urgent, same week, medical or neurology assessment with a formal clinical EEG. Possible interictal epileptiform discharges, persistent focal slowing, a new episodic spell pattern, or new unexplained diffuse slowing.

Routine, coordinate with the prescriber. Everything else, including poor data quality, artifact burden, and drowsiness that clears on arousal.

A resting QEEG cannot exclude epilepsy, nonconvulsive seizures, or toxic-metabolic encephalopathy. A record that looks acceptable is not neurologic clearance.

Q2: Confound dominance. Does the client have an active factor that plausibly produces the same direction as the primary finding? Use the shortlist: stimulant timing / benzodiazepine or Z-drug / antipsychotic or mood stabilizer / cannabis or alcohol / opioid / sleep deprivation / OSA or drowsiness / TBI or post-viral / pain medication / OTC antihistamine. If yes: assign the interaction mode (masking / mimicry / exaggeration / transformation) and lower confidence accordingly.

Q3: State stability. Was the recording obtained under a stable, representative state? (Usual medication timing, no acute illness, no hangover, no unusual caffeine loading, no withdrawal, adequate sleep.) If not: label the recording as a state-specific snapshot, not a trait baseline.

Q4: Forward confidence. Given Q1-Q3, what is the confidence level for the primary phenotype? High (no dominant confounds, stable state, clean data) / Moderate (one confound, documented) / Reduced (multiple confounds or unstable state) / Substantially Reduced / Not interpretable. Write this explicitly in the report.

Q5: Next action. Based on confidence: (a) High/Moderate confidence: proceed with full interpretation. (b) Reduced confidence: write a conditional report naming the limiting factors. (c) Substantially Reduced: schedule a follow-up recording after state stabilization. (d) Not interpretable: defer and refer. If the clinical question requires higher confidence than this recording permits, say so before writing the phenotype section.

The five-question pass takes three minutes on a familiar case and five on a complex one. It replaces the less disciplined habit of seeing a pattern and writing to it.

Appendix C: Pre-recording Intake Form Template

Complete before QEEG acquisition and review again on recording day.

Governing recording-state rule. Record the state relevant to the referral question, ordinarily the person's stable prescribed and habitual functional state. Do not change a prescribed medication schedule solely for QEEG. Any deliberately altered medication-state comparison must be patient-specific and initiated or explicitly designed by the treating prescriber. This applies to all prescribed medications, including psychostimulants. It also applies to habitual substance patterns: a daily caffeine user's caffeinated state, a dependent smoker's nicotine-maintained state, a nightly cannabis user's habitual pattern, and a routine drinker's ordinary pattern are all part of the person's functional baseline. Manufacturing withdrawal to obtain a "clean" recording substitutes one confound for a worse one. Prescribed medications are not subject to washout.

Alcohol carries the rule further than the others. Caffeine or cannabis withdrawal produces a worse recording. Alcohol withdrawal in a dependent drinker can produce seizures and delirium, so asking that client to abstain before a session is a medical decision and not the QEEG clinician's to make. Two separate limits sit alongside the rule and are not exceptions to it: do not record a client who is acutely intoxicated, and do not proceed when withdrawal is suspected. Both are reasons to defer the session and involve medical care, not reasons to impose a drinking schedule.

Substance and Medication Timing Reference

The intervals below are pharmacokinetic context for interpreting what a recording captured. They are not instructions to impose on the client. The default is to record the person's habitual functional state and document the timing.

Exposure	Timing context	Interpretation note
Caffeine (coffee, tea, energy drinks, decaf, chocolate)	~5 h half-life; residual effects extend further in slow metabolizers	A recording 2 hours after a large coffee sits near peak exposure and should be read as such. A recording 18+ hours after the last dose captures minimal residual. In habitual users, enforcing abstinence produces a withdrawal-state recording that may be more misleading than the caffeine itself
Psychostimulants (MPH, amphetamine, modafinil)	IR clinical effect ~4-6 h; XR ~10-12 h	A recording near stimulant peak answers a different question than one obtained before the morning dose. Document formulation and last-dose timing. Any off-medication comparison must be initiated by the prescriber
Cannabis (inhaled)	Acute pharmaco-EEG window ~3-4 h for most users	Document last use and frequency. Acute intoxication warrants deferral. In heavy daily users, habitual exposure is the functional state

Exposure	Timing context	Interpretation note
Cannabis (edibles)	11-OH-THC produces longer duration than inhaled	Document product, dose, and timing. Effects may persist into the next morning after high-dose evening use
Alcohol (routine drinkers)	Context-dependent	Heavy prior-night drinking fragments sleep and introduces hangover physiology. Document last drink and sleep quality
Alcohol (non-routine drinkers)	Context-dependent	Any intake within 24 hours may confound spectral interpretation through sleep disruption or residual pharmacology
Nicotine (light/occasional)	Acute effects resolve within hours	Light users are not dependent; same-day abstinence before the session does not create withdrawal and avoids acute arousal shift
Nicotine (habitual/dependent)	Acute effects resolve within hours, but withdrawal begins quickly	In dependent users, abstinence produces a withdrawal-state recording. Document the decision and label the recording state

Exposure	Timing context	Interpretation note
All daily psychotropics	Varies by compound and formulation	Document last dose and timing relative to the usual schedule. The recording captures the exposure state at that moment; label it as peak, trough, or routine accordingly
Recording time	AM preferred when feasible	Reduces circadian variability, but the person's ordinary state takes priority over clock-time preference

The governing rule above already covers habitual-use cases: the person's ordinary functional state is the default. A heavy daily caffeine user, a nightly cannabis user, and a nicotine-dependent smoker are each recorded in their habitual state unless a specific clinical question justifies departure. When the clinician does alter the recording state for a stated reason, that departure and its rationale should be documented and the report labeled accordingly.

Client and Recording Information

Client: ____________ **DOB:** ____________ **Date/Time:** ____________

Reason for QEEG: ______________________________

Medications

List all current prescriptions: psychiatric, neurologic, pain, sleep, hormone, cardiac, GI.

Medication (generic / brand)	Dose	Form	Schedule / PRN	Last dose (date / time)
________	________	________	________	________
________	________	________	________	________
________	________	________	________	________
________	________	________	________	________
________	________	________	________	________
________	________	________	________	________

Form means tablet, capsule, IR or XR, liquid, patch, sublingual, nasal, or injection. Two clients on "20 mg" of the same drug in different formulations are not in the same exposure state at 9 AM.

Medication continuation sheet. The chapters treat route, indication, duration, prescriber, and adherence as first-order metadata rather than background. The table above does not hold them. Copy the block below once for each medication listed.

Medication: ________________________________

Route: oral / sublingual / patch / injection / nasal / inhaled / other:

Indication, in the client's own words: ________________

Prescriber and practice: ________________________

Start date, or time at the current dose: ________________

Taken as prescribed over the last 7 days? yes / missed ____ doses / PRN, used ____ times

Last dose relative to the usual time: usual / earlier / later / skipped

Client-reported effects, wanted and unwanted: ____________

Recent changes (starts, stops, dose changes, tapers, generic switches, missed doses, last 30 days): ________________________

LAI, depot, patch, or infusion? ________________________

Consent to contact the prescriber about recording conditions or dose timing: yes / no

Preferred contact route: ________________________

OTC Medications and Supplements (last 7 days)

Include antihistamines, sleep aids, melatonin, herbals, nootropics, kratom.

Product	Dose	Last use

Substances (recording day / recent)

Caffeine today: none / coffee / tea / energy drink / other: Amount and time: ______

Nicotine last 24 h: none / cigarette / vape / pouch / other: Amount and time: ______

Alcohol last 7 days: none / yes: Last use and amount: ______

Cannabis/THC/CBD last 14 days: none / yes: Product, route, amount, last use: ______

Other substances last 30 days: none / yes: Substance, route, last use:

Procedures

Surgery, anesthesia, sedation, concussion eval, or hospitalization last 90 days? ______

Outpatient ketamine/esketamine? Date of last session: ______

Today's State

Morning dose taken: before recording / after recording / N/A

Recording reflects habitual substance state: yes / no – If not, specify departure and reason: ______

Sleep last night: __ h Quality: poor / fair / good **Night before:** __ h

OSA / CPAP: no / yes / suspected CPAP used last night: yes / no / N/A

Current ratings (0–10): Pain ___ Fatigue ___ Anxiety ___ Alertness ___

Acute illness, migraine, withdrawal, or unusual stress today? ______

Hormonal Context (where relevant)

Cycle status: N/A / regular / irregular / perimenopause / menopause / postpartum

LMP: __________ **Pregnant/possibly pregnant:** no / yes / unsure

Hormonal contraception, HRT, fertility meds, or testosterone/estrogen/progesterone: ______________

Medical History

Concussion, TBI, seizure, syncope, migraine, stroke, or neurologic condition: ______________

Chronic conditions: OSA / Long COVID / ME/CFS / fibromyalgia / chronic pain / thyroid / other: ______________

Symptom ratings (0–10): Attention ___ Mood ___ Anxiety ___ Sleep ___ Brain fog ___ Irritability ___

Clinician Review

Medication/substance factors affecting interpretation: ______

Recording-state factors affecting interpretation: ______

Confidence adjustment: none / mild / moderate / substantial / not interpretable

This intake should be stored with the QEEG record. A missing medication inventory is not a neutral omission: it limits interpretive confidence.

Intake-Questions Master Sheet

Quick-reference cross-tab: by medication class, pull the questions most likely to change interpretation. Use before acquisition, not after.

Stimulants (Ch. 5)

- What exact medication and formulation? (MPH vs amphetamine; IR vs ER/XR)
- When was last dose: is that typical?
- Caffeine, nicotine, cannabis, or sleep aids in last 24 h?
- How stable is the current regimen? (new start / dose change / holiday)
- For adolescents: sleep schedule past 3 nights?

SSRIs / SNRIs (Ch. 6)

- Which antidepressant, dose, and duration?
- Recent dose change, taper, or missed doses?
- Side effects active now: activation, sedation, insomnia, emotional blunting?
- Sleep context: insomnia, hypersomnia, sleep-apnea risk?
- Reproductive-hormone context (female clients): cycle phase, OCP, pregnancy, perimenopause?

TCAs / MAOIs / Atypical Antidepressants (Ch. 7)

- Indication: depression, sleep, pain, migraine, or smoking cessation?
- Sedating, activating, or both: describe current side effects.
- Full anticholinergic burden (include OTC antihistamines, bladder meds)?
- Seizure history, eating-disorder history, or high-dose bupropion?
- Recent starts, switches, or sleep-medication substitutions?

Benzodiazepines (Ch. 8)

- Which benzo, dose, formulation, last dose: usual or unusual timing?
- Duration: acute / intermittent / chronic / tapering / recently stopped?
- Withdrawal symptoms, interdose symptoms, missed doses, or dose reductions?

- Alcohol, opioids, cannabis, antihistamines, OSA risk?
- Paradoxical reactions: agitation, disinhibition, worsened anxiety?

Typical Antipsychotics (Ch. 9) / Atypical Antipsychotics (Ch. 10)

- Which compound, dose, route (oral / IM / LAI), last dose?
- For LAI: last injection date and usual interval?
- EPS, akathisia, tremor, rigidity, sedation, cognitive fog?
- Anticholinergic burden; full adjunct list (benzodiazepines, mood stabilizers, sleep meds)?
- Current clinical state: stable / recent hospitalization / acute episode?

Anticonvulsants / Mood Stabilizers (Ch. 11)

- Indication: epilepsy / bipolar / migraine / pain / fibromyalgia / augmentation?
- Dose change, missed doses, or recent taper?
- Seizure history, aura, syncope, or paroxysmal events?
- Sedation, cognitive slowing, tremor, word-finding difficulty?
- Pregnancy/postpartum (especially lamotrigine): dosing changes or serum monitoring?

Anesthetics (Ch. 12)

- Procedure and date: how many days since anesthesia?
- Anesthesia type if known: propofol / volatile / dexmedetomidine / ketamine / midazolam?
- Complications: delirium, prolonged confusion, ICU stay, hypoxia?
- Post-op medications: opioids, benzodiazepines, antiemetics, steroids?
- Current sleep, pain, and cognition status?

Ketamine / Esketamine (Ch. 13)

- Route and protocol: IV / IM / intranasal / compounded / recreational?
- Last session date, time, and induction vs. maintenance phase?
- Dissociation, blood pressure, sleep, and next-day function after last session?
- Co-medications: benzodiazepines, antidepressants, cannabis, alcohol?

- QEEG goal: baseline / treatment-state monitoring / neurofeedback planning?

Opioids (Ch. 14)

- Which opioid or antagonist, dose, route, and indication?
- Last dose: stable or unusual timing?
- Withdrawal symptoms, intoxication, craving, relapse, recent overdose/naloxone?
- Co-medications: benzodiazepines, alcohol, cannabis, gabapentinoids, sleep meds?
- Pain, sleep, breathing, and daytime alertness today?

Z-Drugs / Sleep Meds (Ch. 15)

- What sleep medication was taken last night and when?
- Hours slept and current level of rest?
- Skipped, tapered, or changed a usual sleep medication?
- OSA screening: snoring, witnessed apneas, CPAP, morning headache, excessive daytime sleepiness?
- Next-day grogginess, memory gaps, or complex sleep behaviors?

OTC / Non-Psychotropic (Ch. 16)

- Any allergy, sleep, cold, pain, or PM medications in last 48 h (especially diphenhydramine, hydroxyzine, pseudoephedrine)?
- Paradoxical reactions to antihistamines?
- Chronic non-psychotropic prescriptions: statins, PPIs, beta-blockers, steroids?
- Current infection, fever, hypoglycemia, or medication toxicity concern?
- OTC combination products: ask for photos or labels?

Nutraceuticals / Herbals (Ch. 17)

- What supplements, blends, powders, teas, or nootropics?
- Dose and timing: especially caffeine-theanine, melatonin, kava, valerian, magnesium, kratom, phenibut?
- Withdrawal or dependence concerns: kratom, phenibut, tianeptine, sedative herbals?
- Indication: sleep / anxiety / cognition / stimulant substitute?
- Prescription interactions: SSRIs, opioids, anticoagulants?

For full context, refer to the Intake questions section of each Part II chapter. The questions above are extraction shortcuts for clinical intake, not substitutes for the chapter-level confidence adjustments.

Appendix D: Glossary

QEEG Terms

Absolute power: The amount of EEG power in a frequency band, usually expressed in microvolts squared or log-transformed values. Absolute power can be altered by medication, drowsiness, artifact, reference choice, and age.

Relative power: The proportion of total EEG power represented by a frequency band. Relative power can rise because that band increased, because other bands decreased, or both. Interpret relative power with absolute power.

Z-score: A standardized score showing how far a client's value deviates from a normative database mean for age and recording condition. It depends on the database, reference, montage, artifact procedure, and feature definition used to compute it.

Individual alpha peak frequency (iAPF): The dominant frequency within the alpha range for an individual, often measured during eyes-closed rest. iAPF can vary with age, vigilance, medication state, menstrual cycle factors, and neurodevelopmental or neurologic context.

Theta/beta ratio (TBR): A ratio comparing theta power to beta power, commonly discussed in ADHD assessment. TBR is not specific to ADHD and can be affected by sleepiness, age, medication, stimulant timing, anxiety, artifact, and analytic pipeline.

Coherence: A measure of the degree to which activity at two scalp sites shows stable phase or amplitude relationship at a given frequency. Coherence can be influenced by volume conduction, reference choice, montage, age, artifact, and medication effects on arousal.

Asymmetry: A left-right difference in EEG power or another feature. Frontal alpha asymmetry is often discussed in mood research, but its clinical meaning varies by method, state, reference, and medication context.

Aperiodic exponent: A measure of the slope of the broadband EEG power spectrum, separate from oscillatory peaks. Related to excitation-inhibition balance, arousal, aging, and medication effects.

Currently best treated as an exploratory measure alongside oscillatory features in individual QEEG interpretation.

Oscillatory activity: Rhythmic EEG activity concentrated around a frequency band, such as alpha or beta. Oscillatory findings should be distinguished from broad spectral slope changes when possible.

Source localization: A computational estimate of where scalp-recorded activity may originate in the brain. LORETA and related methods depend on model assumptions, electrode density, artifact handling, and the same medication and state factors that affect scalp EEG.

Normative database: A reference dataset used to compare an individual's EEG to expected values for age and condition. Database mismatch can produce apparent abnormalities that reflect method differences rather than physiology.

Reference: The electrode or mathematical reference against which EEG channels are measured. Linked ears, average reference, mastoids, Laplacian, and other choices can change topography and connectivity estimates.

Artifact: Non-brain signal contaminating the EEG, including eye movement, muscle tension, cardiac activity, electrode noise, movement, sweat, and environmental interference. Some medication effects, such as activation, sedation, tremor, or akathisia, can increase artifact risk.

Montage: The arrangement used to display or compute EEG channels. Different montages can make the same underlying activity appear more focal, diffuse, symmetric, or asymmetric.

Band edge: The frequency boundary used to define a band such as theta, alpha, or beta. Small band-edge differences can change power estimates, especially near iAPF or medication-related slowing.

Pharmaco-EEG Terms

Pharmaco-EEG: The study of medication and substance effects on EEG. In clinical QEEG, pharmaco-EEG evidence helps adjust interpretation confidence but does not prove medication causation in an individual client.

Bispectral index (BIS): A processed EEG index used mainly in anesthesia monitoring to estimate depth of anesthesia or sedation. BIS is not a routine outpatient QEEG measure, but anesthesia literature is useful for understanding strong drug effects on cortical rhythms.

Burst suppression: A pattern of alternating high-amplitude bursts and low-amplitude suppressed periods, typically associated with deep anesthesia, severe encephalopathy, hypothermia, or other major brain-state changes. It is a safety-relevant raw EEG pattern, not a routine phenotype label.

Paroxysmal abnormality: A sudden, transient EEG event such as spike, sharp wave, spike-wave discharge, or other epileptiform-appearing pattern. Paroxysmal findings require clinical caution and appropriate referral rather than routine neurofeedback interpretation.

Vigilance: The brain's wakefulness or arousal state during recording. Drowsiness can increase theta and slow activity, change alpha, reduce task engagement, and mimic medication or phenotype effects.

Reactivity: A change in EEG with condition or task, such as eyes opening, eyes closing, hyperventilation, photic stimulation, or cognitive load. Medication effects may be more visible in one state than another.

Alpha blocking: Reduction of alpha activity when the eyes open or attention shifts. Reduced, exaggerated, or inconsistent alpha blocking may reflect state, medication, attention, fatigue, or neurologic factors.

Photic driving: EEG entrainment or response to rhythmic visual stimulation. It can be affected by medication, vigilance, migraine tendency, seizure risk, and recording method.

Hyperventilation response: EEG change during or after hyperventilation, often involving slowing. Response varies by age, physiology, anxiety, medications, and clinical context.

Event-related potential (ERP): A time-locked EEG response to a stimulus or task event. ERP findings can show drug effects on attention, processing speed, or inhibition that may not appear in resting QEEG.

Clinical Pharmacology Terms

Half-life: The time required for blood concentration of a drug to decrease by half. Half-life helps estimate exposure duration but does not fully describe clinical effect, active metabolites, brain exposure, or withdrawal risk.

Steady state: A condition in which drug input and elimination are approximately balanced after repeated dosing. Many medications require several half-lives to approach steady state.

Peak concentration: The approximate time when drug concentration is highest after a dose. EEG recorded near peak concentration may differ from EEG recorded at trough.

Trough: The low point in drug concentration before the next dose. Long-acting formulations and depot preparations may still have substantial drug exposure at trough.

CYP polymorphism: Genetic variation in cytochrome P450 enzymes that can alter drug metabolism. CYP2D6 and CYP2C19 variation can change exposure to many psychiatric medications and may contribute to unusually strong, weak, delayed, or paradoxical responses.

Anticholinergic load: The cumulative burden of medications with anticholinergic effects. Higher load can affect cognition, sedation, delirium risk, and EEG interpretation, especially in older adults.

IR/XR: Immediate-release and extended-release formulations. IR products tend to produce faster peaks and shorter exposure windows, while XR products produce more prolonged exposure. Timing must be recorded.

LAI (long-acting injectable) / Depot: A formulation that releases medication slowly over time, typically by injection. Commonly used for some antipsychotics. EEG interpretation should consider position in the injection cycle.

Drug holiday: Planned or informal interruption of medication, often discussed with stimulants. Drug holidays can alter symptoms, sleep, withdrawal state, and QEEG interpretation.

Active metabolite: A drug breakdown product that has its own biologic effect. Active metabolites can prolong EEG-relevant exposure beyond the parent compound's apparent half-life.

Withdrawal: Physiologic or psychological symptoms after reduction or discontinuation of a substance or medication. Withdrawal can create EEG findings that are not equivalent to an unmedicated baseline.

Discontinuation syndrome: Symptoms after stopping or reducing certain medications, especially some antidepressants. EEG usually cannot distinguish discontinuation from relapse without clinical context.

Tolerance: Reduced response after repeated exposure. Tolerance can change the relationship between dose and EEG effect.

Sensitization: Increased response after repeated exposure or repeated withdrawal episodes. Sensitization is relevant to substances, stimulants, alcohol, and some stress-related presentations.

Confounder Terms

Confounder: A factor that can alter QEEG findings or their interpretation independent of the target phenotype. Confounders include medications, substances, sleep, pain, medical conditions, age, hormone state, and pipeline choices.

POCD: Postoperative cognitive dysfunction, a cognitive decline described after surgery and anesthesia, especially in older or medically vulnerable adults. Recent anesthesia should be documented before QEEG interpretation.

POD: Postoperative delirium, an acute fluctuating disturbance of attention and awareness after surgery or medical illness. POD is a clinical safety issue, not a routine phenotype.

Kindling: A process in which repeated withdrawals or neurologic excitations may increase future vulnerability, commonly discussed in alcohol withdrawal and seizure-risk contexts.

Medication mimicry: A medication or substance effect that resembles a clinical phenotype, such as drug-related slowing resembling underarousal.

Masking: A medication effect that hides or reduces visibility of an underlying phenotype.

Exaggeration: A medication or confounder effect that amplifies an existing pattern.

Transformation: A case in which medication, state, comorbidity, or pipeline context changes the apparent meaning of a finding rather than increasing or decreasing it.

Developmental variant: A respectful term for neurodevelopmental differences or populations when the point is variation in development or neurobiology, not pathology framing.

Pipeline confound: A measurement or analysis choice that changes the observed QEEG result, including reference, filters, artifact rejection, segment selection, database, and feature extraction.

Clinical portability: The degree to which a finding from one study, device, montage, database, or pipeline can be applied to another. Medication signatures often have limited portability unless methods are comparable.

Confidence adjustment: A structured change in interpretive confidence based on medication, substance, state, condition, or pipeline context. Confidence adjustment does not erase the finding; it changes how strongly the finding can be attributed to a stable phenotype.

Recording state: The client's physiologic and behavioral condition during acquisition, including eyes open or closed, alertness, sleep pressure, pain, medication timing, caffeine timing, withdrawal state, and task demands.

Trait-state distinction: The difference between relatively stable physiology and temporary state-dependent physiology. Medication-aware QEEG interpretation depends on not mistaking a temporary state for a durable trait.

Appendix E: Pharmacogenetics and Individual Differences

Medication-aware QEEG interpretation has to account for a basic fact: the same dose does not mean the same brain exposure in every client. Two clients can take the same medication at the same nominal dose and still differ in blood levels, receptor occupancy, side-effect burden, withdrawal vulnerability, and EEG expression. Some of that difference is explained by age, sex, body composition, liver function, renal function, smoking status, drug interactions, adherence, formulation, and timing. Some is explained by pharmacogenetics.

For the QEEG clinician, pharmacogenetics is not a diagnostic shortcut. A QEEG map cannot determine CYP2D6 status, CYP2C19 status, or any other genotype. The practical use is narrower: when a medication effect looks unusually strong, unusually weak, delayed, inconsistent with dose, or paradoxical, individual metabolism becomes part of the confidence adjustment.

CYP450 Metabolism

The cytochrome P450 system is one of the main pathways by which the body metabolizes many psychiatric and neurologic medications. The most clinically relevant enzymes for this book are CYP2D6, CYP2C19, CYP1A2, CYP3A4, and CYP3A5. Their activity varies across people due to genetic polymorphisms, medication interactions, smoking status, hepatic function, age, and other physiologic factors.

Pharmacogenetic reports often classify metabolism into categories such as poor metabolizer, intermediate metabolizer, normal or extensive metabolizer, rapid metabolizer, and ultrarapid metabolizer. The exact terminology varies by testing vendor and guideline, but the clinical logic is similar. A poor metabolizer may have higher exposure at a standard dose for medications dependent on that pathway. An ultrarapid metabolizer may have lower exposure or shorter effective duration.

For QEEG interpretation, the chain of reasoning is indirect:

1. Genotype and interacting factors can alter metabolism.
2. Metabolism can alter plasma level and active exposure.
3. Exposure can alter receptor occupancy and circuit effects.
4. Circuit effects can alter EEG state, spectral power, vigilance, reactivity, or artifact risk.

That chain is plausible and clinically useful, but there is little literature linking CYP phenotype directly to pharmaco-EEG outcomes. Most clinical use remains a workflow heuristic: a mechanistic confidence modifier, not a proven individual QEEG biomarker. The same logic applies to all CYP pathways discussed below: a QEEG map cannot determine genotype, and the clinician should not interpret metabolic pathways as prescribing advice. The correct move is documentation and, when relevant, communication with the prescriber.

CYP2D6

CYP2D6 is relevant for many antidepressants, stimulants and stimulant-like agents, antipsychotics, beta-blockers, opioids, and other medications. Fluoxetine and paroxetine can inhibit CYP2D6, which may increase exposure to other CYP2D6 substrates. A client whose medication list appears moderate on paper may be functionally more exposed if one medication inhibits the metabolism of another.

In QEEG terms, this matters when the map looks more medication-shaped than the nominal dose suggests. A low or moderate dose could still be associated with marked slowing, beta change, sedation, activation, tremor, or cognitive dulling if exposure is higher than expected. Weak or absent EEG change is still compatible with a real medication effect; low exposure or rapid metabolism can be one explanation.

Examples include a client taking an SSRI that inhibits CYP2D6 while also taking another psychotropic metabolized by the same pathway, or a client on codeine or tramadol whose opioid response depends partly on CYP2D6 conversion.

CYP2C19

CYP2C19 is especially relevant to several SSRIs and other psychotropics. CPIC guidelines for CYP2D6 and CYP2C19 have made genotype-informed dosing more visible in psychiatry, including for selective serotonin reuptake inhibitors. From a QEEG perspective, CYP2C19 variation can help explain why two clients on the same SSRI dose may show different levels of drowsiness, activation, sleep disruption, frontal asymmetry change, or cognitive side effects.

If a client reports unusual sensitivity, poor tolerability, or repeated unexpected responses, pharmacogenetic variability belongs in the clinical differential.

CYP1A2, Smoking, and Caffeine

CYP1A2 is relevant to caffeine and some antipsychotics, including clozapine and olanzapine. Smoking can induce CYP1A2 activity. Stopping smoking can reduce induction and raise exposure to medications metabolized by CYP1A2. Heavy caffeine use, caffeine withdrawal, nicotine exposure, and antipsychotic dosing can therefore interact in ways that matter for QEEG interpretation.

This is one reason caffeine and nicotine questions belong on the intake form. They are not lifestyle trivia. They can change arousal, vigilance, sleep, medication exposure, and the interpretation of beta, alpha, and slowing findings.

CYP3A4 and CYP3A5

CYP3A pathways metabolize many medications and are vulnerable to drug-drug interactions. Some antibiotics, antifungals, anticonvulsants, HIV medications, grapefruit products, and other agents can inhibit or induce CYP3A activity. In a polypharmacy case, CYP3A interactions may contribute to unexpected sedation, activation, altered sleep, or increased side-effect burden.

A map recorded during a complex interaction state should not be interpreted as a clean trait baseline.

Phase II Metabolism: UGT1A4 and Lamotrigine

CYP enzymes handle Phase I oxidative metabolism, but some medications bypass or supplement that with Phase II conjugation pathways. The most clinically relevant Phase II enzyme for this book is UGT1A4 (UDP-glucuronosyltransferase 1A4), which is the primary metabolic pathway for lamotrigine.

UGT1A4 activity varies with genetic polymorphism, hormonal state, drug interactions, and pregnancy. Lamotrigine clearance can increase by two- to threefold during pregnancy due to estrogen-mediated UGT1A4 induction, producing a dramatic drop in plasma levels even when the dose is unchanged. Postpartum, clearance falls rapidly as estrogen drops, potentially leading to lamotrigine toxicity if the pregnancy-adjusted dose is not reduced promptly. These pharmacokinetic shifts are well documented and have direct implications for any QEEG recorded during pregnancy or the postpartum period: the same lamotrigine dose can produce different brain exposure at different reproductive stages.

Valproate inhibits lamotrigine glucuronidation, roughly doubling lamotrigine levels. Hormonal contraceptives containing ethinyl estradiol can also induce UGT1A4, lowering lamotrigine exposure. Pill-free weeks can then raise levels transiently. These interactions are prescriber-managed, but the QEEG clinician should document oral contraceptive use, pregnancy status, and valproate co-prescription when interpreting a lamotrigine-treated recording.

The same exposure-to-EEG logic from the CYP framework applies. A lamotrigine-treated client whose recording looks surprisingly medication-shaped (or surprisingly clean) may be reflecting a Phase II metabolism shift rather than dose effect alone. Document reproductive state, valproate co-prescription, and hormonal contraceptive use in the intake.

HLA Pharmacogenomic Markers

CYP enzymes govern how much drug reaches the brain. HLA markers govern whether certain drugs trigger rare but life-threatening immune reactions. For two anticonvulsants in this book: carbamazepine and oxcarbazepine: HLA genotyping is a recognized safety standard backed by an FDA boxed warning and CPIC Level A recommendations.

HLA-B*15:02 and Stevens-Johnson Syndrome / Toxic Epidermal Necrolysis. Carriage of HLA-B*15:02 confers a roughly 50- to 100-fold or greater increased risk of carbamazepine-induced SJS/TEN, with near-perfect negative predictive value in Han Chinese cohorts. The allele is most prevalent in Southeast and East Asian populations (Han Chinese 5–15%, Thai 8–27%, Malay 12–15%) and rare in Japanese, Korean, South Asian, and European ancestry groups (<2%). The FDA added a boxed warning to the carbamazepine label in 2007, requiring

HLA-B*15:02 screening for patients of at-risk ancestry before initiating therapy. CPIC's 2017 guideline extends the same recommendation to oxcarbazepine and classifies the evidence as Level A (strong). Patients testing positive should not start carbamazepine or oxcarbazepine unless the benefit outweighs the risk.

HLA-A*31:01 and Drug Reaction with Eosinophilia and Systemic Symptoms (DRESS). HLA-A*31:01 predisposes to a broader spectrum of carbamazepine hypersensitivity including maculopapular exanthema, DRESS, and SJS/TEN in European, Japanese, Korean, and some North African populations. Allele frequency is roughly 2–4% in Europeans, 7–12% in Japanese, and 5–6% in Koreans. The FDA label now mentions HLA-A*31:01 as a risk factor, and CPIC recommends testing with a moderate (Level B) recommendation: avoid carbamazepine in carriers when alternatives are available.

Other anticonvulsant–HLA associations. Phenytoin and lamotrigine also carry associations with HLA-B*15:02 and SJS/TEN, but the effect sizes are smaller than for carbamazepine and no boxed warning currently applies. HLA-A*24:02 has been reported as a risk factor for lamotrigine-induced cutaneous adverse reactions in some Asian cohorts, but evidence is heterogeneous and no consensus guideline recommends routine HLA screening before lamotrigine initiation.

Medication	HLA marker	Reaction	Strength	Regulatory status
Carbamazepine, oxcarbazepine	HLA-B*15:02	SJS/TEN	CPIC Level A	FDA boxed warning
Carbamazepine	HLA-A*31:01	DRESS, MPE, SJS/TEN	CPIC Level B	FDA label mention
Phenytoin	HLA-B*15:02	SJS/TEN	Moderate association	No boxed warning
Lamotrigine	HLA-B*15:02, HLA-A*24:02	SJS/TEN, rash	Weaker/heterogeneous	No guideline

Why this matters for QEEG clinicians. The neurofeedback practitioner does not prescribe, but may see clients on carbamazepine who were started without HLA testing, especially outside East and Southeast Asia or before 2007 guideline uptake. If a client develops rash, fever, mucosal lesions, or encephalopathic symptoms in the first two to three months of carbamazepine and the QEEG shows new diffuse slowing, treat this as a red flag and advise urgent medical evaluation. SJS/TEN and DRESS are medical emergencies. If carbamazepine must be discontinued abruptly because of a serious dermatologic reaction, seizure threshold may fall acutely, with implications for subsequent QEEG recordings and neurofeedback safety.

Age Effects

Age changes both baseline EEG and medication response. Children, adolescents, adults, and older adults do not share a single expected EEG background. Developmental maturation affects alpha frequency, theta power, beta expression, sleep pressure, and attention-state stability. Adult aging can slow iAPF, change alpha magnitude, alter aperiodic slope, increase vulnerability to drowsiness, and change cognitive reserve.

Age also changes pharmacology. Older adults often have reduced clearance, higher anticholinergic burden, more polypharmacy, greater sensitivity to benzodiazepines, Z-drugs, antipsychotics, opioids, and sedating antihistamines, and higher delirium risk. The absence of strong age-specific pharmaco-EEG studies is itself a clinical warning. A spectral effect demonstrated in a young adult sample should not be assumed to have the same magnitude or meaning in a 75-year-old with polypharmacy and cognitive complaints.

Pediatric and adolescent cases raise the opposite problem. Much of the stimulant EEG literature comes from children with ADHD, but adult clients on long-term stimulant therapy are not scaled-up pediatric subjects. Puberty, cortical maturation, chronic exposure, sleep schedules, caffeine, cannabis, vaping, anxiety, and adherence patterns all change interpretation. For adolescents and emerging adults, medication-aware QEEG should be development-aware QEEG.

Sex, Hormones, and Reproductive State

Sex differences in pharmaco-EEG remain under-studied, and many foundational samples are male-skewed or do not report sex-stratified results. Some evidence suggests sex-specific medication effects or predictors, including findings around SSRI response and frontal alpha asymmetry, benzodiazepine and sleep-medication response, stimulant dopamine effects, and antipsychotic outcomes. These findings should be treated cautiously but not ignored.

Hormonal state can also matter. Menstrual cycle phase, hormonal contraception, pregnancy, postpartum status, perimenopause, menopause, and polycystic ovary syndrome can influence sleep, arousal, mood, migraine, medication exposure, and EEG features such as iAPF or alpha expression. Chapter 29 covers these factors in more detail. The practical rule: if the factor may change physiology or medication handling, document it.

Pharmacogenetic Testing

Commercial pharmacogenetic testing is now common, and some results are clinically useful for medication selection or dosing discussions. The QEEG clinician should treat these reports as medical information, not as independent authority for changing treatment. Results may be incomplete, vendor categories may differ, and genotype does not determine response by itself.

When a client has a pharmacogenetic report, the most useful QEEG workflow is to record the relevant metabolizer information, note interacting medications, and use the information to refine interpretation confidence. A poor-metabolizer result may help explain a strong medication-shaped EEG effect. An ultrarapid-metabolizer result may help explain weak effect or short duration. Either way, the finding belongs in communication with the prescriber if it affects clinical interpretation.

Interaction Review

Pharmacogenetics should be read together with the medication list, not separately from it. A normal metabolizer can function like a poor metabolizer if a strong inhibitor is present. A smoker may metabolize some CYP1A2 substrates differently than a nonsmoker, and that exposure can shift again after smoking cessation. A client taking multiple serotonergic, sedating, anticholinergic, stimulant, or anticonvulsant agents may show an EEG pattern that reflects cumulative exposure rather than a single compound.

For that reason, the intake form should capture start dates, dose changes, last-dose timing, missed doses, recent additions, discontinued medications, over-the-counter agents, supplements, caffeine, nicotine, cannabis, and alcohol. The QEEG report does not need to become a pharmacology consult, but it should not hide the fact that drug handling may be unstable.

Repeat Recordings

When medication exposure, genotype information, or interaction status is clinically important, repeat recordings can be more informative than a single map. A follow-up QEEG after medication stabilization, sleep improvement, withdrawal resolution, or substance-use change can help separate stable features from state-dependent features. This approach is most useful when the acquisition method, recording condition, artifact procedure, and analytic pipeline are kept consistent.

Repeat recording does not prove causation, but it can improve confidence. If a pattern resolves after stabilization of sleep and medication timing, state attribution becomes more plausible. If the pattern persists across different medication states, trait interpretation becomes more plausible.

Practical Interpretation Rule

Pharmacogenetics should be invoked when it changes the confidence of the report, not to decorate a standard interpretation. Example:

"Interpretive confidence is reduced because the client reports unusual medication sensitivity and is taking medications with CYP-mediated exposure variability; pharmacogenetic and medication-interaction factors may affect the degree to which this QEEG reflects a stable baseline."

Appendix F: Recording and Pipeline Considerations

The governing principle here is that the instrument is not the amplifier. The instrument is the whole chain: amplifier, electrodes, reference, filters, artifact handling, segment selection, normative database, and the state the client was in while the data were collected. Every one of those is a choice, and a change in any of them between two recordings can produce a difference that looks exactly like a medication effect.

That principle is easy to agree with and easy to skip. What follows is the operational version, which is the part that does the work: the minimum you write down so that a second reader, or you in eight months, can tell whether a difference between two maps belongs to the client or to the method.

The QEEG Field Guide (Hill, in press) is the methodological companion to this book and goes further on acquisition, reference schemes, ICA-based artifact correction, and database selection. This book does not wait on it. What a clinician needs to record and read a medicated client's map at the standard this book asks for is in this appendix.

The Minimum Acquisition and Processing Record

Keep this block with the raw file and reproduce it in the report. It is short enough to sit in a template and specific enough that someone else can check it.

Acquisition

- Amplifier make and model, channel count, and cap or electrode type
- Sampling rate
- Online reference and ground
- Impedance or contact-quality values as your system reports them, and the threshold you accepted
- Conditions collected and the order they ran in: eyes closed, eyes open, task, hyperventilation, photic

- Clock time of the recording, plus last-dose times for everything on the medication and substance list

Data accepted

- Usable minutes per condition after artifact handling, not minutes recorded
- How alert and drowsy segments were separated, and how many usable minutes came from each
- Whether the vigilance trajectory across the run was inspected, and what it showed
- Artifact method, its settings, and what came out: number of ICA components rejected and what each was judged to be, amplitude-rejection thresholds, any ASR parameters
- Residual artifact burden after cleaning, stated rather than implied. Frontal ocular activity and temporalis or frontalis EMG are the two that move band-power conclusions most often
- Who reviewed the raw data, and whether that is the same person who wrote the report

Processing

- Offline reference and montage, stated per feature. A linked-ear power map and a Laplacian coherence estimate are not the same montage and should not be reported as though they were
- High-pass, low-pass, and notch settings
- Band edges in Hz for every band you name. "Beta" is not a frequency range until you say what it is, and beta boundaries differ across platforms by enough to move a z-score on their own
- Any transform applied before comparison: log, relative power, ratio measures, periodic and aperiodic decomposition

Normative comparison

- Database name and version
- Age range covered and the age model used
- Whether the database's acquisition matches yours on sampling rate, reference, montage, and filter settings, and what you did about it if it did not

- The medication status of the normative sample, where the vendor states it. Most databases were not built from a drug-free population, and it is worth knowing which comparison you are actually making
- Reliability and test-retest information the vendor publishes, and the retest interval if this recording is a repeat

Two Rules That Follow From the Record

A longitudinal comparison requires matched conditions. A within-person comparison is interpretable only when the second recording matches the first on acquisition system, database and database version, recording condition, artifact pipeline, medication clock time, sleep and circadian state, and usable segment length. If any of those changed, name the change and stop treating the difference as a change in the client. A database version that updated between sessions is a pipeline change, whatever the difference map shows.

Connectivity and source estimates carry a lower portability ceiling than power. Coherence, phase measures, and source-localized estimates depend more heavily on reference, volume conduction, artifact handling, and head model than well-characterized power features do. They are more sensitive to the pipeline choices listed above and they travel less well between systems. Weight them accordingly, and be slower to build a medication argument on them.

What a Z-Score Is

A z-score is a comparison between this client's processed data and a reference distribution built under specific assumptions. It is a database-relative statistic. It is not a confidence level, it is not a diagnosis, and it is not a phenotype.

Two cautions follow. A full head map across bands and metrics runs to hundreds of comparisons, and some will land in the tails by arithmetic alone, so an isolated deviation with nothing around it is weak evidence for anything. And an extreme z-score is more often a data problem than a physiological finding. Before it goes in a report, return to the raw trace and confirm it is not an electrode, a muscle, or a drowsy stretch.

A finding earns narrative weight when it is visible in the raw record, coherent across neighboring sites, stable across the conditions you collected, and convergent with the clinical picture. Isolated deviations get documented. They do not get a paragraph.

Cross-References

See Appendix C for pre-recording substance and timing protocols, Chapter 4 for the evidence framework used throughout this book, and Chapter 26 for the ten-step reading workflow that this record feeds.

Appendix G: Cross-Book Phenotype Name Crosswalk

This appendix maps phenotype names across the three-book series. The **clinical name** is shared between this book and *The QEEG Field Guide* (FG taxonomy v1.1.0). The **consumer name** is the variant used in *Neurofeedback, Explained* Appendix G where applicable. The **G&T Character** references the pedagogical archetype from *Gifted & Tortured* (Hill, 2026) where mapped.

FG taxonomy codes (e.g., `frontal_theta_high`) appear in the Field Guide Chapter 6 taxonomy table and the shared data files. Not all phenotypes appear in all three books. The Field Guide documents 41 entries; this book documents 45 (41 shared + 4 medication-prediction-specific); *Neurofeedback, Explained* documents 20 consumer-relevant entries.

Individual Phenotypes (31)

Clinical Name	NFB Consumer Name	G&T Character
FAA (Left > Right, Approach Deficit)	n/a	Grumpy Old Man
Frontal Alpha Excess	Frontal Alpha Excess	Happy Little Kid
FAA (Right > Left, Withdrawal)	Frontal Alpha Asymmetry	n/a
Elevated Frontal High Beta	Frontal High Beta	Problem Child
Posterior Cingulate Hyperactivation	Posterior Cingulate Hyperactivation	Lifeguard
Elevated Frontal Theta	Frontal Theta Excess	Grumpy Old Man
Suppressed Frontal Theta	n/a	n/a

Clinical Name	NFB Consumer Name	G&T Character
Frontal Slowing (Delta + Theta)	n/a	Grumpy Old Man
Low SMR (12–15 Hz)	Low SMR	Supervisor
Elevated SMR (12–15 Hz)	n/a	n/a
Elevated Theta/Beta Ratio	Theta-Beta Ratio Elevation	n/a
Low-Voltage Fast EEG	Low-Voltage Fast	Fog & the Tide
Elevated Midline Theta (ACC/DMN)	n/a	CEO
Elevated Temporal Beta	Temporal Beta	Bard
Elevated Mu Rhythm (Central Alpha)	n/a	Stabilizer
Elevated Left Temporal Alpha	Left Temporal Alpha	Interpreter
Elevated High Beta (Global Hyperarousal)	Global High Beta Excess	Princess & the Pea
Elevated Posterior Alpha (Hypoarousal)	Excess Alpha	n/a
Deficient Posterior Alpha (Hypervigilance)	PDR Suppression	Princess & the Pea
Slow iAPF	Slowed Alpha Peak Frequency	Timekeeper
Fast iAPF	n/a	n/a
Beta Spindling (Cortical Irritability)	n/a	n/a
Deficient Mu Rhythm	Mu Rhythm Suppression	n/a
Low Central Beta	n/a	Supervisor
Posterior Slowing (Delta + Theta)	n/a	Timekeeper

Clinical Name	NFB Consumer Name	G&T Character
Globally Low Beta (Underactivation)	n/a	n/a
Global Hypercoherence	Coherence Anomalies	n/a
Frontal Hypocoherence	Coherence Anomalies	n/a
Diffuse Slowing (Elevated Delta)	Diffuse Slowing	Fog & the Tide
Mixed Fast-Slow (Encephalopathic)	Mixed Fast-Slow	n/a
Temporal Theta Dysrhythmia	Temporal Dysrhythmia	Bard

Composite Signatures (10)

Clinical Name	NFB Consumer Name	G&T Character
Hyperarousal Constellation	High Beta with Alpha Suppression	Princess & the Pea
Classic Attention Constellation	n/a	Grumpy Old Man + Supervisor
Sensory Sensitivity Composite	n/a	Princess & the Pea
ADHD Excess-Beta Subtype	n/a	Problem Child
ADHD Excess-Alpha Subtype	n/a	n/a
Frontal Disconnect (TBI Pattern)	n/a	n/a
Rumination Constellation	n/a	Lifeguard + Happy Little Kid
Encephalopathic Composite	n/a	Fog & the Tide
OCD Signature Composite	n/a	CEO + Problem Child

Clinical Name	NFB Consumer Name	G&T Character
Slowed-Modality Composite (Brainmarker-I)	n/a	Timekeeper + Grumpy Old Man

BoD-Only Entries (4)

These entries appear in Chapter 21 but have no counterpart in the Field Guide phenotype atlas or *Neurofeedback, Explained,* because they are medication-prediction constructs rather than standalone phenotypes.

BoD Entry	Description
GABAergic Response Patterns	Benzodiazepine / anticonvulsant-specific spectral signatures
Theta Cordance (Early SSRI Response Predictor)	Leuchter cordance metric for antidepressant response prediction
Limited-Response Signatures	Patterns associated with poorer pharmacotherapy outcomes
Right Temporal Alpha	Assessed only in medication-response context

Naming Conventions

- **Clinical context (FG / BoD):** Use the full clinical name with parenthetical descriptor when present. Short form (e.g., "Elevated Frontal Theta") is sufficient after first use.
- **Consumer context (NFB):** Consumer names deliberately omit "Elevated / Deficient" clinical framing in favor of accessible descriptors.
- **G&T Characters:** Used as clinical mnemonics and teaching aids, not diagnostic labels. See *Gifted & Tortured* (Hill, 2026) for the full character model.

Appendix H: Worked Complete Reports

Five composite clinical reports, each with a weak version followed by a stronger version. All clients are composites; no identifying information represents any real individual. The stronger versions apply the ten-step decision framework from Chapter 26 and the confidence language from Appendix B.

What these examples show is the interpretive half of a report. A real one also carries the acquisition and processing record from Appendix F, and the z-values and peak frequencies quoted below are readable only against a named database and version. Where a number appears here without one, that is compression for the page and not a model to copy.

Report 1: Clean Medication Picture (Stimulant + SSRI, Stable)

Clinical context. David, 29, referred for QEEG-guided neurofeedback for persistent attention difficulties and residual low mood despite two years on lisdexamfetamine (Vyvanse) 50 mg QAM and escitalopram 10 mg QD. Both medications stable for 14 months. No dose changes. Recorded AM, 90 minutes after the lisdexamfetamine dose, 3 hours after the escitalopram dose. Slept 7.5 hours. No caffeine. No other substances. Clean EEG. No drowsiness. 7/10 alertness.

QEEG findings. Frontal theta (Fz/F3) at +1.5 SD, posterior alpha amplitude mid-range at iAPF of 10.1 Hz, mild beta excess (high beta band, 22–28 Hz) bilateral frontal, no asymmetry, intact alpha reactivity EC→EO.

Acquisition. 19 channels at 256 Hz, linked ears, eyes closed 8 usable minutes of 10 recorded, eyes open 4 of 5, 3 ICA components removed (2 ocular, 1 cardiac), residual artifact burden low. Band edges and database version per Appendix F.

Weak report:

"QEEG findings consistent with inattentive ADHD phenotype. Elevated frontal theta with high beta excess suggests cortical hypoarousal with compensatory arousal mechanism. Stimulant appears insufficient to normalize the theta/beta ratio. Recommend continued neurofeedback targeting frontal SMR and posterior alpha protocol."

Stronger report:

"Recording obtained 90 minutes after the AM lisdexamfetamine dose under stable dual-medication conditions (14 months escitalopram + lisdexamfetamine, no recent changes). This is a deliberate treated-state recording, labeled as such: the goal was to evaluate the medicated phenotype under current stimulant coverage, not to obtain an unmedicated baseline. Ninety minutes post-dose is near peak stimulant exposure; this is a treated-state recording, not an off-medication comparison. Alertness rated 7/10; no drowsiness or artifact. Sleep was adequate.

Primary findings: frontal theta slightly elevated at Fz/F3 (+1.5 SD), with mid-range posterior alpha amplitude and intact reactivity. High-beta excess (22–28 Hz) is present bilaterally frontal at approximately +1.3 SD.

Confidence assessment: phenotype inference for the frontal theta. Lisdexamfetamine can mask unmedicated theta under full medication exposure, and this recording was obtained during peak coverage. The theta elevation may represent a residual trait feature that persists despite stimulant coverage, but it may also represent a reduced-masking signal in a client whose unmedicated baseline would show more prominent theta. Confidence in this phenotype as a stable treatment target is moderate, not high.

High-beta excess interpretation requires additional context. This degree of high-beta elevation is consistent with SSRI activation or anxiety in this range; it may also reflect stimulant-class contribution. Without an off-medication comparison recording, causal attribution is not supportable.

Summary: Moderate confidence for an attention-related phenotype. The frontal theta finding is clinically useful as a monitoring baseline under current stable medication conditions. A follow-up recording after a prescriber-initiated off-medication interval would increase confidence in phenotype characterization, if clinically appropriate.

The QEEG cannot determine whether medication should be changed, supplemented, or maintained. Those decisions belong with the prescribing clinician."

Report 2: Stacked Polypharmacy (Antipsychotic + Mood Stabilizer + Benzo + Cannabis)

Clinical context. Renata, 36, bipolar disorder with anxiety. Current medications: quetiapine 150 mg QHS, lamotrigine 200 mg BID, clonazepam 0.5 mg QHS PRN (used 4–5 nights per week), low-dose escitalopram 5 mg QAM added 6 weeks ago. Also uses cannabis (edible, ~5 mg THC) 3–4 nights per week, most recently 48 hours before the recording. Recording at 9 AM; took quetiapine at 10 PM the night before and lamotrigine at 8 AM. Slept 8 hours but reports persistent morning grogginess. No caffeine.

QEEG findings. Diffuse mild slowing (elevated delta and theta broadly), reduced posterior alpha amplitude, slowed iAPF to 8.8 Hz, poor alpha reactivity EC→EO, no asymmetry, sparse artifact, mild drowsiness noted in second half of recording.

Acquisition. 19 channels at 500 Hz, linked ears, eyes closed 6 usable minutes of 10 recorded (drowsiness onset in second half confirmed by slow rolling eye movements; alert and drowsy segments separated), eyes open 3 of 4, 4 ICA components removed (2 ocular, 1 cardiac, 1 EMG), residual frontal ocular burden low. Band edges and database version per Appendix F.

Weak report:

"QEEG findings suggest hypoarousal phenotype with slowed alpha peak, broadly elevated delta and theta. Pattern may indicate cognitive dysregulation consistent with bipolar disorder or ongoing mood episode. Recommend neurofeedback targeting posterior alpha normalization."

Stronger report:

"Recording obtained in a stacked polypharmacy context: quetiapine 150 mg (10 hours post-dose), lamotrigine 200 mg (1 hour post-dose), escitalopram 5 mg (6 weeks), clonazepam PRN (4–5 nights per week, most recent use estimated 48 hours prior), and edible cannabis (5 mg THC, 48 hours prior). Edible cannabis 48 hours prior approaches the tail of 11-OH-THC duration; cannabinoid residual effects remain plausible at this interval.

Primary findings: diffuse mild slowing, reduced posterior alpha amplitude, slowed iAPF (8.8 Hz), poor alpha reactivity, and drowsiness in the second half of recording.

Confidence assessment: Substantially reduced for phenotype labeling. The sedative-medication stack (quetiapine, clonazepam, cannabis) and morning grogginess are dominant confounds for the diffuse slowing and iAPF findings. Quetiapine at this dose is clinically sedating, but direct resting-QEEG quantification is limited (Chapter 10), so it is a documented confound for the delta, theta, and iAPF findings rather than a quantified source of them. Lamotrigine runs in the other direction: the audited source reports reduced delta and theta power with alpha mean frequency preserved (Chapter 11), so it does not account for the slowing here and should not be named for the alpha finding. Clonazepam residual contributes to beta and vigilance instability. Cannabis edibles at 48 hours sit at the boundary of the acute pharmaco-EEG window rather than cleanly past it. Drowsiness noted during recording is an additional source of theta and slowed-reactivity.

The iAPF of 8.8 Hz is in the slow range, but this finding cannot be interpreted as a trait slow-alpha phenotype under these conditions. Medication-stack effects, cannabis residual, and drowsiness can each slow iAPF, and this recording cannot apportion the finding among them. This is a clinical measurement of a heavily medicated brain in a drowsy state, not a stable individual trait baseline.

Summary: This recording is clinically useful as a documentation of the current medication state. Phenotype labeling or neurofeedback protocol selection should be deferred until the prescriber has reviewed the recording context. A follow-up recording after stable titration, a cleaner cannabis interval, and confirmed AM alertness would improve confidence. The QEEG findings do not indicate any medication adjustment."

Report 3: Post-Concussive Client with Caffeine

Clinical context. Marco, 47, former semi-professional soccer player. Three documented concussions between ages 22 and 31, the last requiring four weeks of cognitive rest. Current medications: bupropion 300 mg XL QAM (depression), gabapentin 300 mg QHS (chronic neck pain). Also uses caffeine (one large coffee, 5 hours before recording, usual practice). Works third shift; recording at 11 AM after sleeping

6 hours. Reports persistent cognitive fog and word-finding difficulty since his last concussion.

QEEG findings. Posterior theta elevation (P3/P4/Pz, +1.8 SD), mildly reduced posterior alpha amplitude, iAPF 9.5 Hz, intermittent frontal slowing, mild beta excess temporal bilaterally.

Acquisition. 19 channels at 250 Hz, linked ears, eyes closed 6 usable minutes of 9 recorded, eyes open 4 of 6, 5 ICA components removed (2 ocular, 2 temporal EMG, 1 cardiac), residual temporalis EMG moderate. Band edges and database version per Appendix F.

Weak report:

"QEEG findings show posterior theta elevation and mild frontal slowing, consistent with executive dysfunction and underarousal. Alpha peak within normal limits for age. Recommend frontal theta-reduction protocol with posterior alpha augmentation."

Stronger report:

"Recording obtained under the following documented conditions: bupropion 300 mg XL (approximately 3 hours post-dose), gabapentin 300 mg (approximately 11 hours post-dose), caffeine (1 large coffee, 5 hours prior), third-shift worker sleeping 6 hours before recording, with post-concussive history including 3 documented injuries over 9 years.

Primary findings: posterior theta elevation (+1.8 SD), mildly reduced posterior alpha amplitude, iAPF 9.5 Hz, intermittent frontal slowing, and mild temporal beta excess.

Confidence assessment: Reduced for phenotype labeling. At least five concurrent factors can produce the observed pattern:

1. Post-concussive physiology (posterior theta, connectivity changes, cognitive fatigue). This client has a history of three documented concussions, with the most recent requiring 4 weeks cognitive rest and leaving persistent word-finding complaints. Post-concussive contribution is a primary interpretive frame here, not a footnote.

2. Sleep restriction (6 hours, shift worker). Posterior theta elevation and slowed reactivity are expected consequences of sleep restriction independent of any medication or injury.

3. Gabapentin residual (11 hours post-dose, nightly use). Gabapentinoids are read through drowsiness and condition overlap rather than as a compound-specific spectral fingerprint (Chapter 11). Reduced vigilance is the route by which they can add slow activity to a record like this one.

4. Bupropion. Direct resting-QEEG evidence for a bupropion spectral signature is limited (Chapter 7), so it is not carried here as a source of the slowing and should not be named as the source of the temporal beta either. That beta sits in a client taking bupropion with caffeine and restricted sleep, and arousal state and muscle artifact are live alternatives.

5. Caffeine (1 large coffee, 5 hours before recording) places this recording near peak caffeine exposure. Recent caffeine can shift arousal and elevate beta, and it lowers interpretive confidence for the temporal beta excess in particular.

These factors stack. Narrowing the picture would require a recording under more controlled conditions: adequate sleep, a stable or documented caffeine state, and a morning recording during the peak bupropion window. The gabapentin contribution cannot be separated out this way. Gabapentin is prescribed, and prescribed medications are not withheld for a recording (Appendix C), so the workable step is to hold its dose timing constant across sessions and document it rather than to seek a gabapentin-free comparison.

Summary: Moderate confidence that the QEEG reflects a real physiological state. Low confidence in any specific phenotype attribution. This recording is best used as a current-state documentation baseline for a client with multiple concurrent contributions to the pattern. Neurofeedback protocol selection should account for the post-concussive history alongside the medication and caffeine contributions rather than treating any one of them as the settled explanation. The word-finding and cognitive-fog complaints have at least three live candidate contributors here, and this recording does not separate them. Naming which one drives the symptoms is a clinical question for the treating team, not something the trace decides.

Refer for sleep hygiene support. OSA screening is warranted given the shift-work schedule, snoring history (if present), and gabapentin use. The QEEG cannot direct medication changes."

Report 4: Perimenopausal Client on HRT + SSRI

Clinical context. Vivienne, 51. Perimenopausal symptoms for 3 years. Current medications: sertraline 100 mg QD (depression and perimenopausal anxiety, 2 years), estradiol patch 0.1 mg twice weekly +

oral progesterone 200 mg QHS cyclically (most recent progesterone dose 3 days ago, off-cycle week). Sleep is inconsistent (5–7 hours). Recording at 8:30 AM, 2 hours after sertraline, on the second day after her last estradiol patch change. No caffeine. Alertness 6/10.

QEEG findings. Frontal alpha asymmetry (right > left, approximately 15% ratio), mild theta elevation (Fz/F3 at +1.2 SD), posterior alpha amplitude mid-range (iAPF 10.3 Hz), intact reactivity.

Acquisition. 19 channels at 512 Hz, linked ears, eyes closed 7 usable minutes of 10 recorded, eyes open 4 of 5, 3 ICA components removed (2 ocular, 1 EMG), residual artifact burden low. Band edges and database version per Appendix F.

Weak report:

"QEEG shows frontal alpha asymmetry (right-greater-than-left) consistent with SSRI-responder phenotype per Bruder et al. 2001 findings. This pattern may indicate antidepressant responsiveness. Frontal theta elevation consistent with attention or mood regulation difficulty. Recommend continued monitoring."

Stronger report:

"Recording obtained under the following documented conditions: sertraline 100 mg (2 hours post-dose, 2 years stable), transdermal estradiol (second day after patch change), oral progesterone cyclically (most recent dose 3 days ago, currently off-cycle), inconsistent sleep (range 5–7 hours), alertness 6/10.

Primary findings: frontal alpha asymmetry (right-greater-than-left, approximately 15% ratio), mild frontal theta elevation, mid-range posterior alpha amplitude, intact reactivity. iAPF 10.3 Hz.

Confidence assessment for the FAA finding: Reduced. The frontal alpha asymmetry finding requires the following qualifications before any medication-response interpretation is applied:

1. The source finding is narrower than the weak report implies: Bruder and colleagues located the responder/nonresponder alpha asymmetry difference at occipital rather than frontal sites, with the hemispheric difference stronger among women in their earlier, more female samples. The 2025 meta-analysis (Luo et al.) then found a near-zero pooled FAA effect in depression overall, with high heterogeneity and no convincing subgroup rescue. The FAA as an

SSRI-response biomarker is no longer supported at the population level and should not be used as a primary clinical rationale.

2. Reproductive-hormone context. Resting alpha power and alpha frequency shift with cycle phase and with exogenous hormone exposure (Chapter 29), so the hormonal state is a documented and uncontrolled variable in this recording. No asymmetry-specific effect of estradiol or of oral progesterone at this dose is established, so the point is that the state is unaccounted for, not that it explains the asymmetry. This recording was obtained 3 days after the last progesterone dose, in the off-cycle week; a recording during the progesterone week is a different exposure state.

3. SSRI exposure changes what an FAA value means. Chapter 6 treats a woman on an SSRI and an unmedicated woman as different clinical objects for this measure, and no sertraline-specific asymmetry direction or magnitude is established.

Summary: This asymmetry finding cannot be used to infer antidepressant responsiveness or guide treatment recommendations. It is a valid measurement of the current hormonal-medication state. If serial monitoring is the goal, all future recordings should document cycle phase, HRT cycle position, and sertraline timing consistently. Phenotype comparisons across recordings are only interpretable when those variables are held constant. This QEEG does not indicate a need for medication change."

Report 5: Tapering Benzodiazepine

Clinical context. Cecile, 44. Long-term clonazepam 1.5 mg QHS (9 years) being tapered under prescriber supervision at 0.125 mg per 4 weeks. Currently at 1.25 mg QHS, 3 weeks into this dose step. Reports intermittent insomnia, morning anxiety, mild derealization on some mornings. Recording at 9 AM; last dose 11 hours ago. Sleep was 5 hours. Alertness 5/10. Current adjunct: trazodone 50 mg QHS for sleep (not sedating at this dose for this client per her report).

QEEG findings. Elevated beta (bilateral, 14–30 Hz, +2.1 SD), poor alpha reactivity EC→EO, intermittent theta bursts, low posterior alpha amplitude, occasional artifact consistent with autonomic instability.

Acquisition. 19 channels at 256 Hz, linked ears, eyes closed 5 usable minutes of 11 recorded (2 minutes excluded for suspected microsleep, 2 for movement artifact), eyes open 3 of 5, 6 ICA components removed

(2 ocular, 2 EMG, 1 cardiac, 1 movement), residual frontal EMG burden moderate. Band edges and database version per Appendix F.

Weak report:

"QEEG shows significant beta excess with poor alpha organization consistent with anxiety and hyperarousal phenotype. May reflect trait hyperarousal or medication-related activation. Recommend posterior alpha augmentation neurofeedback. Consider whether current SSRI augmentation is appropriate."

Stronger report:

"Recording obtained during active benzodiazepine taper under prescriber supervision: clonazepam 1.25 mg QHS (3 weeks at this dose, tapering from 1.5 mg after 9 years of use, 11 hours since last dose). Client reports intermittent insomnia, morning anxiety, and mild derealization consistent with benzodiazepine discontinuation symptoms. Trazodone 50 mg QHS for sleep support. Sleep was 5 hours; alertness rated 5/10.

Primary findings: elevated beta (14–30 Hz, +2.1 SD bilaterally), poor alpha reactivity, intermittent theta bursts, low posterior alpha amplitude, occasional autonomic artifact.

Confidence assessment: Substantially reduced for phenotype labeling. This recording cannot be interpreted as a stable trait baseline under any standard phenotype framework for the following reasons:

1. Benzodiazepine withdrawal state. After 9 years of therapeutic clonazepam use, a 3-week taper at 0.125 mg steps produces a gradual neuroadaptive shift. The nervous system is in a continuous withdrawal-adjustment state. Beta rebound is a described feature of benzodiazepine withdrawal, most clearly after abrupt reductions, and reduced GABAergic tone is the usual mechanistic account of it. The withdrawal literature this book relies on is clinical rather than a controlled QEEG trial (Chapter 8), so withdrawal state is a competing explanation for this beta and not a signature that identifies it. It cannot be scored as endogenous anxiety beta either; this recording does not separate the two.

2. The symptomatic picture (insomnia, derealization, morning anxiety) is consistent with a discontinuation syndrome that directly shapes the EEG state.

3. Sleep restriction (5 hours) independently elevates slow activity and reduces alpha amplitude.

Summary: This recording is a documentation of a nervous system in active withdrawal adjustment. The beta excess, poor alpha reactivity, and intermittent theta are consistent with a brain adapting to reduced GABAergic support. Interpreting this as a trait anxiety or hyperarousal phenotype would misattribute a taper state to a stable endogenous characteristic.

Clinical use of this recording: document current taper-state EEG for longitudinal tracking. After taper completion and a period of post-taper stability, a repeat recording would provide a valid comparison. Neurofeedback protocol selection should await post-taper stabilization.

Important: benzodiazepine tapering carries seizure risk and must be supervised medically. Nothing in this report comments on the taper schedule, which was set by the prescribing clinician. If withdrawal symptoms worsen or if new neurological symptoms emerge, contact the prescribing clinician immediately. This QEEG does not indicate a need to modify the taper schedule."

Report-Language Pairs: Extended Reference

Six additional Weak/Stronger dyads covering specialized scenarios. These complement dyads 1–6 in Chapter 26.

7. Slow iAPF in a polypharmacy client - Weak: "Slow individual alpha peak frequency (9.1 Hz) suggests underarousal phenotype." - Stronger: "Individual alpha peak frequency is slow-normal at 9.1 Hz. Cannabis use within 48 hours and sleep restriction are both active factors that can slow iAPF, and quetiapine's clinical sedation adds a further state confound, though direct resting-QEEG quantification for quetiapine is limited. Phenotype confidence for 'slow-alpha underarousal' is reduced to low under these conditions. A recording under stable conditions with substance timing documented and habitual state confirmed would be needed for valid iAPF phenotyping."

8. Post-viral fatigue and medication attribution - Weak: "Posterior theta and reduced alpha amplitude are consistent with SSRI effect." - Stronger: "Posterior theta elevation and reduced alpha amplitude are present. The client has documented post-COVID illness onset predating the SSRI start by 4 months. Post-viral illness and SSRI exposure are both plausible contributors, and the SSRI evidence does not fix a direction for either finding. Attribution to the SSRI alone is not supportable given the clinical timeline."

9. Withdrawal-state recording - Weak: "Beta excess and poor alpha reactivity consistent with anxiety phenotype. Consider augmentation." - Stronger: "Recording was obtained 11 hours after the last dose of clonazepam during an active prescriber-supervised taper. The beta excess (+2.3 SD) and poor alpha reactivity are consistent with GABAergic withdrawal hyperexcitability, and this recording cannot separate that from an endogenous anxiety phenotype. This recording is a taper-state measurement. Phenotype interpretation should be deferred until taper completion and stabilization."

10. Follow-up change after medication start - Weak: "Follow-up QEEG shows improvement in alpha organization, consistent with antidepressant response." - Stronger: "Follow-up recording shows increased posterior alpha amplitude and improved reactivity compared to baseline. Between recordings, the client started sertraline 50 mg and also increased sleep consistency from approximately 5.5 to 7 hours per night. The spectral change is documented but cannot be attributed exclusively to the antidepressant. Sleep improvement, time, and therapy are concurrent changes that independently contribute to alpha organization."

11. Seizure-risk medication and slow activity - Weak: "Diffuse slowing is likely from mood disorder and should be targeted with neurofeedback." - Stronger: "Diffuse delta and theta elevation is present. The client takes levetiracetam (Keppra) 500 mg BID for post-traumatic seizure prophylaxis. Direct resting-QEEG evidence for levetiracetam is limited, so its contribution here is a documented gap rather than a quantified effect, and the head-injury history that prompted the prophylaxis is itself a plausible contributor. Attributing the slowing to mood disorder without naming either would be clinically misleading. If neurofeedback training is planned, the treating neurologist should be consulted about the interaction of training targets with seizure prophylaxis medication."

12. Pre-recording protocol deviation - Weak: "QEEG shows elevated TBR and frontal theta consistent with attention phenotype." - Stronger: "Elevated frontal theta and theta/beta ratio are present. The recording was obtained 30 minutes after the stimulant dose and 2 hours after a large caffeinated beverage, placing both near peak exposure. Near-peak stimulant and caffeine exposure reduce interpretive confidence for frontal theta and TBR. This recording documents a caffeinated-and-recently-medicated state and should be interpreted as such rather than as an unmedicated phenotype baseline."

Appendix I: For Prescribers

What This Appendix Is For

Occasionally a prescriber receives a QEEG report and wants to understand what the clinician was doing and how to interpret it. This appendix is written for that reader. It is also useful for QEEG clinicians who want to explain their work to prescribers they collaborate with.

What Is a QEEG?

A quantitative EEG (QEEG) is not a separate instrument. An EEG is acquired from sensors placed on the scalp, usually for 15 to 20 minutes, and quantitative methods are then applied to the segments of that recording a clinician selects as usable. The analysis describes oscillatory patterns in different frequency ranges (delta, theta, alpha, beta, gamma) across the scalp surface and compares them against a normative database to identify features outside the usual range. The distinction matters: the numbers in a QEEG report are a product of the raw recording and the processing choices together, so both belong in the report.

Neurofeedback practice uses QEEG to identify patterns thought to be associated with attention, mood, arousal, and cognitive function. The method is not a diagnostic test in the medical sense and does not diagnose ADHD, depression, anxiety, or any other condition by itself.

What QEEG Can and Cannot Do

QEEG can: - Identify spectral patterns (elevated theta, reduced alpha reactivity, beta excess, slowed peak frequency) relative to a normative reference - Document how those patterns change across sessions or conditions - Contribute hypothesis-generating context to a clinical conversation - Support neurofeedback protocol selection and monitoring

QEEG cannot: - Diagnose any psychiatric or neurological condition - Exclude epilepsy, nonconvulsive seizures, or toxic-metabolic encephalopathy; a resting recording of this length is not a diagnostic EEG, and a normal-looking QEEG is not neurologic clearance - Identify which medication is "causing" a finding with certainty - Predict individual treatment response (although some group-level associations exist in the research literature) - Recommend starting, stopping, adjusting, or substituting any medication
The clinician's role is to interpret what the brain looks like under current conditions and to communicate that interpretation with appropriate confidence. Your role is to determine what to do about it.

What the Report Is Telling You

A well-written QEEG report contains several layers:
What was observed. The spectral measurements: frequency-band amplitudes, symmetry, peak frequency, coherence. These are the measured data.

What factors were active during the recording. Medications, substances, sleep state, clinical conditions, recording protocol. These are the measurement context. A QEEG is not a photograph of trait physiology; it is a recording of a brain in a specific state at a specific time.
What confidence level the clinician assigns to the phenotype interpretation. High confidence means the measurement is stable and the active factors do not plausibly explain the finding. Reduced confidence means one or more factors could produce the same spectral change. The report should state this explicitly.
What the clinician recommends for next steps. Usually: documentation, monitoring, neurofeedback protocol selection, repeat recording under different conditions, or coordination with prescribers. A good QEEG report does not recommend medication changes.

Questions Worth Asking Back

If you receive a QEEG report and it is unclear, these questions will help:

1. **"Under what medication state was this recording obtained?"** Stimulants, benzodiazepines, antipsychotics, gabapentinoids, and cannabis all alter QEEG findings measurably. The report should document this.

2. **"What is the confidence level for this finding?"** If the report does not distinguish between high-confidence and reduced-confidence findings, ask. A finding that "cannot be attributed to medication" carries different weight than a finding where medication effects are a plausible contributor.

3. **"What would change your interpretation?"** A thoughtful QEEG clinician can tell you what a follow-up recording under different conditions would clarify.

4. **"Is this finding stable across sessions?"** A single QEEG recording is a snapshot. Patterns that appear consistently across multiple sessions under similar conditions carry more weight.

5. **"Is this report recommending any medication change?"** It should not be. If it appears to be, ask for clarification. QEEG is not a prescribing instrument.

The One Thing This Book Wants You to Know

Most QEEG interpretation in clinical neurofeedback practice does not adequately account for medication effects. A client on an antidepressant, a benzodiazepine, a stimulant, and nightly cannabis is not presenting a "baseline" brain to the recording electrode. The recording is real and clinically useful, but it has to be interpreted as what it is: a layered measurement of a brain under multiple concurrent influences.

When a QEEG clinician mentions that medication context reduces interpretive confidence, they are doing their job correctly: honest measurement, not a failure of the technology.

When a QEEG Report Is Useful to You

A QEEG report is most useful to a prescriber when:

- It documents the client's current neurophysiological state under stable medication conditions as a baseline for monitoring
- It identifies patterns associated with neurofeedback training targets that can be monitored over time
- It contributes context to a treatment question you are already considering, by naming what the group-level research literature suggests about phenotype-medication associations (with appropriate uncertainty)
- It identifies non-drug confounders (untreated OSA, TBI, post-viral fatigue, sleep restriction) that you may not have been aware of and that could affect treatment response

A QEEG report is less useful when:

- It arrives as a single recording without documented medication timing or recording conditions
- It attributes all findings to medication without separating state-related from trait-related patterns
- It makes treatment recommendations without consultation with your clinical judgment
- It uses phenotype language ("ADHD phenotype," "depression phenotype") without qualifying what medication effects may have contributed

---

Shared Language

A few terms used in QEEG reports and this book:

Masking. A medication suppresses the brain pattern the clinician was looking for. Stimulants can reduce theta in attention-phenotype clients; a medicated recording near stimulant peak may look more "normal" than the unmedicated state.

Mimicry. A medication produces a pattern that looks like a clinical phenotype. Benzodiazepines increase beta activity, which can look like anxiety-related beta. The report should name this.

Exaggeration. A medication and a clinical condition both push the same spectral feature in the same direction. A client with untreated sleep apnea on a sedating antipsychotic will show more slowing than either factor alone.

Transformation. A medication changes what a spectral feature means. A high-beta pattern under benzodiazepine exposure carries different clinical implications than the same pattern in an unmedicated anxious client.

Spectral effect / phenotype inference / workflow heuristic. The claim types used through most of this book label the kind of statement being made, not the quality of the study behind it. A spectral effect is a claim about what a drug does to the EEG itself. A phenotype inference is an interpretation: what that spectral effect means for a phenotype reading. A workflow heuristic is a rule of clinical practice. Evidence quality varies within all three and is stated in the text rather than carried by the label, so a spectral-effect label is not by itself a reason to believe something.

In Part III, where the question runs backward from phenotype to treatment response, the same labels apply: a phenotype inference names an empirical association between a measured pattern and a treatment outcome; a workflow heuristic names a clinical reasoning convention. Evidence quality, replication status, and individual-level limits are discussed in the text of each entry rather than carried by the label. Most phenotype-to-medication-response claims in QEEG practice are phenotype inferences or workflow heuristics. None of them is a basis for a prescribing decision.

This appendix is part of Your Brain on Drugs: A Clinician's Guide to Medications, Substances, and Confounded QEEG Brain Maps. *For prescribers who want a deeper introduction to the evidence base, Chapter 26 (The Decision Framework) and Chapter 18 (Patterns Across Substances) are the most accessible starting points.*

References

Akeju, O. et al. (2014a). A comparison of propofol- and dexmedetomidine-induced electroencephalogram dynamics using spectral and coherence analysis. *Anesthesiology, 121*(5), 978–989. https://doi.org/10.1097/ALN.0000000000000419

Akeju, O. et al. (2014b). Age-dependency of sevoflurane and propofol electroencephalogram dynamics. *Anesthesiology, 121*(5), 990–998. https://doi.org/10.1097/ALN.0000000000000436

Akeju, O. et al. (2016). Electroencephalogram signatures of ketamine anesthesia-induced unconsciousness. *Clinical Neurophysiology, 127*(6), 2414–2422. https://doi.org/10.1016/j.clinph.2016.03.005

Armitage, R. (1996). Effects of antidepressant treatment on sleep EEG in depression. *Journal of Psychopharmacology, 10*, 22–25. https://doi.org/10.1177/026988119601001S01

Arns, M. (2012). EEG-based personalized medicine in ADHD: Individual alpha peak frequency as an endophenotype associated with nonresponse. *Journal of Neurotherapy, 16*(2), 123–141. https://doi.org/10.1080/10874208.2012.677664

Arns, M., Conners, C. K., & Kraemer, H. C. (2013). A decade of EEG theta/beta ratio research in ADHD: A meta-analysis. *Journal of Attention Disorders, 17*(5), 374–383. https://doi.org/10.1177/1087054712460087

Arns, M., Gunkelman, J., Breteler, R., & Spronk, D. (2008). EEG phenotypes predict treatment outcome to stimulants in children with ADHD. *Journal of Integrative Neuroscience, 7*(3), 421–438. https://doi.org/10.1142/s0219635208001897

Ashton, H. (2002). *Benzodiazepines: How they work and how to withdraw.*

Babiloni, C. et al. (2024). Resting state electroencephalographic alpha rhythms are sensitive to Alzheimer's disease mild cognitive impairment progression at a 6-month follow-up. *Neurobiology of Aging, 137*, 19–37. https://doi.org/10.1016/j.neurobiolaging.2024.01.013

Baradits, M., Spitzberg, A., Davani, A. J., Csukly, G., Arcaro, N., Joanlanne, A., Vodovozov, W., Malhotra, A. K., & Argyelan, M. (2026). Individual alpha peak predicts clinical response in TMS therapy for depression: An independent replication. *Psychiatry Research, 355*, 116828. https://doi.org/10.1016/j.psychres.2025.116828

Bares, M., Brunovsky, M., Kopecek, M., Novak, T., Stopkova, P., Kozeny, J., Sos, P., Krajca, V., & Hoschl, C. (2008). Early reduction in prefrontal theta QEEG cordance predicts response to venlafaxine treatment in patients with resistant depressive disorder. *European Psychiatry, 23*(5), 350–355. https://doi.org/10.1016/j.eurpsy.2008.03.001

Bares, M., Brunovsky, M., Kopecek, M., Stopkova, P., Novak, T., Kozeny, J., & Hoschl, C. (2007). Changes in QEEG prefrontal cordance as a predictor of response to antidepressants in patients with treatment resistant depressive disorder: A pilot study. *Journal of Psychiatric Research, 41*(3–4), 319–325. https://doi.org/10.1016/j.jpsychires.2006.06.005

Barker, M. J., Greenwood, K. M., Jackson, M., & Crowe, S. F. (2004). Persistence of cognitive effects after withdrawal from long-term benzodiazepine use: A meta-analysis. *Archives of Clinical Neuropsychology, 19*(3), 437–454. https://doi.org/10.1016/S0887-6177(03)00096-9

Barry, R. J., Clarke, A. R., Hajos, M., McCarthy, R., Selikowitz, M., & Bruggemann, J. M. (2009). Acute atomoxetine effects on the EEG of children with attention-deficit/hyperactivity disorder. *Neuropharmacology, 57*(7–8), 702–707. https://doi.org/10.1016/j.neuropharm.2009.08.003

Barry, R. J., Clarke, A. R., Johnstone, S. J., Magee, C. A., & Rushby, J. A. (2007). EEG differences between eyes-closed and eyes-open resting conditions. *Clinical Neurophysiology, 118*(12), 2765–2773. https://doi.org/10.1016/j.clinph.2007.07.028

Barry, R. J., Rushby, J. A., Wallace, M. J., Clarke, A. R., Johnstone, S. J., & Zlojutro, I. (2005). Caffeine effects on resting-state arousal. *Clinical Neurophysiology, 116*(11), 2693–2700. https://doi.org/10.1016/j.clinph.2005.08.008

Bauer, L. O. (2001). Predicting relapse to alcohol and drug abuse via quantitative electroencephalography. *Neuropsychopharmacology, 25*(3), 332–340. https://doi.org/10.1016/S0893-133X(01)00236-6

Becker, D., Creutzfeldt, O. D., Schwibbe, M., & Wuttke, W. (1982). Changes in physiological, EEG and psychological parameters in women during the spontaneous menstrual cycle and following oral contraceptives. *Psychoneuroendocrinology, 7*(1), 75–90. https://doi.org/10.1016/0306-4530(82)90057-9

Bemmel, A. L. van, Havermans, R. G., & Diest, R. van. (1992). Effects of trazodone on EEG sleep and clinical state in major depression. *Psychopharmacology, 107*(4), 569–574. https://doi.org/10.1007/BF02245272

Bigdely-Shamlo, N., Mullen, T., Kothe, C., Su, K. A., & Robbins, K. A. (2015). The PREP pipeline: Standardized preprocessing for large-scale EEG analysis. *Frontiers in Neuroinformatics, 9*, 16. https://doi.org/10.3389/fninf.2015.00016

Bodenmann, S., & Landolt, H.-P. (2010). Effects of modafinil on the sleep EEG depend on Val158Met genotype of COMT. *Sleep, 33*(8), 1027–1035. https://doi.org/10.1093/sleep/33.8.1027

Boxum, M., Voetterl, H., Dijk, H. van, Gordon, E., DeBeus, R., Arnold, L. E., & Arns, M. (2024). Challenging the diagnostic value of theta/beta ratio: Insights from an EEG subtyping meta-analytical approach in ADHD. *Applied Psychophysiology and Biofeedback, 50*, 655–666. https://doi.org/10.1007/s10484-024-09649-y

Bresnahan, S. M., Anderson, J. W., & Barry, R. J. (1999). Age-related changes in quantitative EEG in attention-deficit/hyperactivity disorder. *Biological Psychiatry, 46*(12), 1690–1697. https://doi.org/10.1016/s0006-3223(99)00042-6

Brötzner, C. P., Klimesch, W., Doppelmayr, M., Zauner, A., & Kerschbaum, H. H. (2014). Resting state alpha frequency is associated with menstrual cycle phase, estradiol and use of oral contraceptives. *Brain Research, 1577*, 36–44. https://doi.org/10.1016/j.brainres.2014.06.034

Brown, E. N., Lydic, R., & Schiff, N. D. (2010). General anesthesia, sleep, and coma. *New England Journal of Medicine, 363*(27), 2638–2650. https://doi.org/10.1056/NEJMra0808281

Bruder, G. E., Sedoruk, J. P., Stewart, J. W., McGrath, P. J., Quitkin, F. M., & Tenke, C. E. (2008). Electroencephalographic alpha measures predict therapeutic response to a selective serotonin reuptake inhibitor antidepressant: Pre- and post-treatment findings. *Biological Psychiatry, 63*(12), 1171–1177. https://doi.org/10.1016/j.biopsych.2007.10.009

Bruder, G. E., Stewart, J. W., Tenke, C. E., McGrath, P. J., Leite, P., Bhattacharya, N., & Quitkin, F. M. (2001). Electroencephalographic and perceptual asymmetry differences between responders and nonresponders to an SSRI antidepressant. *Biological Psychiatry, 49*(5), 416–425. https://doi.org/10.1016/S0006-3223(00)01016-7

Brunner, D. P., Dijk, D.-J., Munch, M., & Borbely, A. A. (1991). Effect of zolpidem on sleep and sleep EEG spectra in healthy young men. *Psychopharmacology, 104*(1), 1–5. https://doi.org/10.1007/BF02244546

Buzsaki, G., & Draguhn, A. (2004). Neuronal oscillations in cortical networks. *Science, 304*(5679), 1926–1929. https://doi.org/10.1126/science.1099745

Cajochen, C., Brunner, D. P., Krauchi, K., Graw, P., & Wirz-Justice, A. (1995). Power density in theta/alpha frequencies of the waking EEG progressively increases during sustained wakefulness. *Sleep, 18*(10), 890–894. https://doi.org/10.1093/sleep/18.10.890

Carhart-Harris, R. L. et al. (2014). The entropic brain: A theory of conscious states informed by neuroimaging research with psychedelic drugs. *Frontiers in Human Neuroscience, 8*, 20. https://doi.org/10.3389/fnhum.2014.00020

Cavanagh, J. F., & Frank, M. J. (2014). Frontal theta as a mechanism for cognitive control. *Trends in Cognitive Sciences, 18*(8), 414–421. https://doi.org/10.1016/j.tics.2014.04.012

Cecchetti, G. et al. (2022). Cognitive, EEG, and MRI features of COVID-19 survivors: A 10-month study. *Journal of Neurology, 269*(7), 3400–3412. https://doi.org/10.1007/s00415-022-11047-5

Centorrino, F., Price, B. H., Tuttle, M., Bahk, W.-M., Hennen, J., Albert, M. J., & Baldessarini, R. J. (2002). EEG abnormalities during treatment with typical and atypical antipsychotics. *American Journal of Psychiatry, 159*(1), 109–115. https://doi.org/10.1176/appi.ajp.159.1.109

Chabot, R. J., & Serfontein, G. (1996). Quantitative electroencephalographic profiles of children with attention deficit disorder. *Biological Psychiatry, 40*(10), 951–963. https://doi.org/10.1016/0006-3223(95)00576-5

Choi, J.-B., Lee, Y.-J. G., & Jeong, D.-U. (2017). Transdermal nicotine patch effects on EEG power spectra and heart rate variability during sleep of healthy male adults. *Psychiatry Investigation, 14*(4), 499–506. https://doi.org/10.4306/pi.2017.14.4.499

Chouinard, G., & Jones, B. D. (1980). Neuroleptic-induced supersensitivity psychosis: Clinical and pharmacologic characteristics. *American Journal of Psychiatry, 137*(1), 16–21. https://doi.org/10.1176/ajp.137.1.16

Clarke, A. R., Barry, R. J., Bond, D., McCarthy, R., & Selikowitz, M. (2002). Effects of stimulant medications on the EEG of children with attention-deficit/hyperactivity disorder. *Psychopharmacology, 164*(3), 277–284. https://doi.org/10.1007/s00213-002-1205-0

Clarke, A. R., Barry, R. J., McCarthy, R., & Selikowitz, M. (2001). EEG-defined subtypes of children with attention-deficit/hyperactivity disorder. *Clinical Neurophysiology, 112*(11), 2098–2105. https://doi.org/10.1016/s1388-2457(01)00668-x

Clarke, A. R., Barry, R. J., McCarthy, R., Selikowitz, M., & Johnstone, S. J. (2002). EEG differences between good and poor responders to methylphenidate in boys with the inattentive type of attention-deficit/hyperactivity disorder. *Clinical Neurophysiology, 113*(8), 1191–1198. https://doi.org/10.1016/s1388-2457(02)00147-5

Clemens, B., Menes, A., Piros, P., Bessenyei, M., Altmann, A., Jerney, J., Kollar, K., Rosdy, B., Rozsavolgyi, M., Steinecker, K., & Hollody, K. (2006). Quantitative EEG effects of carbamazepine, oxcarbazepine, valproate, lamotrigine, and possible clinical relevance of the findings. *Epilepsy Research, 70*(2–3), 190–199. https://doi.org/10.1016/j.eplepsyres.2006.05.003

Clinical Pharmacogenetics Implementation Consortium. (2019). CPIC guideline for atomoxetine therapy and CYP2D6 genotype. *Clinical Pharmacology and Therapeutics, 106*(1), 94–102. https://doi.org/10.1002/cpt.1409

Cohen, M. X. (2011). Error-related medial frontal theta activity predicts cingulate-related structural connectivity. *NeuroImage, 55*(3), 1373–1383. https://doi.org/10.1016/j.neuroimage.2010.12.072

Cole, S. R., & Voytek, B. (2017). Brain oscillations and the importance of waveform shape. *Trends in Cognitive Sciences, 21*(2), 137–149. https://doi.org/10.1016/j.tics.2016.12.008

Czobor, P., Kakuszi, B., Fullajtar, M., & Bitter, I. (2026). High-density EEG study in patients with schizophrenia treated with cariprazine. *International Journal of Neuropsychopharmacology, 29*(4), pyag008. https://doi.org/10.1093/ijnp/pyag008

Davidson, R. J. (2004). What does the prefrontal cortex "do" in affect: Perspectives on frontal EEG asymmetry research. *Biological Psychology, 67*(1–2), 219–234. https://doi.org/10.1016/j.biopsycho.2004.03.008

Davidson, R. J., & Fox, N. A. (1982). Asymmetrical brain activity discriminates between positive and negative affective stimuli in human infants. *Science, 218*(4578), 1235–1237. https://doi.org/10.1126/science.7146906

De Gennaro, L., Ferrara, M., & Bertini, M. (2001). The boundary between wakefulness and sleep: Quantitative electroencephalographic changes during the sleep onset period. *Neuroscience, 107*(1), 1–11. https://doi.org/10.1016/S0306-4522(01)00309-8

De la Fuente, J. M., Tugendhaft, P., & Mavroudakis, N. (1998). Electroencephalographic abnormalities in borderline personality disorder. *Psychiatry Research, 77*(2), 131–138. https://doi.org/10.1016/s0165-1781(97)00149-2

Dias Alves, M., Micoulaud-Franchi, J.-A., Simon, N., & Vion-Dury, J. (2018). Electroencephalogram modifications associated with atypical strict antipsychotic monotherapies. *Journal of Clinical Psychopharmacology, 38*(6), 555–562. https://doi.org/10.1097/JCP.0000000000000953

Dijk, D.-J., Roth, C., Landolt, H.-P., Werth, E., Aeppli, M., Achermann, P., & Borbély, A. A. (1995). Melatonin effect on daytime sleep in men: Suppression of EEG low frequency activity and enhancement of spindle frequency activity. *Neuroscience Letters, 201*(1), 13–16. https://doi.org/10.1016/0304-3940(95)12118-N

Donoghue, T., Haller, M., Peterson, E. J., Varma, P., Sebastian, P., Gao, R., Noto, T., Lara, A. H., Wallis, J. D., Knight, R. T., Shestyuk, A., & Voytek, B. (2020). Parameterizing neural power spectra into periodic and aperiodic components. *Nature Neuroscience, 23*, 1655–1665. https://doi.org/10.1038/s41593-020-00744-x

Ehlers, C. L., Gilder, D. A., Wall, T. L., Phillips, E., Feiler, H., & Wilhelmsen, K. C. (2010). EEG alpha phenotypes: Linkage analyses and relation to alcohol dependence in an american indian community study. *BMC Medical Genetics, 11*(1), 43. https://doi.org/10.1186/1471-2350-11-43

Fallon, N., Chiu, Y., Nurmikko, T., & Stancak, A. (2018). Altered theta oscillations in resting EEG of fibromyalgia syndrome patients. *European Journal of Pain, 22*(1), 49–57. https://doi.org/10.1002/ejp.1076

Frei, E., Gamma, A., Pascual-Marqui, R., Lehmann, D., Hell, D., & Vollenweider, F. X. (2001). Localization of MDMA-induced brain activity in healthy volunteers using low resolution brain electromagnetic tomography (LORETA). *Human Brain Mapping, 14*(3), 152–165. https://doi.org/10.1002/hbm.1049

Galderisi, S., Mucci, A., Bucci, P., Mignone, M. L., & Maj, M. (1996). Multilead quantitative EEG profile of clozapine in resting and vigilance-controlled conditions. *Psychiatry Research, 67*(2), 113–122. https://doi.org/10.1016/0925-4927(96)02883-1

Gilbert, J. R., & Zarate, C. A. (2020). Electrophysiological biomarkers of antidepressant response to ketamine in treatment-resistant depression: Gamma power and long-term potentiation. *Pharmacology, Biochemistry, and Behavior, 189*, 172856. https://doi.org/10.1016/j.pbb.2020.172856

Glass, P. S. A., Bloom, M., Kearse, L., Rosow, C., Sebel, P., & Manberg, P. (1997). Bispectral analysis measures sedation and memory effects of propofol, midazolam, isoflurane, and alfentanil in healthy volunteers. *Anesthesiology, 86*(4), 836–847. https://doi.org/10.1097/00000542-199704000-00014

Gomez-Ramirez, M., Kelly, S. P., Montesi, J. L., & Foxe, J. J. (2009). The effects of L-theanine on alpha-band oscillatory brain activity during a visuo-spatial attention task. *Brain Topography, 22*(1), 44–51. https://doi.org/10.1007/s10548-008-0068-z

Guirguis, V., Korsapathy, S., Pupillo, F., McClure, R. K., Zarzar, D., Zhang, M., Frohlich, F., & Schwippel, T. (2025). Esketamine disinhibits brain networks in depression: Evidence from oscillatory and aperiodic activity. *Progress in Neuro-Psychopharmacology and Biological Psychiatry, 140*, 111438. https://doi.org/10.1016/j.pnpbp.2025.111438

Gunkelman, J. D., & Johnstone, J. (2005). Neurofeedback and the brain. *Journal of Adult Development, 12*(2–3), 93–98. https://doi.org/10.1007/s10804-005-7024-x

Haneef, Z., Levin, H. S., Frost, J. D., & Mizrahi, E. M. (2013). Electroencephalography and quantitative electroencephalography in mild traumatic brain injury. *Journal of Neurotrauma, 30*, 653–656. https://doi.org/10.1089/neu.2012.2585

He, B. J. (2014). Scale-free brain activity: Past, present, and future. *Trends in Cognitive Sciences, 18*(9), 480–487. https://doi.org/10.1016/j.tics.2014.04.003

Hill, A. (2026). Drowsiness as an under-measured confound in clinical QEEG phenotype classification. In *NeuroRegulation*.

Hoekzema, E. et al. (2017). Pregnancy leads to long-lasting changes in human brain structure. *Nature Neuroscience, 20*(2), 287–296. https://doi.org/10.1038/nn.4458

Hyun, J., Baik, M. J., & Kang, U. G. (2011). Effects of psychotropic drugs on quantitative EEG among patients with schizophrenia-spectrum disorders. *Clinical Psychopharmacology and Neuroscience, 9*(2), 78–85. https://doi.org/10.9758/cpn.2011.9.2.78

Ibrahim, K., & Donyai, P. (2015). Drug holidays from ADHD medication: International experience over the past four decades. *Journal of Attention Disorders, 19*, 551–568. https://doi.org/10.1177/1087054714548035

Ilan, A. B., Smith, M. E., & Gevins, A. (2004). Effects of marijuana on neurophysiological signals of working and episodic memory. *Psychopharmacology, 176*(2), 214–222. https://doi.org/10.1007/s00213-004-1868-9

International Pharmaco-EEG Society. (2012). Guidelines for the recording and evaluation of pharmaco-EEG data in man: The international pharmaco-EEG society (IPEG). *Neuropsychobiology, 66*(4), 201–220. https://doi.org/10.1159/000343478

Itil, T. M., Cora, R., Hsu, W., Gig, E., & Saletu, B. (1972). Clinical, toxicological and electroencephalographical effects of a new tricyclic antidepressant, OI-77. *Arzneimittel-Forschung,* 22(12), 2063–2066.

Jacobus, J., & Tapert, S. F. (2014). Effects of cannabis on the adolescent brain. *Current Pharmaceutical Design, 20*(13), 2186–2193. https://doi.org/10.2174/13816128113199990426

Johnstone, J., & Gunkelman, J. (2003). Use of databases in QEEG evaluation. *Journal of Neurotherapy, 7*(3–4), 31–52. https://doi.org/10.1300/J184v07n03_02

Johnstone, J., Gunkelman, J., & Lunt, J. (2005). Clinical database development: Characterization of EEG phenotypes. *Clinical EEG and Neuroscience, 36*(2), 99–107. https://doi.org/10.1177/155005940503600209

Kalechstein, A. D., De la Garza, R., Newton, T. F., Green, M. F., Cook, I. A., & Leuchter, A. F. (2009). Quantitative EEG abnormalities are associated with memory impairment in recently abstinent methamphetamine-dependent individuals. *Journal of Neuropsychiatry and Clinical Neurosciences, 21*(3), 254–258. https://doi.org/10.1176/jnp.2009.21.3.254

Keane, M. A., & James, J. E. (2008). Effects of dietary caffeine on EEG, performance and mood when rested and sleep restricted. *Human Psychopharmacology, 23*(8), 669–680. https://doi.org/10.1002/hup.987

Kerson, C. (Ed.). (2023). *Drug effects on the EEG* (2nd ed.). International Society for Neuroregulation; Research.

Kim, S.-H., Byeon, J.-Y., Kim, Y.-H., Lee, C.-M., Lee, Y. J., Jang, C.-G., & Lee, S.-Y. (2018). Physiologically based pharmacokinetic modelling of atomoxetine with regard to CYP2D6 genotypes. *Scientific Reports, 8*(1), 12405. https://doi.org/10.1038/s41598-018-30841-8

Klimesch, W. (1999). EEG alpha and theta oscillations reflect cognitive and memory performance: A review and analysis. *Brain Research Reviews, 29*(2–3), 169–195. https://doi.org/10.1016/S0165-0173(98)00056-3

Knott, V. J. (1989). Brain electrical imaging: The dose-response effects of cigarette smoking. *Neuropsychobiology, 22*(4), 236–242. https://doi.org/10.1159/000118623

Knott, V. J. et al. (1999). Transdermal nicotine: Single dose effects on mood, EEG, performance, and event-related potentials. *Pharmacology Biochemistry and Behavior, 63*(2), 253–261. https://doi.org/10.1016/S0091-3057(99)00006-4

Knott, V. J., Mahoney, C., Kennedy, S., & Evans, K. (2000). Pre-treatment EEG and its relationship to depression severity and paroxetine treatment outcome. *Pharmacopsychiatry, 33*(6), 201–205.

Knott, V., Labelle, A., Jones, B., & Mahoney, C. (2001). Quantitative EEG in schizophrenia and in response to acute and chronic clozapine treatment. *Schizophrenia Research, 50*(1–2), 41–53. https://doi.org/10.1016/s0920-9964(00)00165-1

Kopanska, M. et al. (2022). Comparison of QEEG findings before and after onset of post-COVID-19 brain fog symptoms. *Sensors, 22*(17), 6606. https://doi.org/10.3390/s22176606

Kuate, C., Gélisse, P., Baldy-Moulinier, M., & Crespel, A. (2004). Bupropion-induced epileptic seizures. *Revue Neurologique, 160*(6–7), 701–703. https://doi.org/10.1016/s0035-3787(04)71021-8

Kwan, P., & Brodie, M. J. (2001). Effectiveness of first antiepileptic drug. *Epilepsia, 42*(10), 1255–1260. https://doi.org/10.1046/j.1528-1157.2001.04501.x

Lee, D. Y. et al. (1999). Pharmacokinetic-pharmacodynamic modeling of risperidone effects on EEG in healthy volunteers. *Psychopharmacology, 144*(3), 272–278. https://doi.org/10.1007/s002130051003

Lees, T., Scott, J. N., Boyle, B. W., Esfand, S. M., Linton, S. R., Miller, C., Li, M., Woronko, S. E., Dunayev, R., Bogdanov, M., Bolton, P., Li, S., Meisner, R. C., & Pizzagalli, D. A. (2026). Modulatory effects of ketamine on EEG source-based resting state connectivity in treatment resistant depression. *Translational Psychiatry, 16*(1), 22. https://doi.org/10.1038/s41398-026-03928-4

Leon, J. de, & Nikoloff, D. M. (2008). Paradoxical excitation on diphenhydramine may be associated with being a CYP2D6 ultrarapid metabolizer: Three case reports. *CNS Spectrums, 13*(2), 133–135. https://doi.org/10.1017/s109285290001628x

Leuchter, A. F., Cook, I. A., Lufkin, R. B., Dunkin, J., Newton, T. F., Cummings, J. L., Mackey, J. K., & Walter, D. O. (1994). Cordance: A new method for assessment of cerebral perfusion and metabolism using quantitative electroencephalography. *NeuroImage, 1*(3), 208–219. https://doi.org/10.1006/nimg.1994.1006

Leuchter, A. F., Cook, I. A., Marangell, L. B., Gilmer, W. S., Burgoyne, K. S., Howland, R. H., Trivedi, M. H., Zisook, S., Jain, R., McCracken, J. T., Fava, M., Iosifescu, D., & Greenwald, S. (2009). Comparative effectiveness of biomarkers and clinical indicators for predicting outcomes of SSRI treatment in major depressive disorder: Results of the BRITE-MD study. *Psychiatry Research, 169*(2), 124–131. https://doi.org/10.1016/j.psychres.2009.06.004

Li, G., Huang, B., Wang, Y., Zhou, B., Hu, F., & Wang, L. (2026). Neurophysiological mechanisms and predictive modeling of SSRI treatment response in depression disorder based on multidimensional EEG features. *Journal of Affective Disorders, 393*(Pt B), 120424. https://doi.org/10.1016/j.jad.2025.120424

Linton, S. R., Murphy, M., Schroder, H. S., Breiger, M., Iturra-Mena, A. M., Kangas, B. D., Bergman, J., & Carlezon, W. A. (2022). Effects of modafinil on electroencephalographic microstates in healthy adults. *Psychopharmacology, 239*(8), 2573–2584. https://doi.org/10.1007/s00213-022-06149-x

Loo, S. K., & Barkley, R. A. (2005). Clinical utility of EEG in attention deficit hyperactivity disorder. *Applied Neuropsychology, 12*(2), 64–76. https://doi.org/10.1207/s15324826an1202_2

Lukas, S. E., Mendelson, J. H., Benedikt, R. A., & Jones, B. (1986). EEG alpha activity increases during transient episodes of ethanol-induced euphoria. *Pharmacology Biochemistry and Behavior, 25*(4), 889–895. https://doi.org/10.1016/0091-3057(86)90403-X

Lunsford-Avery, J. R., Kollins, S. H., Kansagra, S., Wang, K. W., & Engelhard, M. M. (2022). Impact of daily caffeine intake and timing on electroencephalogram-measured sleep in adolescents. *Journal of Clinical Sleep Medicine, 18*(3), 877–884. https://doi.org/10.5664/jcsm.9736

Luo, Y., Tang, M., & Fan, X. (2025). Meta-analysis of resting frontal alpha asymmetry as a biomarker of depression. *Npj Mental Health Research, 4*(1), 5. https://doi.org/10.1038/s44184-025-00117-x

Mahjoory, K., Nikulin, V. V., Botrel, L., Linkenkaer-Hansen, K., Fato, M. M., & Haufe, S. (2017). Consistency of EEG source localization and connectivity estimates. *NeuroImage, 152*, 590–601. https://doi.org/10.1016/j.neuroimage.2017.02.076

Mancuso, C. E., Tanzi, M. G., & Gabay, M. (2004). Paradoxical reactions to benzodiazepines: Literature review and treatment options. *Pharmacotherapy, 24*, 1177–1185. https://doi.org/10.1592/phco.24.13.1177.38089

Mandema, J. W., Tuk, B., Steveninck, A. L. van, Breimer, D. D., Cohen, A. F., & Danhof, M. (1992). Pharmacokinetic-pharmacodynamic modeling of the central nervous system effects of midazolam and its main metabolite alpha-hydroxymidazolam in healthy volunteers. *Clinical Pharmacology and Therapeutics, 51*(6), 715–728. https://doi.org/10.1038/clpt.1992.84

Martins, S., Tramontina, S., Polanczyk, G., Eizirik, M., Swanson, J. M., & Rohde, L. A. (2004). Weekend holidays during methylphenidate use in ADHD children: A randomized clinical trial. *Journal of Child and Adolescent Psychopharmacology, 14*(2), 195–206. https://doi.org/10.1089/1044546041649066

Mazaheri, A., & Jensen, O. (2010). Rhythmic pulsing: Linking ongoing brain activity with evoked responses. *Frontiers in Human Neuroscience, 4*, 177. https://doi.org/10.3389/fnhum.2010.00177

Modarres, M. H., Kuzma, N. N., Kretzmer, T., Pack, A. I., & Lim, M. M. (2017). EEG slow waves in traumatic brain injury: Convergent findings in mouse and man. *Neurobiology of Sleep and Circadian Rhythms, 2*, 59–70. https://doi.org/10.1016/j.nbscr.2016.06.001

Mohler, H. (2006). GABA(A) receptor diversity and pharmacology. *Cell and Tissue Research, 326*(2), 505–516. https://doi.org/10.1007/s00441-006-0284-3

Mojtabai, R., & Olfson, M. (2010). National trends in psychotropic medication polypharmacy in office-based psychiatry. *Archives of General Psychiatry, 67*(1), 26–36. https://doi.org/10.1001/archgenpsychiatry.2009.175

Monastra, V. J. et al. (1999). Assessing attention deficit hyperactivity disorder via quantitative electroencephalography: An initial validation study. *Neuropsychology, 13*(3), 424–433. https://doi.org/10.1037/0894-4105.13.3.424

Moore, T. J., & Mattison, D. R. (2017). Adult utilization of psychiatric drugs and differences by sex, age, and race. *JAMA Internal Medicine, 177*(2), 274–275. https://doi.org/10.1001/jamainternmed.2016.7507

Muthukumaraswamy, S. D. et al. (2013). Broadband cortical desynchronization under psilocybin. *Journal of Neuroscience, 33*(38), 15171–15183. https://doi.org/10.1523/JNEUROSCI.2063-13.2013

Naguy, A., Pridmore, S., & Alamiri, B. (2024). Letter: Paradoxical sedation on methylphenidate in a child with attention-deficit/hyperactivity disorder. *Journal of Child and Adolescent Psychopharmacology, 34*(6), 271–272. https://doi.org/10.1089/cap.2024.0031

Nestler, E. J., Hyman, S. E., Holtzman, D. M., & Malenka, R. C. (2020). *Molecular neuropharmacology: A foundation for clinical neuroscience* (4th ed.). McGraw-Hill Education.

Newton, T. F., Cook, I. A., Kalechstein, A. D., Duran, S., Monroy, F., & Ling, W. (2003). Quantitative EEG abnormalities in recently abstinent methamphetamine dependent individuals. *Clinical Neurophysiology, 114*(3), 410–415.

Nobre, A. C., Rao, A., & Owen, G. N. (2008). L-theanine, a natural constituent in tea, and its effect on mental state. *Asia Pacific Journal of Clinical Nutrition, 17*(Suppl. 1), 167–168.

Oberman, L. M. et al. (2005). EEG evidence for mirror neuron dysfunction in autism spectrum disorders. *Cognitive Brain Research, 24*(2), 190–198. https://doi.org/10.1016/j.cogbrainres.2005.01.014

Ogrim, G., & Hestad, K. (2013). Effects of neurofeedback versus stimulant medication in attention-deficit/hyperactivity disorder: A randomized pilot study. *Journal of Child and Adolescent Psychopharmacology, 23*(7), 448–457. https://doi.org/10.1089/cap.2012.0090

Ogrim, G., Kropotov, J., & Hestad, K. (2012). The quantitative EEG theta/beta ratio in attention deficit/hyperactivity disorder and normal controls: Sensitivity, specificity, and behavioral correlates. *Psychiatry Research, 198*(3), 482–488. https://doi.org/10.1016/j.psychres.2011.12.041

Olbrich, S. et al. (2009). EEG-vigilance and BOLD effect during simultaneous EEG/fMRI measurement. *NeuroImage, 45*(2), 319–332. https://doi.org/10.1016/j.neuroimage.2008.11.014

Owen, G. N., Parnell, H., De Bruin, E. A., & Rycroft, J. A. (2008). The combined effects of L-theanine and caffeine on cognitive performance and mood. *Nutritional Neuroscience, 11*(4), 193–198. https://doi.org/10.1179/147683008X301513

Papakostas, G. I. et al. (2007). Treatment of anxious depression with bupropion versus selective serotonin reuptake inhibitors. *Journal of Psychiatric Research, 42*(2), 134–140. https://doi.org/10.1016/j.jpsychires.2007.05.012

Pascual-Marqui, R. D. (2002). Standardized low-resolution brain electromagnetic tomography (sLORETA): Technical details. *Methods and Findings in Experimental and Clinical Pharmacology, 24*(Suppl D), 5–12.

Perucca, P., & Gilliam, F. G. (2012). Adverse effects of antiepileptic drugs. *The Lancet Neurology, 11*(9), 792–802. https://doi.org/10.1016/S1474-4422(12)70153-9

Pfurtscheller, G., & Lopes da Silva, F. H. (1999). Event-related EEG/MEG synchronization and desynchronization: Basic principles. *Clinical Neurophysiology, 110*(11), 1842–1857. https://doi.org/10.1016/S1388-2457(99)00141-8

Pickworth, W. B., Herning, R. I., & Henningfield, J. E. (1986). Electroencephalographic effects of nicotine chewing gum in humans. *Pharmacology Biochemistry and Behavior, 25*(4), 879–882. https://doi.org/10.1016/0091-3057(86)90401-6

Pineda, J. A. (2005). The functional significance of mu rhythms: Translating "seeing" and "hearing" into "doing". *Brain Research Reviews, 50*(1), 57–68. https://doi.org/10.1016/j.brainresrev.2005.04.005

Pinto, J., Cera, N., & Pignatelli, D. (2024). Psychological symptoms and brain activity alterations in women with PCOS and their relation to the reduced quality of life: A narrative review. *Journal of Endocrinological Investigation, 47*(7), 1–22. https://doi.org/10.1007/s40618-024-02329-y

Prashad, S., Dedrick, E. S., & Filbey, F. M. (2018). Cannabis users exhibit increased cortical activation during resting state compared to non-users. *NeuroImage, 179*, 176–186. https://doi.org/10.1016/j.neuroimage.2018.06.031

Prashad, S., Paek, A. Y., & Fournier, L. R. (2026). Longer chronic cannabis use in humans is associated with impaired implicit motor learning and supranormal resting state cortical activity. *PLOS One, 21*(1), e0338082. https://doi.org/10.1371/journal.pone.0338082

Privitera, M. D. et al. (2017). Bioequivalence between generic and branded lamotrigine in people with epilepsy: The EQUIGEN randomized clinical trial. *JAMA Neurology, 74*(8), 919–926. https://doi.org/10.1001/jamaneurol.2017.0497

Purdon, P. L., Pierce, E. T., Mukamel, E. A., Prerau, M. J., Walsh, J. L., Wong, K. T., Salazar-Gomez, A. F., Harrell, P. G., Sampson, A. L., Cimenser, A., Ching, S., Kopell, N. J., Tavares-Stoeckel, C., Habeeb, K., Merhar, R., & Brown, E. N. (2013). Electroencephalogram signatures of loss and recovery of consciousness from propofol. *Proceedings of the National Academy of Sciences of the United States of America, 110*(12), E1142–E1151. https://doi.org/10.1073/pnas.1221180110

Raichle, M. E. et al. (2001). A default mode of brain function. *Proceedings of the National Academy of Sciences, 98*(2), 676–682. https://doi.org/10.1073/pnas.98.2.676

Rampil, I. J. (1998). A primer for EEG signal processing in anesthesia. *Anesthesiology, 89*(4), 980–1002. https://doi.org/10.1097/00000542-199810000-00023

Rangaswamy, M. et al. (2002). Beta power in the EEG of alcoholics. *Biological Psychiatry, 52*(8), 831–842. https://doi.org/10.1016/S0006-3223(02)01362-8

Reeves, R. R., Struve, F. A., & Patrick, G. (2001). Does EEG predict response to valproate versus lithium in patients with mania? *Annals of Clinical Psychiatry, 13*(2), 69–73. https://doi.org/10.1023/a:1016611506740

Ruiz, N. V. (2018). Deciding when less is more: The crossroads of withdrawing antiepileptic drugs. *Epilepsy Currents, 18*(1), 21–23. https://doi.org/10.5698/1535-7597.18.1.21

Russell, J. K., Conley, A. C., Boyd, B. D., Begnoche, J. P., Schlossberg, R., Stranick, A., Rosenberg, A. J., Acosta, L. M. Y., Martin, D., Neal, Y., Kanel, P., Albin, R. L., Rafii, M. S., Dumas, J., & Newhouse, P. A. (2025). Differences in cholinergic terminal density in adults with down syndrome compared to neurotypical controls measured by [18f]-fluoroethoxybenzovesamicol positron emission tomography imaging. *Neurobiology of Aging, 148*, 50–60. https://doi.org/10.1016/j.neurobiolaging.2025.01.008

Saletu, B., Anderer, P., & Saletu-Zyhlarz, G. M. (2006). EEG topography and tomography (LORETA) in the classification and evaluation of depression. *Clinical EEG and Neuroscience, 37*(2), 66–80. https://doi.org/10.1177/155005940603700205

Saletu, B., Anderer, P., Saletu-Zyhlarz, G. M., & Pascual-Marqui, R. D. (2002). EEG topography and tomography in diagnosis and treatment of mental disorders: Evidence for a key-lock principle. *Methods and Findings in Experimental and Clinical Pharmacology, 24*(Suppl. D), 97–106.

Saletu, B., Grunberger, J., & Linzmayer, L. (1986). On central effects of serotonin re-uptake inhibitors: Quantitative EEG and psychometric studies with sertraline and zimelidine. *Journal of Neural Transmission, 67*(3-4), 241–266. https://doi.org/10.1007/BF01243351

Saletu, M. T., Anderer, P., Saletu-Zyhlarz, G. M., Mandl, M., Arnold, O., Nosiska, D., Zeitlhofer, J., & Saletu, B. (2005). EEG-mapping differences between narcolepsy patients and controls and subsequent double-blind, placebo-controlled studies with modafinil. *European Archives of Psychiatry and Clinical Neuroscience, 255*(1), 20–32. https://doi.org/10.1007/s00406-004-0530-1

Santamaria, J., & Chiappa, K. H. (1987). The EEG of drowsiness in normal adults. *Journal of Clinical Neurophysiology, 4*(4), 327–382. https://doi.org/10.1097/00004691-198710000-00002

Schenberg, E. E. et al. (2015). Acute biphasic effects of ayahuasca. *PLoS ONE, 10*(9), e0137202. https://doi.org/10.1371/journal.pone.0137202

Schomer, D. L., & Lopes da Silva, F. H. (Eds.). (2017). *Niedermeyer's electroencephalography: Basic principles, clinical applications, and related fields* (7th ed.). Oxford University Press.

Schuld, A., Kühn, M., Haack, M., Kraus, T., Hinze-Selch, D., Lechner, C., & Pollmächer, T. (2000). A comparison of the effects of clozapine and olanzapine on the EEG in patients with schizophrenia. *Pharmacopsychiatry, 33*(3), 109–111. https://doi.org/10.1055/s-2000-7976

Schulz, C., Mavrogiorgou, P., Schröter, A., Hegerl, U., & Juckel, G. (2000). Lithium-induced EEG changes in patients with affective disorders. *Neuropsychobiology, 42*(Suppl. 1), 33–37. https://doi.org/10.1159/000054850

Sigl, J. C., & Chamoun, N. G. (1994). An introduction to bispectral analysis for the electroencephalogram. *Journal of Clinical Monitoring, 10*, 392–404. https://doi.org/10.1007/BF01618421

Singh, A., Arun, P., Singh, G. P., Kaur, D., & Kaur, S. (2024). QEEG predictors of treatment response in major depressive disorder. *Clinical EEG and Neuroscience, 55*(2), 176–184. https://doi.org/10.1177/15500594221142396

Skosnik, P. D., Sloshower, J., Safi-Aghdam, H., Pathania, S., Syed, S., Pittman, B., & D'Souza, D. C. (2023). Sub-acute effects of psilocybin on EEG correlates of neural plasticity in major depression: Relationship to symptoms. *Journal of Psychopharmacology*, *37*(7), 687–697. https://doi.org/10.1177/02698811231179800

Small, J. G., Milstein, V., Small, I. F., Miller, M. J., Kellams, J. J., & Corsaro, C. J. (1987). Computerized EEG profiles of haloperidol, chlorpromazine, clozapine and placebo in treatment resistant schizophrenia. *Clinical EEG*, *18*(3), 124–135.

Snyder, S. M., & Hall, J. R. (2006). A meta-analysis of quantitative EEG power associated with attention-deficit hyperactivity disorder. *Journal of Clinical Neurophysiology*, *23*(5), 441–456. https://doi.org/10.1097/01.wnp.0000221363.12503.78

Solis-Ortiz, S., Guevara, M. A., & Corsi-Cabrera, M. (2004). Performance in a test demanding prefrontal functions is favored by early luteal phase progesterone: An electroencephalographic study. *Psychoneuroendocrinology*, *29*(8), 1047–1057. https://doi.org/10.1016/j.psyneuen.2003.10.007

Solowij, N., Broyd, S. J., Beale, C., Prick, J.-A., Greenwood, L., Hell, H. van, Suo, C., Galettis, P., Pai, N., Fu, S., Croft, R. J., Martin, J. H., & Yucel, M. (2018). Therapeutic effects of prolonged cannabidiol treatment on psychological symptoms and cognitive function in regular cannabis users: A pragmatic open-label clinical trial. *Cannabis and Cannabinoid Research*, *3*(1), 21–34. https://doi.org/10.1089/can.2017.0043

Soltanzadeh, M., Wang, Z., Allohverdi, S. G., Charlton, C. E., Schmidt, A., Vollenweider, F. X., & Diaconescu, A. O. (2025). Divergent effects of ketamine and psilocybin on EEG power spectral density in a mismatch negativity paradigm. *Psychopharmacology*. https://doi.org/10.1007/s00213-025-06952-2

Srivastava, A., Sanyal, S., Jaiswal, S., & Srivastava, S. (2024). Meta-analysis on QEEG changes to antidepressant treatment among patients with depression. *Indian Journal of Psychological Medicine*, *48*(1), 16–25. https://doi.org/10.1177/02537176241271716

Stahl, S. M. (2021). *Stahl's essential psychopharmacology: Neuroscientific basis and practical applications* (5th ed.). Cambridge University Press.

Steriade, M., McCormick, D. A., & Sejnowski, T. J. (1993). Thalamocortical oscillations in the sleeping and aroused brain. *Science*, *262*(5134), 679–685. https://doi.org/10.1126/science.8235588

Sterman, M. B. (1996). Physiological origins and functional correlates of EEG rhythmic activities: Implications for self-regulation. *Biofeedback and Self-Regulation*, *21*(1), 3–33. https://doi.org/10.1007/bf02214147

Strauß, M., Reif, A., Ulke, C., Paucke, M., Sander, C., Hegerl, U., Weber, H., Heupel, J., Kopf, J., & Kittel-Schneider, S. (2020). Is brain arousal regulation a predictor of response to psychostimulant therapy in adult ADHD patients? *European Archives of Psychiatry and Clinical Neuroscience*, *270*(8), 1073–1076. https://doi.org/10.1007/s00406-019-01085-y

Strijkstra, A. M., Beersma, D. G. M., Drayer, B., Halbesma, N., & Daan, S. (2003). Subjective sleepiness correlates negatively with global alpha (8–12 Hz) and positively with central frontal theta (4–8 Hz) frequencies in the human resting awake electroencephalogram. *Neuroscience Letters*, *340*(1), 17–20. https://doi.org/10.1016/S0304-3940(03)00033-8

Struve, F. A., Straumanis, J. J., Patrick, G., Leavitt, J., Manno, J. E., & Manno, B. R. (1999). Topographic quantitative EEG sequelae of chronic marihuana use: A replication using medically and psychiatrically screened normal subjects. *Drug and Alcohol Dependence*, *56*(3), 167–179. https://doi.org/10.1016/s0376-8716(99)00029-0

Strzelczyk, D., Vetsch, A., & Langer, N. (2026). Theta-beta ratio in attention deficit hyperactivity disorder: A multiverse analysis. *eLife*, *15*, RP111114. https://doi.org/10.7554/elife.111114

Suffin, S. C., & Emory, W. H. (1995). Neurometric subgroups in attentional and affective disorders and their association with pharmacotherapeutic outcome. *Clinical Electroencephalography*, *26*(2), 76–83. https://doi.org/10.1177/155005949502600204

Surova, G., Ulke, C., Schmidt, F. M., Hensch, T., Sander, C., & Hegerl, U. (2021). Fatigue and brain arousal in patients with major depressive disorder. *European Archives of Psychiatry and Clinical Neuroscience, 271*(3), 527–536. https://doi.org/10.1007/s00406-020-01216-w

Szponar, M., Dzianok, P., Gmaj, B., Jernajczyk, W., & Kamiński, J. (2026). Brainwaves under medication: Revealing class-specific neural signatures of psychotropic medication from 24,000 EEGs. *eBioMedicine, 130*, 106375. https://doi.org/10.1016/j.ebiom.2026.106375

Tarokh, L., & Carskadon, M. A. (2010). Developmental changes in the human sleep EEG during early adolescence. *Sleep, 33*(6), 801–809. https://doi.org/10.1093/sleep/33.6.801

Tatum, W. O., Selioutski, O., Ochoa, J. G., Munger Clary, H., Cheek, J., Drislane, F., & Tsuchida, T. N. (2016). American clinical neurophysiology society guideline 7: Guidelines for EEG reporting. *Journal of Clinical Neurophysiology, 33*(4), 328–332. https://doi.org/10.1097/WNP.0000000000000319

Thatcher, R. W. (2010). Validity and reliability of quantitative electroencephalography. *Journal of Neurotherapy, 14*(2), 122–152. https://doi.org/10.1080/10874201003773500

Thatcher, R. W., Walker, R. A., Gerson, I., & Geisler, F. H. (1989). EEG discriminant analyses of mild head trauma. *Electroencephalography and Clinical Neurophysiology, 73*(2), 94–106. https://doi.org/10.1016/0013-4694(89)90188-0

Timmermann, C. et al. (2019). Neural correlates of the DMT experience assessed with multivariate EEG. *Scientific Reports, 9*(1), 16927. https://doi.org/10.1038/s41598-019-51974-4

Ting, T. Y., Jiang, W., Lionberger, R., Wong, J., Jones, J. W., Kane, M. A., Krumholz, A., Temple, R., & Polli, J. E. (2015). Generic lamotrigine versus brand-name Lamictal bioequivalence in patients with epilepsy: A field test of the FDA bioequivalence standard. *Epilepsia, 56*(9), 1415–1424. https://doi.org/10.1111/epi.13095

Traynelis, S. F., Wollmuth, L. P., McBain, C. J., Menniti, F. S., Vance, K. M., Ogden, K. K., Hansen, K. B., Yuan, H., Myers, S. J., & Dingledine, R. (2010). Glutamate receptor ion channels: Structure, regulation, and function. *Pharmacological Reviews, 62*(3), 405–496. https://doi.org/10.1124/pr.109.002451

Vanneste, S., Ost, J., Van Havenbergh, T., & De Ridder, D. (2017). Resting state electrical brain activity and connectivity in fibromyalgia. *PLOS ONE, 12*(6), e0178516. https://doi.org/10.1371/journal.pone.0178516

Voetterl, H., Sack, A. T., Olbrich, S., Stuiver, S., Rouwhorst, R., Prentice, A., Pizzagalli, D. A., Vinne, N. van der, Waarde, J. A. van, Brunovsky, M., Oostrom, I. van, Reitsma, B., Fekkes, J., Dijk, H. van, & Arns, M. (2023). Alpha peak frequency-based Brainmarker-I as a method to stratify to pharmacotherapy and brain stimulation treatments in depression. *Nature Mental Health, 1*, 1023–1032. https://doi.org/10.1038/s44220-023-00160-7

Voetterl, H., Wingen, G. van, Michelini, G., Griffiths, K. R., Gordon, E., DeBeus, R., Korgaonkar, M. S., Loo, S. K., Palmer, D., Breteler, R., Denys, D., Arnold, L. E., Jour, P. du, Ruth, R. van, Jansen, J., Dijk, H. van, & Arns, M. (2023). Brainmarker-I differentially predicts remission to various attention-deficit/hyperactivity disorder treatments: A discovery, transfer, and blinded validation study. *Biological Psychiatry: Cognitive Neuroscience and Neuroimaging, 8*(1), 52–60. https://doi.org/10.1016/j.bpsc.2022.02.007

Wang, D., Bai, X. X., Williams, S. C., Hua, S. C., Kim, J.-W., Marshall, N. S., D'Rozario, A., & Grunstein, R. R. (2015). Modafinil increases awake EEG activation and improves performance in obstructive sleep apnea during continuous positive airway pressure withdrawal. *Sleep, 38*(8), 1297–1303. https://doi.org/10.5665/sleep.4912

Wang, G. Y., Kydd, R., Wouldes, T. A., Jensen, M., & Russell, B. R. (2015). Changes in resting EEG following methadone treatment in opiate addicts. *Clinical Neurophysiology, 126*(5), 943–950. https://doi.org/10.1016/j.clinph.2014.08.021

Wang, W. W., Li, X., & Wu, X. (2003). Quantitative EEG effects of topiramate. *Clinical Electroencephalography, 34*(2), 80–84. https://doi.org/10.1177/155005940303400208

Williams, L. M., Rush, A. J., Koslow, S. H., Wisniewski, S. R., Cooper, N. J., Nemeroff, C. B., Schatzberg, A. F., & Gordon, E. (2011). International Study to Predict Optimized Treatment for Depression (iSPOT-D), a randomized clinical trial: rationale and protocol. *Trials, 12*, 4. https://doi.org/10.1186/1745-6215-12-4

Winterer, G., Kloppel, B., Heinz, A., Ziller, M., Dufeu, P., Schmidt, L. G., & Herrmann, W. M. (1998). Quantitative EEG (QEEG) predicts relapse in patients with chronic alcoholism and points to a frontally pronounced cerebral disturbance. *Psychiatry Research, 78*(1–2), 101–113. https://doi.org/10.1016/s0165-1781(97)00148-0

Yadav, R., & Garg, B. (2025). Methylphenidate and the paradox of sedation: A case report. *Indian Journal of Psychological Medicine, 47*(2), 216–218. https://doi.org/10.1177/02537176251332231

Zandstra, T. E. et al. (2023). Associations between psychotropic drugs and rsEEG connectivity and network characteristics: A cross-sectional study in hospital-admitted psychiatric patients. *Frontiers in Neuroscience, 17*, 1176825. https://doi.org/10.3389/fnins.2023.1176825

Zinn, M. A., Zinn, M. L., Valencia, I., Jason, L. A., & Montoya, J. G. (2018). Cortical hypoactivation during resting EEG suggests central nervous system pathology in patients with chronic fatigue syndrome. *Biological Psychology, 136*, 87–99. https://doi.org/10.1016/j.biopsycho.2018.05.016